Fitz Simons

Maternal-Newborn Nursing

Clinical Handbook

Sally B. Olds, RNC, MS

Marcia L. London, RNC, MSN, NNP

Patricia W. Ladewig, PhD, RNC, NP

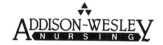

A Division of The Benjamin/Cummings Publishing Company, Inc.

Redwood City, California • Menlo Park, California
Reading, Massachusetts • New York • Don Mills, Ontario
Wokingham, U.K. • Amsterdam • Bonn • Sydney
Singapore • Tokyo • Madrid • San Juan

Sponsoring Editor: Patti Cleary
Production Editor: Cathy Lewis
Assistant Editor: Bradley Burch
Book Designer: Richard Kharibian
Cover Designer: Yvo Riezebos
Cover Quilt: *The Tide* by Miwako Kimura
Photographers: Suzanne Arms Wimberley, Elizabeth Elkin,
and Amy Snyder
Illustrators: Elizabeth Morales Denney (medical),
Merry Finley (technical)
Copy Editor: Jennifer Pulsipher
Proofreader: Holly McLean-Aldis
Indexer: William Richardson Associates
Manufacturing Supervisor: Casimira Kostecki
Composition: G & S Typesetters, Inc.

Care has been taken to confirm the accuracy of information presented
in this book. The authors, editors, and publisher, however, cannot accept any responsibility for errors or omissions or for consequences
from application of the information in this book and make no war-
ranty, express or implied, with respect to its contents.

The authors and publisher have exerted every effort to ensure that
drug selections and dosages set forth in this text are in accord with
current recommendations and practice at the time of publication.
However, in view of ongoing research, changes in government regula-
tions, and the constant flow of information relating to drug therapy
and drug reactions, the reader is urged to check the package inserts of
all drugs for any change in indications of dosage and for added warn-
ings and precautions. This is particularly important when the recommended agent is a new and/or infrequently employed drug. Mention
of a particular generic or brand name drug is not an endorsement, nor
an implication that it is preferable to other named or unnamed agents.

ISBN 0-8053-5588-X
2 3 4 5 6 7 8 9 10–MW–95 94 93 92

Addison-Wesley Nursing
A Division of the Benjamin/Cummings Publishing Company, Inc.
390 Bridge Parkway
Redwood City, California 94065

PREFACE

You are a student (or a nurse new to the maternal-child area) and are assigned to work on the Postpartum unit. Over the next 12 hours you will be responsible for providing care for a 22-year-old who had her first baby four hours ago and seems well prepared; a 35-year-old who has Pregnancy Induced Hypertension and gave birth to full-term twins last night; a 25-year-old who, after ten weeks of treatment for preterm labor, has now given birth to a preterm baby that is in the Neonatal Intensive Care Nursery; and a 15-year-old who gave birth yesterday, is breast-feeding and is planning to care for her baby by herself without any support.

As you organize your thoughts for today, what are your priorities? What special assessments and interventions will be needed for the woman who has PIH? How will you assist the breast-feeding mother? What are the critical assessments and interventions for any postpartum woman? How will you translate maternal-child nursing theory into this practice setting? How can you assure that you are giving safe nursing care?

The *Maternal-Newborn Nursing Clinical Handbook* has been created to help you in situations just like these. The *Handbook* provides succinct, pertinent information regarding the antepartum, intrapartum, newborn and postpartum client. Each content area includes key information regarding medical therapy and nursing care information which is organized around the nursing process. Critical nursing assessments and interventions are identified, and specific suggestions are given regarding documentation of care. In many sections, a special "Alert" heading signals the reader to watch for specific signs and symptoms.

In addition to serving as a resource for normal and selected complications of childbearing, the *Handbook* includes practical features that will assist the nurse. Nursing care plans are located together and can be quickly referenced for additional information or may guide the development of a care plan on the clinical unit. Procedures specific to the maternal-child clinical area are also included to assist the nurse in providing care. Commonly used medications are presented in the Drug Guides. The Resource Guide contains an overview of many agencies available to assist childbearing clients.

Although the *Handbook* addresses each subject area in a condensed manner in comparison to a comprehensive textbook, critical aspects of nursing practice have been presented. It is our hope that maternal-newborn nursing practice will be enhanced and that safe, competent nursing care will be provided to all mothers and babies.

We would like to express our appreciation to Linda Culotta, Zeone DeMarrais, Christine Milhollan, Marilyn Rowe, and Aubrey Wade for their careful review of the manuscript. Each one of them is involved in current nursing practice and was able to give us many suggestions regarding content. As always, we are deeply grateful to the talented Addison-Wesley team for their encouragement, support and assistance: Cathy Lewis, Production Editor; Bradley Burch, Assistant Editor; and Jennifer Pulsipher, freelance Copy Editor. A special salute is reserved for our editor Patti Cleary. She has nudged, encouraged, and cajoled us to take our *Clinical Handbook* in a new direction and once again she is the essence of the inspiration. Finally, we would like to extend our heartfelt appreciation to our students who brighten each day. It is in being with them that we are able to gain an understanding of the struggle that comes with translating what seems like mountains of information into a single clinical day.

S.B.O
P.W.L
M.L.L.

BRIEF CONTENTS

CONTENTS

CHAPTER 8   The At-risk Postpartal Client   202

DRUG GUIDES

PROCEDURES

NURSING CARE PLANS

APPENDICES

RESOURCE DIRECTORY 500

(space)

PHOTOGRAPHIC CREDITS

CHAPTER 5

Figures 5–5 and 5–6: Reprinted by permission of V. Dubowitz, M.D., Hammersmith Hospital. London, England. Figure 5–9: Elizabeth D. Elkin. Figure 5–10: From Smith D.W.: *Recognizable Patterns of Human Deformation.* Philadelphia: W.B. Saunders, 1981.

CHAPTER 7

Figure 7–3: © William Thompson

CHAPTER 8

Figure 8–5: Amy H. Snyder

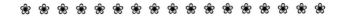

CHAPTER 1

The Antepartum Client

OVERVIEW

Pregnancy generally lasts about nine calendar months, ten lunar months, 40 weeks, or 280 days. The woman's due date (date on which baby is expected) is calculated from the first day of her last menstrual period (LMP). In reality, conception actually occurs about 14 days before the start of her next menstrual period. Thus the actual time she is pregnant is about two weeks less, or 266 days.

Typically, pregnancy is discussed in terms of trimesters, which each last three calendar months. During the first trimester, the woman usually learns she is pregnant and may seek prenatal care. The first trimester is the time of primary organ development for the fetus.

The second trimester is considered the most tranquil for the pregnant woman. Morning sickness passes and quickening (feeling the baby move) occurs.

In the third trimester the woman becomes anxious for the pregnancy to end. She may feel awkward because of her increasing weight and the physical and psychologic changes she experiences.

During the antepartal period nursing interventions focus primarily on client teaching and ongoing monitoring of the woman so that any potential complications are detected promptly. Teaching typically focuses on nutrition, on interventions to deal with the common discomforts of pregnancy, and on self-care activities indicated throughout pregnancy.

NORMAL PHYSICAL CHANGES OF PREGNANCY

Uterus

- Dramatic increase in size and weight.
- **Braxton Hicks contractions** begin by the end of the first trimester. These are rhythmic contractions of the uterus that are painless initially but become noticeable, and sometimes uncomfortable, toward term (the end of pregnancy). They are then referred to as "false labor." Braxton Hicks contractions are palpable during bimanual exam by the fourth month and palpable abdominally by the 28th week.

Cervix

- Glandular tissue increases in number and becomes hyperactive.
- Mucous plug is formed in cervix, which acts as a barrier to prevent ascending infection.
- Increased blood flow to cervix leads to softening (Goodell's sign) and bluish coloration (Chadwick's sign) (visible on speculum examination).

Ovaries

- Ovum production ceases.
- Corpus luteum persists and secretes hormones until weeks 10–12.

Vagina

- Increased vascularity produces bluish color (Chadwick's sign).
- Epithelium hypertrophies.

Breasts

- Increased size and nodularity; some increased tenderness.
- Superficial veins prominent.
- Increased pigmentation of areola and nipple.
- Colostrum is usually produced by week 12. (Colostrum is

the antibody-rich forerunner of mature breast milk.)
Women who are not visibly secreting colostrum need re-
assurance that they are producing it even if it is not evident.

Respiratory System

- Some hyperventilation occurs as pregnancy progresses.
- Increased tidal volume, decreased airway resistance.
- Diaphragm elevated, substernal angle increased.
- Breathing changes from abdominal to thoracic.

Cardiovascular System

- Blood volume increases about 45%.
- Decreased systemic and pulmonary vascular resistance.
- Increased pulse rate.
- BP decreases slightly by second trimester; near prepregnant levels at term.
- Pressure of enlarging uterus on vena cava can interfere
with blood return to the heart and cause dizziness, pallor,
clamminess, and lowered BP. This condition is called vena
caval syndrome or supine hypotensive syndrome and is
corrected by having woman lie on her side or with a
wedge under the right hip.
- RBC and hemoglobin levels increase as does plasma level.
Because plasma volume increases more, a **physiologic
anemia of pregnancy** results, evident in an apparent decrease in hematocrit (Hct). Hct levels of 32% to 44% are
considered normal.
- Leukocyte production increases to levels of 10,000–11,000/
mm^3. Levels may reach 25,000/mm^3 during labor.
- Increased fibrin, fibrinogen, factors VII, VIII, IX, X.

Gastrointestinal System

- Nausea common; vomiting occurs occasionally.
- Ptyalism (excessive salivation) is an occasional problem.
- Intestines and stomach are displaced by uterus.
- Relaxed cardiac sphincter leads to reflux of acidic secre-
tions, resulting in heartburn.
- Delayed gastric emptying leads to constipation.
- Hemorrhoids may develop.

Urinary Tract

- Increased pressure on the bladder from the growing uterus during the first and third trimesters leads to urinary frequency.
- Glomerular filtration rate (GFR) and renal plasma flow (RPF) increased.
- Increased incidence of glycosuria, which may be normal or may indicate gestational diabetes mellitus (see Chapter 2).

Skin and Hair

- Increased pigmentation of areola, nipples, vulva, linea nigra.
- Facial chloasma, a butterfly-shaped area of pigmentation over the face, may develop. Usually fades after childbirth. Called the "mask of pregnancy."
- Striae or stretch marks may develop on the abdomen, also on breasts and thighs.
- Vascular spider nevi, small, bright red elevations of the skin radiating from central body, may develop.
- Rate of hair growth may decrease.

Musculoskeletal System

- Joints of pelvis relax somewhat.
- Waddling gait develops due to changed center of gravity and accentuated lumbosacral curve.
- Separation of rectus abdominis muscle may occur, called diastasis recti.

PSYCHOLOGIC RESPONSES OF THE MOTHER TO PREGNANCY

Unless the following responses are extreme or exaggerated, they are considered normal. In most cases the nurse can reassure the woman of the normality of the response and explain that it is related to hormonal changes and to the body's efforts to prepare for childbirth and parenting.

1. **Ambivalence.** Initially, even if pregnancy is planned, the mother may have mixed feelings about it. She may have concerns about her career, her relationship with her part-

ner, financial implications, and role change. She may make comments such as "I thought I wanted a baby but now that I'm pregnant, I'm not so sure."

2. **Acceptance of pregnancy.** As the woman begins to accept the reality of the pregnancy she shows a high degree of tolerance for the discomforts she may experience in the first trimester. In the second trimester she may begin wearing maternity clothes. At about 17 to 21 weeks she will begin to perceive movement. She may make comments such as, "Feeling the baby move makes it all seem real" or "It's finally sinking in that I'm going to be a mother."

3. **Introversion.** The expectant woman typically becomes more inwardly focused, less interested in outside activities. She is using this time to plan and adjust. Her partner may see this as excluding him. She may say, "I never used to like to be alone but now I like having time to myself just to think and plan."

4. **Mood swings.** Mood swings from joy to sadness are common and difficult for the woman and her family. The woman often feels a great need for love and affection, but her partner, confused by her emotional changes, may react by withdrawing. She may say, "I'm not usually so emotional but lately any little thing can set me off."

5. **Changes in body image.** Typically the woman tends to feel somewhat negative about her body as pregnancy progresses. Her increasing abdomen coupled with the waddling gait of pregnancy may cause a woman to feel ungainly and unattractive. She may say, "I can't even see my feet anymore" or "I feel big as a house."

PSYCHOLOGIC TASKS OF THE MOTHER

Rubin (1984) identified the following developmental tasks of the mother:

1. **Ensuring safe passage through pregnancy, labor, and birth.** To meet this task she seeks competent prenatal care, practices good health behaviors and self-care activities, reads about childbirth, and gathers information.

2. **Seeking acceptance of this child by others.** The expectant woman seeks to gain support for the coming child from her partner and family. She will also work to help her other children accept the coming baby.

3. **Seeking of commitment and acceptance of self as mother to the infant (binding-in).** After she perceives fetal movement (quickening) the mother begins to form bonds of attachment to the child and he/she becomes more real. The woman may talk about the child as a separate person: "The baby was so active today! I don't think he (or she) appreciated the pizza last night."

4. **Learning to give of one's self on behalf of one's child.** The woman begins to develop patterns of self-denial and delayed personal gratification to meet the needs of her child. She may, for example, give up smoking or alcohol, and make plans to adjust her personal schedule to spend more time with her child.

ANTEPARTAL ASSESSMENT

Critical Terms

Gravida: any pregnancy, regardless of duration.

Primigravida: a woman who is pregnant for the first time.

Multigravida: a woman who is pregnant for her second or any subsequent pregnancy.

Para: birth after 20 weeks' gestation, regardless of whether infant is alive or dead.

Multipara: a woman who has had two or more births at more than 20 weeks' gestation.

Note: in clinical practice care givers often refer to a woman who is pregnant for the first time as a primip (short for primipara). In reality the correct term would actually be nulligravida, but it is seldom used. A woman becomes a primipara after she has had one birth of more than 20 weeks' gestation. Thus the term could be used on postpartum.

Stillbirth: a fetus born dead after 20 weeks' gestation.

Client History

1. **Current pregnancy.** A form of notation is used to quickly describe a woman's pregnancy history. For example, a woman pregnant for the first time would be gravida 1 para 0 (or G1 P0). A woman pregnant for the second time who

has one living child born at term and had one miscarriage (also called spontaneous abortion) would be gravida 2 para 1 abortion 1 (G2 P1 Ab1).

Some agencies use a more detailed approach: Gravida means the same as in the previous example; para refers to the number of infants but is further divided to identify the number of **t**erm, **p**reterm, **a**bortions, and **l**iving children (TPAL). The woman pregnant for the first time would be gravida 1 para 0000 (sometimes listed as 10000, 1 for gravida, 0000 for para). The second woman would be gravida 2 para 1011, i.e., one term infant, no preterm, one abortion, one living child (21011).

Other critical information:
- LMP: first day of last normal menstrual period (helps to date pregnancy)
- Presence of any problems or complications such as bleeding
- Any discomforts, concerns, questions

2. **History of past pregnancies.** Number of pregnancies, abortions (spontaneous or therapeutic), living children, complications. This information helps care givers avoid unintentionally hurtful comments and alerts them to potential problems. For example, a woman with a history of preterm labor is at increased risk for preterm labor.

3. **Gynecologic history.** Detailed gynecologic history is obtained. Critical information includes information on contraceptive history (For example, an intrauterine device [IUD] in place is usually removed because it could cause spontaneous abortion. Also, a woman who becomes pregnant while on birth control pills may have difficulty identifying LMP); history of sexually transmitted infections (history of herpes, for example, might influence route for childbirth); history of abnormal pap smears.

4. **Current and past medical history.** Provides information about woman's general state of health and health habits, any medical/surgical conditions that might impact the pregnancy, such as diabetes, heart disease, sickle cell anemia. Also notes use of alcohol, cigarettes, drugs, exposure to teratogens, allergies, current medications, blood type and Rh factor, record of immunizations, especially rubella.

5. **Religious/cultural/occupational history.** Gives information about any cultural influences and any workplace hazards.

Partner's History

Information is obtained about the partner's age; health; current and past medical history; use of substances including alcohol, cigarettes, social drugs, etc; blood type and Rh factor; occupation; and attitude about the pregnancy.

High-risk Pregnancy

Certain factors in the woman's history place her at increased risk for complications during her current pregnancy. These include smoking, maternal age less than 20, previous preterm birth, and so forth. Preexisting medical conditions such as maternal diabetes automatically place the woman in a higher risk category. After the history is obtained, most agencies use a form to rate the number of risk factors and obtain a score. **Women who fall into a high-risk category are monitored more closely for potential complications.**

Initial Prenatal Physical Examination

Critical nursing actions   The nurse is responsible for the following assessments at the initial prenatal examination:

- Vital signs, including temperature, pulse, respirations, and blood pressure (some agencies omit temperature)
- Height and weight

The nurse also obtains the following:

- Urinalysis (to detect proteinuria, glycosuria, hematuria, etc)
- Blood for CBC, including hematocrit (to detect anemia) and differential, VDRL, ABO and Rh typing, Rubella titer (to detect whether the woman is immune to German measles), sickle cell screen for black clients, other lab tests as ordered

The nurse then remains in the room to assist the examiner with the physical exam, including the pelvic exam (see Procedure 16: Pelvic Exam: Nursing Responsibilities).

Critical elements of the initial physical examination

1. **Skin.** Color noted (to detect anemia, cyanosis, jaundice); edema noted (may be normal or could indicate pregnancy-induced hypertension); changes normally associated with pregnancy noted, such as chloasma, linea nigra, spider nevi.

2. **Neck.** Thyroid assessed; may enlarge slightly during pregnancy; marked enlargement, nodules, etc, could indicate hyperthyroidism or goiter and are assessed further.

3. **Lungs.** Inspection, palpation, auscultation should be normal with no adventitious sounds.

4. **Breasts.** Inspection and palpation performed. Normal changes of pregnancy noted; orange-peel skin, palpable nodule suggest possible carcinoma; redness indicates mastitis.

5. **Heart.** Rate, rhythm, and heart sounds noted; should be normal. Short systolic murmur common due to increased blood volume.

6. **Abdomen.** Inspection and palpation performed. Liver and spleen not palpable. Shows changes of pregnancy including enlargement, striae.

   a. Fundus (upper portion of uterus) palpable as follows:

   - 10–12 weeks—slightly above symphysis
   - 16 weeks—halfway between symphysis and umbilicus
   - 20 weeks—at umbilicus
   - 28 weeks—three fingerbreadths above umbilicus
   - 36 weeks—just below ensiform cartilage

   b. Fetal heartbeat auscultated as follows:

   - 10–12 weeks—heard with Doppler (rate 120–160 beats/min)
   - 17–20 weeks—heard with stethoscope

   c. Fetal movement can be palpated by examiner at 20 weeks' gestation.

7. **Reflexes.** At least brachial and patellar assessed. Hyperreflexia could indicate developing PIH (see Procedure 3: Deep Tendon Reflexes and Clonus Assessment; PIH is discussed in Chapter 2).

8. **Pelvic exam.** External and internal genitalia inspected, pap obtained; gonorrhea culture (and sometimes chlamydia screen) obtained; changes of pregnancy noted, including Chadwick's sign, Goodell's sign. Uterine size evaluated to determine whether size seems appropriate for length of gestation. Ovaries palpated. Pelvic dimensions assessed to estimate whether pelvic size adequate for a vaginal birth.

The following dimensions are considered necessary for vaginal birth (See Figures 1–1 to 1–3):

- Pelvic inlet: Diagonal conjugate (extends from lower border of symphysis pubis to sacral promontory) at least 11.5 cm.
- Pelvic outlet: Anteroposterior diameter (from lower border of symphysis pubis to tip of sacrum) 9.5–11.5 cm.
- Pelvic outlet: Transverse diameter (measured by placing a fist between the ischial tuberosities) (Figure 1–2).
- Subpubic angle: Obtained by palpating bony structure externally, normally 85–90 degrees (Figure 1–3).

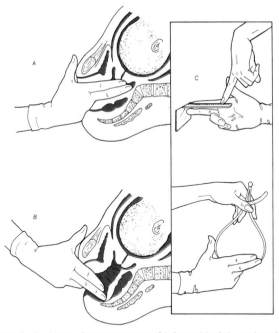

Figure 1–1 Manual measurement of inlet, midpelvis, and outlet:
A, *Estimation of diagonal conjugate, which extends from lower border of symphysis pubis to sacral promontory.* B, *Estimation of anteroposterior diameter of the outlet, which extends from lower border of the symphysis pubis to the tip of the sacrum.* C, *Methods that may be used to check manual estimation of anteroposterior measurements.*

Figure 1–2   Use of closed fist to measure outlet. Examiner should know the distance between first and last proximal knuckles.

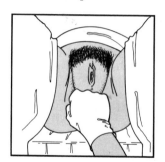

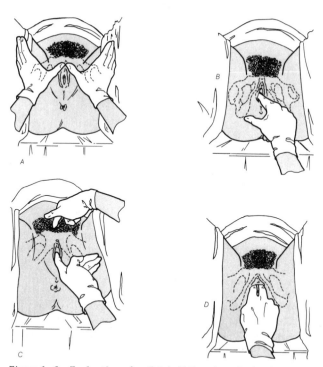

Figure 1–3   Evaluation of outlet: A, *Estimation of subpubic angle.* B, *Estimation of length of pubic ramus.* C, *Estimation of depth and inclination of pubis.* D, *Estimation of contour of subpubic angle.*

- Mobility of coccyx assessed by pressing on coccyx; it should be mobile.

9. **Rectal exam.** Rashes, lumps, hemorrhoids noted; woman with hemorrhoids should be assessed for problems with constipation.

Determination of Due Date

The due date (date around which childbirth will occur) helps the care giver determine if the fetus is growing appropriately and whether the start of labor occurs at the correct time or prematurely. The due date, also called the EDB (estimated date of birth), EDD (estimated date of delivery), or EDC (estimated date of confinement) is calculated using a formula called Nägele's Rule. To use this formula one begins with the first day of the woman's last menstrual period (LMP), subtracts three months, and adds seven days. For example:

First day of LMP	November 21
Subtract 3 months	−3 months
	August 21
Add 7 days	+7 days
EDB	August 28

Due date can also be calculated using a gestational wheel. Some women do not have regular menstrual cycles or may not keep track of their menses. Thus, other methods are also used to date the pregnancy. These include the following:

1. **Uterine assessment, or sizing the uterus.** A skilled examiner can determine by bimanual examination if the size of the uterus is appropriate for the weeks of pregnancy. This is an especially valuable technique in the first trimester.

2. **Measurement of fundal height.** After the first trimester the uterus is palpable in the abdomen. Its height can be measured by using a centimeter tape measure to measure the distance from the top of the symphysis pubis to the top of the fundus. Fundal height corresponds well with weeks of gestation, especially between 20 and 31 weeks. For example, 24 cm would suggest 24 weeks' gestation.

3. **Quickening (perception of fetal movement by the mother).** This almost always occurs by 19 to 20 weeks'

gestation. Because quickening may occur any time from 16 to 22 weeks, this is a less specific measure.

4. **Fetal heartbeat.** The heartbeat can be detected with a Doppler by 10–12 weeks' gestation and with a fetoscope by 19–20 weeks' gestation.

5. **Ultrasound.** This procedure can be used to detect a gestational sac in early pregnancy and to determine specific fetal measurements such as biparietal diameter. These measurements are useful in determining gestational age.

Frequency of Prenatal Visits in Normal Pregnancy

- Every four weeks for first 28 weeks of gestation
- Every two weeks to week 36
- After week 36, weekly until birth

Initial Psychosocial Assessment

The psychosocial assessment helps to determine the woman's attitude about the pregnancy, her teaching needs, the support systems she has available to her, her cultural or religious preferences, economic status, and living conditions. The following critical nursing assessments require further evaluation and intervention:

- Marked anxiety, apathy, fear, or anger about the pregnancy
- Isolated home environment without support systems available
- Language barriers
- Cultural practices that might endanger the child
- Long-term family problems
- Unstable or limited economic status; limited prenatal care
- Crowded or questionable living conditions

Regular Prenatal Visits

Critical nursing responsibilities

1. Weigh woman. During first trimester woman gains 2–4 lb; during second and third trimesters she gains about 1 lb/ week. Thus, when she is seen every four weeks a 4-lb gain is normal.

Be alert for:
- Inadequate gain—evaluate reasons, counsel on nutrition
- Excessive gain—often first sign of developing pregnancy-induced hypertension (PIH), a major complication of pregnancy (See Chapter 2 for further assessments.)

2. Vital signs. Pulse may increase slightly. BP usually decreases slightly toward midpregnancy and gradually returns to normal. Temperature and respirations may be omitted unless adverse symptoms are present.

Be alert for:
- Rapid pulse—could indicate anxiety or cardiac problem. Report findings
- Elevated BP—a cardinal sign of PIH (See Chapter 2 for further assessments.)

3. Assess for edema. Some edema of ankles and feet is normal, especially in last trimester.

Be alert for:
- Edema of hands, face, and legs—usually related to weight gain and may indicate PIH (See Chapter 2 for further assessments.)

4. Dipstick urine specimen.

Be alert for:
- Proteinuria 1+. Could indicate PIH (See Chapter 2.)
- Glycosuria—slight glycosuria may be normal but requires further assessment. Might indicate gestational diabetes mellitus (GDM) (See Chapter 2 for further assessments.)

5. Between 24–28 weeks' gestation a one-hour glucose screen is done. Plasma glucose levels > 140 mg/dL indicate GDM. Woman should be referred to physician.

6. Ask whether woman is experiencing any of the danger signs of pregnancy (see following discussion). Ask about the common discomforts of pregnancy and provide appropriate information (see page 18).

Certified nurse-midwife, nurse practitioner, or physician completes remainder of exam, which includes:

1. Review of history and findings

2. Assessment of uterine size, measurement of fundal height
3. Assessment of fetal heartbeat (normal 120–160 bpm) and position
4. Assessment of deep tendon reflexes (DTRs), clonus (see Procedure 3: Deep Tendon Reflexes and Clonus Assessment)
5. Vaginal exam not repeated until last weeks of pregnancy

Danger Signs of Pregnancy and Their Possible Causes

Table 1–1 identifies the danger signs of pregnancy and their possible causes. These findings indicate a potentially serious problem and require further assessment. The nurse reviews these signs, and stresses to the woman the importance of reporting them immediately should they occur. **Discuss them at each prenatal visit.**

PRENATAL NUTRITION

General Guidelines

1. Recommended dietary allowance (RDA) for most nutrients increases.
2. For a woman of normal weight the American College of Obstetricians and Gynecologists recommends a 26–35-lb gain; others feel this is too high and recommend a 24–32-lb gain.
3. Pattern of weight gain:

    • First trimester: 2–5 lb (1–2.3 kg)
    • Second and third trimester: about 1 lb per week
    • Caloric increase: **only 300 kcal day.** Idea that woman is "eating for two" can lead to excessive weight gain

4. Overweight women should **not** diet during pregnancy.
5. In second and third trimesters, further evaluation indicated for the following:

    • Inadequate gain (less than 2.2 lb [1 kg]/month)
    • Excessive gain (more than 6.6 lb [3 kg]/month)

Table 1–1 Danger Signs in Pregnancy

The woman should report the following danger signs in pregnancy immediately:

Danger Sign	Possible Cause
1. Sudden gush of fluid from vagina	Premature rupture of membranes
2. Vaginal bleeding	Abruptio placentae, placenta previa, lesions of cervix or vagina, "bloody show"
3. Abdominal pain	Premature labor, abruptio placentae
4. Temperature above 38.3°C (101°F) and chills	Infection
5. Dizziness, blurring of vision, double vision, spots before eyes	Hypertension, preeclampsia
6. Persistent vomiting	Hyperemesis gravidarum
7. Severe headache	Hypertension, preeclampsia
8. Edema of hands, face, legs, and feet	Preeclampsia
9. Muscular irritability, convulsions	Preeclampsia, eclampsia
10. Epigastric pain	Preeclampsia-ischemia in major abdominal vessels
11. Oliguria	Renal impairment, decreased fluid intake
12. Dysuria	Urinary tract infection
13. Absence of fetal movement	Maternal medication, obesity, fetal death

Critical Information in Counseling About Nutrition

1. Stress four basic food groups, including the following:
   Dairy: Adults need two servings (one serving = 1 c milk or yogurt, 1.5 oz hard cheese, 2 c cottage cheese, 1 c pudding made with milk)

Grains: Adults need four servings (one serving = 1 slice bread, 1 oz dry cereal, ½ hamburger roll, 1 tortilla, ½ c pasta, ½ c rice or grits)

Fruits/vegetables: Adults need four servings; one should be a good source of vitamin C (one serving = 1 medium-size piece of fruit; ½ c cooked vegetables; 1 c raw vegetables; ½ c juice; 1 c green, leafy vegetables)

Meats and alternates: Adults need at least two servings (one serving = 2 oz cooked lean meat, poultry or fish; 2 eggs; ½ c cottage cheese; 1 c cooked legumes [kidney, lima, garbanzo, or soy beans, split peas, etc]; 6 oz tofu; 2 oz nuts or seeds; 4 T peanut butter)

2. To increase diet by 300 kcal, woman should add two milk servings and one meat or alternate.
3. To get maximum benefit without additional calories, use low-fat dairy products, lean cuts of meat, low-fat cooking methods such as baking or broiling instead of frying, etc.
4. Limit extras that have little nutritional value and are high in sugar or fat, such as doughnuts, chips, candy, mayonnaise, etc.

Nutrition for the Pregnant Adolescent

If adolescent is less than four years post-menarche, her nutritional needs include the increase for pregnancy (300 kcal) plus the intake necessary for her anticipated weight gain developmentally during the year she is pregnant. Adolescent diets tend to be deficient in iron and calcium. Iron supplements are used and iron-rich foods are encouraged (see following discussion of nutrition for the woman with anemia). Folic acid supplements are also given. If the adolescent is unwilling or unable to consume sufficient calcium, supplements may be necessary, usually 1200 mg daily.
Note: Many adolescents have a better diet than believed. Thus their eating patterns over several days, not simply one day, should be assessed.

Nutrition for the Pregnant Vegetarian

There are several types of vegetarians. Lacto-ovovegetarians include milk, dairy products, and eggs in their diet. Some also include fish and poultry. Lactovegetarians include dairy products but no eggs. Vegans are "pure" vegetarians who will not eat any food from animal sources.

If her diet permits, a woman can obtain adequate complete proteins from dairy products and eggs. Pure vegans must use complementing proteins such as unrefined grains (brown rice, whole wheat), legumes (beans, split peas, lentils), and nuts and seeds (in large quantities). Vegans should take a daily supplement of 4 gm of vitamin B_{12}. Vegetarian diets also tend to be low in iron and zinc and supplementation is often necessary.

Nutrition for the Woman with Anemia

To correct iron deficiency anemia the woman will be given iron supplements. The nurse should explain to her that she can also help herself by the following dietary practices:

- Regularly eat meat, poultry, and fish, which are good sources of iron.
- Consume iron-fortified cereals and breads.
- Iron absorption is increased when vitamin C is taken with meals. Good sources of vitamin C include citrus fruits, strawberries, tomatoes, cantaloupe, broccoli, peppers, and potatoes.
- Select iron-rich vegetables such as spinach; broccoli; dandelion greens; and other green; leafy vegetables.
- Use iron pots and pans for cooking.

RELIEF OF THE COMMON DISCOMFORTS OF PREGNANCY

Because of the physical and physiologic changes that occur during pregnancy, the woman may experience a variety of discomforts. The nurse has the primary responsibility for teaching the woman self-care measures to help alleviate these discomforts. The following section focuses on common discomforts and identifies interventions that may be effective:

First Trimester

Nausea and vomiting
- Avoid odors or factors that trigger nausea.
- Eat dry toast or crackers before arising.
- Have small but frequent dry meals with fluids between meals.

- Avoid greasy or highly seasoned foods.
- Drink carbonated beverages.

Urinary frequency

- Increase daytime fluid intake; void when the urge is felt.
- Decrease fluid **only** in the evening to decrease nocturia.

Breast Tenderness

- Wear well-fitting, supportive bra.

Increased vaginal discharge

- Bathe daily but avoid douching, nylon panties, and pantyhose.
- Wear cotton underpants.

Nasal stuffiness and epistaxis

- May be unresponsive; cool air vaporizer may help.
- Avoid nasal sprays and decongestants.

Ptyalism

- Use astringent mouthwash, chew gum, suck hard candy.

Second and Third Trimesters

Pyrosis (heartburn)

- Eat small, frequent meals; avoid overeating or lying down afterward.
- Use low-sodium antacids, avoid sodium bicarbonate.

Ankle edema

- Dorsiflex foot frequently; elevate legs when sitting or resting.
- Avoid tight garters or constricting bands.

Varicose veins

- Wear supportive hose and elevate feet frequently.
- Avoid crossing legs at knees, prolonged standing, and garters.

Constipation

- Increase fluid in diet. (Drink at least eight 8-oz glasses daily.)
- Increase fiber. (Increase fruits/vegetables to six servings; choose fresh fruit when possible and include prunes or prune juice; increase grains to six servings and choose unrefined grains, such as whole wheat, brown rice and bran; include legumes in place of meat.)
- Increase daily exercise to promote peristalsis.

Hemorrhoids

- Avoid constipation and straining to defecate.
- Reinsert into rectum if necessary; treat with topical anesthetics, warm soaks or sitz baths, ice packs.

Backache

- Use good body mechanics; do pelvic tilt exercise regularly.
- Avoid uncomfortable working heights, high-heeled shoes, lifting heavy loads, and fatigue.

Leg cramps

- Practice dorsiflexing foot to stretch affected muscle.
- Apply heat to affected muscle.

Faintness

- Avoid prolonged standing in warm area; arise slowly from resting position.

Dyspnea

- Use proper posture when sitting or standing; sleep propped up with pillows if problem occurs at night.

Flatulence

- Chew food thoroughly and avoid gas-forming food.
- Exercise regularly and maintain normal bowel habits.

Carpal tunnel syndrome

- Avoid aggravating hand movements; use splint as prescribed.
- Elevate affected arm.

PROMOTION OF SELF-CARE DURING PREGNANCY

Pregnant women may have questions about a variety of issues, which they will often raise with the prenatal nurse. The following discussion highlights critical information that the nurse should provide about selected topics.

Monitoring Fetal Activity

Vigorous fetal activity indicates fetal well-being, while a marked decrease in fetal activity may indicate fetal compromise and requires immediate evaluation. Fetal activity may be affected by drugs, cigarette smoking, sound, fetal sleep periods, blood glucose levels, and time of day. It has become accepted practice to teach pregnant women to monitor fetal activity daily beginning at about 27 weeks' gestation. Most healthy babies move at least ten times in 12 hours.

The woman begins counting fetal movements at a specified time twice daily, preferably about one hour after eating and while lying on her side. Movements are counted for 20–30 minutes; five to six movements in that time is considered reassuring. If there are fewer than three movements in that time the woman should continue counting for an hour or more. She should contact her care giver if there are fewer than ten movements in a 12-hour period OR no movements in the morning OR less than three fetal movements in eight hours. The care giver will probably order a nonstress test (NST) (see page 24).

Bathing

Daily bathing, by shower or in a tub, is important. The woman should take care to avoid slipping, especially because of her changed center of gravity. A rubber tub mat helps avoid this. **Stress that tub baths are contraindicated in the presence of ruptured membranes or vaginal bleeding to avoid introducing infection.**

Employment

Major problems with employment during pregnancy include exposure to fetotoxic hazards, excessive physical strain, overfatigue, medical or pregnancy-related complications, and, in later pregnancy, difficulty with occupations involving balance. Advise the woman who continues working to use breaks and lunch for rest, preferably on her side. Women who stand in place for long periods should dorsiflex their feet and walk around periodically to avoid problems with varicose veins, phlebitis, and edema.

Travel

If no complications exist, there are no restrictions on travel. Travel by plane or train is preferable for long distances. The woman should walk about periodically to avoid phlebitis. If traveling by car she should plan to stop every two hours and walk around for ten minutes. Seat belts should be worn with the lap belt positioned under the abdomen.

Exercise

The woman is encouraged to exercise at least three times/week. Swimming, cycling, walking, and cross-country skiing are good choices. She should wear a supportive bra and appropriate shoes, should avoid hyperthermia, and should take fluids liberally to avoid dehydration. The woman should exercise for shorter intervals (15 minutes at a time with a maximum heart rate of 140 beats/min. Fit women can exercise for 30 minutes with a maximum pulse rate of 150 beats/min). To avoid supine hypotensive syndrome she should avoid lying flat on her back to exercise after the fourth month. Dizziness, extreme shortness of breath, tingling and numbness, palpitations, abdominal pain, vaginal bleeding, and abrupt cessation of fetal movement should be reported to her care giver.
   Stress the importance of adequate rest.

Exercises in Preparation for Childbirth

Teach abdominal tightening; partial, bent-knee sit-ups; Kegel exercises; and tailor sitting.

Sexual Activity

Change in desire is normal and may vary according to trimester. In the first trimester, fatigue, nausea, and breast tenderness may lead to decreased desire for some women. Other women experience no change. The second trimester may be a time of increased desire. The third trimester may lead to decreased desire. Woman should avoid lying flat on her back for intercourse after the fourth month to avoid vena caval syndrome. If that position is preferred she should place a pillow under her right hip to displace the uterus. Change in position, such as side-lying, female superior, or vaginal rear entry, may become necessary as her uterus enlarges. In the last weeks of pregnancy orgasms may be more intense and may be followed by uterine cramping.

Stress that sexual intercourse is contraindicated once the membranes are ruptured or in the presence of vaginal bleeding to avoid introducing infection. Women with a history of preterm labor may be advised to avoid intercourse in the third trimester because the oxytocin that is released with orgasm or with breast stimulation may trigger contractions. Couples who prefer anal intercourse should avoid going from anal penetration to vaginal penetration because of the risk of introducing infection.

Men may notice a change in their level of desire, too. If a man feels the desire for further sexual release he may need to masturbate, either with his partner or in private.

The couple can also be encouraged to explore other methods of expressing intimacy and affection, such as stroking, cuddling, and kissing.

Medications, Alcohol, Smoking

Women should avoid taking medication when pregnant—both prescribed and over-the-counter medication. If the need for medication arises, the woman should make certain her care giver knows that she is pregnant. Smoking is related to lower birth weight infants and to preterm labor. Women should avoid it as much as possible. Alcohol has been linked to neurologic deficits in newborns and to low birth weight. Heavy drinking may lead to fetal alcohol syndrome. Since it is not clear how much alcohol is problematic it should be avoided. Similarly women should avoid cocaine, crack, marijuana, and all social and street drugs during pregnancy.

CHARTING

Most prenatal records are comprised of a series of columns for making notations succinctly. These columns include height, weight, blood pressure, urine, fetal heart rate, fundal height, edema, fetal movement, clonus, etc. Notations should be made in the "comments" about any deviations from normal, about any teaching that is done, and about any special procedures.

Charting on the prenatal record tends to be especially succinct, as the following example demonstrates:

> Basic four food groups and caloric increases for pregnancy discussed. Handout on prenatal nutrition reviewed and given to client. Reports she is taking prenatal vitamins regularly. States that nausea has decreased and she is walking 2 miles/four times/week. No problems or distress. Will call if symptoms develop. A. Smythe, RN

ASSESSMENT OF FETAL WELL-BEING

Ultrasound

Obstetric ultrasound is generally done transabdominally but a newer transvaginal technique is also available. Ultrasound is noninvasive, painless, nonradiating to the woman and fetus, and has no known harmful effects. Serial studies can be done for assessment and comparison.

Ultrasound can be used for early identification of pregnancy (as early as 5th–6th week after LMP); for identification of more than one fetus; to measure biparietal diameter; to detect fetal anomalies, hydramnios (excess amniotic fluid) or oligohydramnios (too little fluid); to locate and grade the placenta; to observe fetal heart rate, movement, respirations, position and presentation, or fetal death.

Nursing interventions The nurse provides an opportunity for the woman to ask questions and acts as a client advocate.

Nonstress Test

The nonstress test (NST) is used to assess fetal status using an electronic fetal monitor to observe baseline variability and acceleration of fetal heart rate (FHR) with movement. FHR accelerations indicate that the fetal central and autonomic nervous systems have not been affected by decreased oxygen to the fetus.

Procedure NST may be done in a clinic or an inpatient setting. The woman is placed in semi-Fowler's position, in a side-lying position, or in a reclining chair. Two belts are placed on the woman's abdomen: one records the FHR, the other records uterine or fetal movement. The fetal monitor begins recording activity. The woman is instructed to press a button on the monitor (or on the uterine belt) each time she feels the fetus move. This causes a mark on the tracing paper. An assessment can then be made as to whether FHR accelerations occurred with each fetal movement.

Interpretation of NST Results

* **Reactive test** shows at least two accelerations of FHR with fetal movements, of 15 beats/min, lasting 15 seconds or more, over a period of 20 minutes (Figure 1–4).
* **Nonreactive test** is one in which the reactive criteria are not met (Figure 1–5).
* **Unsatisfactory test** is one in which data cannot be interpreted or there is inadequate fetal activity.

A reactive NST usually indicates fetal well-being and the test does not need to be repeated for a week. A nonreactive NST indicates the need for further testing.

Nursing interventions The nurse explains the procedure, administers the NST, interprets the results, and reports the findings to the physician/certified nurse-midwife. If the fetus is not moving well, it is sometimes helpful to have the mother drink a glass of juice to increase her blood glucose level. This seems to result in increased fetal activity.
Note: If any decelerations in FHR occur during the procedure, the physician/nurse-midwife should be notified for further evaluation of fetal status.

Fetal Biophysical Profile

The fetal biophysical profile is a collection of information regarding selected fetal measurements and assessments of the fetus and the amniotic fluid. It includes five variables: fetal breathing movements, body movement, tone, FHR activity, and amniotic fluid volume. Table 1–2 identifies scoring techniques and interpretation. Table 1–3 outlines a management protocol.

Amniotic Fluid Analysis (Amniocentesis)

Amniotic fluid can be withdrawn through a needle inserted through the abdominal wall into the uterus and analyzed to obtain valuable information about fetal status. Amniotic fluid

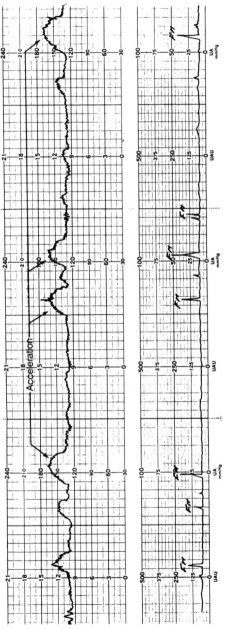

Figure 1—4 Example of a reactive nonstress test (NST). The top portion of the strip is a recording of the FHR. Note that most of the FHR tracing is relatively straight, with some areas that rise from this relatively straight line. These are accelerations. Each small square of the graph paper equals ten seconds, so each of the indicated accelerations is more than 15 seconds in length. Each of the identified accelerations occurs with a fetal movement (FM), which is recorded on the bottom portion of the strip. The criteria for a reactive NST have been met on this tracing.

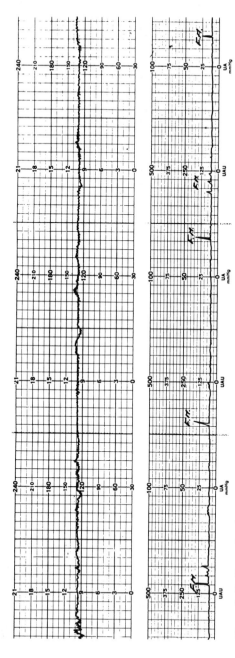

Figure 1–5   Example of a nonreactive NST. There are no accelerations of the FHR with the episodes of fetal movement indicated on the bottom portion of the strip.

Table 1-2 Biophysical Profile Scoring: Technique and Interpretation

Biophysical Variable	Normal (Score = 2)	Abnormal (Score = 0)
1. Fetal breathing movements	≥1 episode of ≥30 sec in 30 min	Absent or no episode of ≥30 sec in 30 min
2. Gross body movements	≥3 discrete body/limb movements in 30 min (episodes of active continuous movement considered as single movement)	≤2 episodes of body/limb movements in 30 min
3. Fetal tone	≥1 episode of active extension with return to flexion of fetal limb(s) or trunk. Opening and closing of hand considered normal tone	Either slow extension with return to partial flexion or movement of limb in full extension or absent fetal movement
4. Reactive fetal heart rate	≥2 episodes of acceleration of ≥15 bpm and of ≥15 sec associated with fetal movement in 20 min	<2 episodes of acceleration of fetal heart rate or acceleration of <15 bpm in 20 min
5. Qualitative amniotic fluid volume	≥1 pocket of fluid measuring ≥1 cm in two perpendicular planes	Either no pockets or a pocket <1 cm in two perpendicular planes

Source: Manning FA et al: Fetal assessment based on fetal biophysical profile scoring: Experience in 12,620 referred high-risk pregnancies. *Am J Obstet Gynecol* 1985; 151(3): 344.

Table 1–3 Biophysical Profile Scoring: Management Protocol

Score	Interpretation	Recommended Management
10	Normal infant, low risk for chronic asphyxia	Repeat testing at weekly intervals. Repeat twice weekly in diabetic patients and patients ≥42 wk
8	Normal infant, low risk for chronic asphyxia	Repeat testing at weekly intervals. Repeat twice weekly in diabetic patients and patients ≥42 wk. Indication for delivery = oligohydramnios
6	Suspected chronic asphyxia	Repeat testing within 24 hr. Indication for delivery = oligohydramnios or persisting ≤6
4	Suspected chronic asphyxia	≥36 wk and favorable cervix. If <36 wk and lecithin/sphingomyelin ratio <2.0, repeat test in 24 hr. Indication for delivery = repeat score ≤6 or oligohydramnios
0–2	Strong suspicion of chronic asphyxia	Extend testing time to 120 min. Indication for delivery = persistent score ≤4, regardless of gestational age

Source: Manning FA et al: Fetal assessment based on fetal biophysical profile scoring: Experience in 12,620 referred high-risk pregnancies. *Am J Obstet Gynecol* 1985; 151(3): 344.

analysis provides genetic information about the fetus and can also be used to determine fetal lung maturity. (See Procedure 1: Amniocentesis: Nursing Responsibilities.)

Fetal lung maturity can be ascertained by determining the ratio of the phospholipids, lecithin and sphingomyelin. These are two components of surfactant, the substance that lowers the surface tension of the alveoli of the lungs when the newborn exhales, thereby preventing lung collapse. Early in pregnancy the sphingomyelin component is greater than the lecithin so that the lecithin to sphingomyelin (L/S) ratio is low. As pregnancy progresses the lecithin increases. Fetal maturity is indicated by an L/S ratio of 2:1 or greater. **Note: delayed lung maturation is often seen in infants born to diabetic mothers. Thus an L/S ratio of 3:1 or higher may be necessary in these infants to ensure lung maturity.**

Another phospholipid, phosphatidylglycerol (PG), appears in the amniotic fluid after about 35 weeks' gestation and the amount continues to increase to term.

Amniotic creatinine progressively increases with the length of pregnancy, apparently because of increasing fetal muscle mass and maturing fetal renal function. Creatinine levels of 2 mg/dL are associated with fetal maturity.

In summary, fetal lung maturity is probable if the following are present:

- L/S ratio of 2:1 or greater
- PG present
- Amniotic creatinine of 2 mg/dL

REFERENCES

Rubin R: *Maternal Identity and the Maternal Experience.* New York: Springer, 1984.

❀ ❀ ❀ ❀ ❀ ❀ ❀ ❀ ❀ ❀ ❀ ❀ ❀ ❀ ❀ ❀ ❀ ❀

CHAPTER 2

The At-risk Antepartal Client

DIABETES MELLITUS

Overview

In diabetes mellitus the pancreas does not produce enough insulin to allow necessary carbohydrate metabolism. Glucose does not enter the cells and they become energy depleted. The physiologic changes of pregnancy can drastically alter insulin requirements. In the first half of pregnancy maternal hormones stimulate increased insulin production by the pancreas and increased tissue response to insulin. In the second half of pregnancy maternal hormones cause increased resistance to insulin. Concurrently, increased amounts of maternal glucose are being diverted to the fetus. Any diabetic potential may be influenced by this increased stress on the β-cells of the pancreas. **Gestational diabetes mellitus (GDM)** refers to diabetes that develops during pregnancy, often in the third trimester. To detect this condition, most women are screened for GDM between 24 and 28 weeks' gestation, using a 50-gram, 1-hour oral glucose screen. Often gestational diabetes can be managed with diet, although some women will receive regular insulin as well.

For women with **pregestational diabetes mellitus** (DM present before conception), the changes in glucose metabolism that result with pregnancy can affect diabetic control and can contribute to possible accelerations of the vascular disease associated with DM. The infant of a diabetic mother (IDM) is at greater risk for mortality or morbidity.

Pregestational diabetes can be type I (insulin dependent) or type II (non–insulin-dependent). Women with pregestational DM are treated with insulin only because oral anti-hyperglycemic agents are teratogenic to the fetus.

Maternal risks with diabetic pregnancy include the following: hydramnios (excessive volume of amniotic fluid), pregnancy-induced hypertension, ketoacidosis, fetal macrosomia leading to dystocia (difficult labor), anemia, monilial vaginitis, urinary tract infection (UTI), and retinopathy.

Fetal-neonatal risks include the following: intrauterine growth retardation (IUGR), macrosomia (large-size infant), hypoglycemia, respiratory distress syndrome, hyperbilirubinemia, and congenital anomalies.

Medical Management

1. **Dietary regulation.** Caloric needs of pregnant women are not altered by diabetes. They need 30 kcal/kg ideal body weight (IBW) during first trimester and 35–36 kcal/kg IBW during second and third trimesters. Fifty to sixty percent of calories should come from complex carbohydrates, 12% to 20% from protein, and 20% to 30% from fat. This is divided among three meals and three snacks. Prebedtime snack is most important because of risk of hypoglycemia during the night and should contain both protein and complex carbohydrates.

2. **Glucose monitoring.** Urine monitoring is seldom used. Many physicians have women come in weekly for assessment of fasting glucose levels and periodic postprandial levels. Most also have the woman do home monitoring of blood glucose levels QID—a fasting level before breakfast and then two hours after each meal. Optimal range, fasting: 60–100 mg/dL, two hours postprandial: 100–140 mg/dL (Ghiloni 1989).

3. **Insulin administration.** The dosage of human insulin is generally divided as follows: ⅔ of total dose taken in AM with a 2:1 ratio of intermediate insulin to regular; remaining ⅓ of dose taken with evening meal in a ratio of 1:1. The amount of insulin needed usually increases during each trimester of pregnancy.
Note: oral hypoglycemics are teratogenic and are never used in pregnancy.

4. **Evaluation of fetal status.** Woman is taught to monitor daily fetal activity (Chapter 1). Nonstress tests (NSTs) (see Chapter 1) are begun weekly at 28 weeks and increase to twice weekly at 32 weeks (Gabbe 1990). Ultrasounds are done at 18 weeks and 28 weeks to establish gestational age and assess for intrauterine growth retardation; biophysical profiles are done in third trimester to evaluate fetal well-being.

Critical Nursing Assessments

1. Assess urine for glucose and ketones at each prenatal visit.
2. Assess results of blood glucose testing for women with diagnosed GDM or pregestational DM.
3. Assess for any signs of UTI (dysuria, urgency, frequency, hematuria) or monilial vaginitis (excessive itching, curdy white discharge, dyspareunia).
4. Assess woman's understanding of her condition, its treatment, and implications.
   Be alert for: hyperglycemia, hypoglycemia, evidence of infection, signs of vascular complications (ulceration of extremities, visual changes, and so forth).

Sample Nursing Diagnoses

1. Knowledge deficit related to the disease and its implications for the woman and her unborn child.
2. Altered family processes related to the client's hospitalization for stabilization of her DM.

Critical Nursing Interventions

1. Obtain serum glucose readings at the specified times (if woman is hospitalized).
2. Administer insulin as prescribed. Have a second nurse verify the dosage before administering the insulin.
3. Monitor for signs of hypoglycemia (Table 2–1). If they occur, immediately check woman's capillary glucose level (and teach her to do the same following discharge). Follow agency policy regarding procedure for correcting hypoglycemia for blood glucose < 60 mg/dL. This may include 8-oz milk or 4-oz orange juice. If woman is not alert enough to swallow, give 1 mg glucagon subq or IM and notify physician. (See Nursing Care Plan 4: Diabetes Mellitus for additional information.)
4. Monitor fetal status including fetal heart rate (FHR) q4h; assist woman with determining fetal movement record daily; do NSTs as ordered while woman is hospitalized.
5. Provide appropriate American Diabetes Association (ADA) diet as indicated. Work with dietitian to ensure appropriate teaching is provided for the woman.

Table 2–1 Comparison of Hypoglycemia and Hyperglycemia

	Hypoglycemia	Hyperglycemia
Causes	Too much insulin Too little food Increased exercise without increased food	Too little insulin Too much food (especially carbohydrate) Emotional stress Infection
Onset	Usually sudden (minutes to half-hour)	Slow (days)
Symptoms in general order of appearance	Nervousness Shakiness Weakness Hunger Sweatiness Cool clammy skin Pallor Blurred or double vision Headache Disorientation	Polyuria Polydipsia Dry mouth Increased appetite Tiredness Nausea Hot flushed skin Abdominal cramps Abdominal rigidity Rapid deep breathing

Chapter 2 ❀ 35

Shallow respirations Irritability Convulsions Coma	Acetone breath Paralysis Headache Soft eyeballs Drowsiness Oliguria or anuria Depressed reflexes Stupor Coma
Laboratory findings:	
Urine	Glucose—negative Acetone—usually negative	Glucose—positive Acetone—positive
Blood	Glucose—60 mg/dL or lower Acetone—negative	Glucose—±250 mg/dL Acetone—usually positive

Treatment: See Nursing Care Plan for Diabetes Mellitus

Other comas: Hyperosmolar coma is most often seen in persons over 60 years of age with type II diabetes. Lactic acidosis coma occurs in advanced stages of diabetes, especially in persons with uremia, arteriosclerotic heart disease, pneumonia, acute pancreatitis, chronic alcoholism, and bacterial infection.

Adapted from Guthrie DW, Guthrie RA: *Nursing Management of Diabetes Mellitus*, 2nd ed. St. Louis: Mosby; 1982.

6. Complete client teaching about the following:

   - Procedure for home monitoring of blood glucose: Wash hands thoroughly before finger puncture. Sides of fingers should be punctured (ends contain more pain sensitive nerves). Hanging arm down for 30 sec before puncture increases blood flow to fingers. Spring-loaded devices are available to make puncture easier. Cleanse finger with alcohol pad first and allow alcohol to air dry. Touch blood droplet, not finger, to test pad on strip. Droplet should completely cover the test pad. If using visual method, wait prescribed time and compare color to color chart. If using a glucose meter, follow directions for use exactly. Record results and bring record sheet to each prenatal visit.

   - Procedure for insulin administration (if woman is not already familiar with it).

   - Signs of hypoglycemia and required treatment (Table 2–1).

   - Signs of hyperglycemia and required treatment (Table 2–1).

   - ADA diet.

7. Review the following critical aspects of the care you have provided:

   - Have I administered the correct doses of insulin at the specified times after first determining blood glucose levels?

   - Have I been alert for any signs of hypoglycemia or hyperglycemia?

   - Have I monitored FHR and fetal activity carefully and discussed with the woman her perceptions of fetal activity?

   - Have I assessed the woman's understanding of her DM and answered her questions? Have I given her opportunities to practice specific skills as necessary?

   - Have I ensured that the woman is eating the appropriate meals?

Evaluation

- The woman clearly understands her condition and its possible impact on her pregnancy.

- The woman participates in developing a health-care regimen to meet her needs and follows it throughout pregnancy.
- The woman avoids developing hypoglycemia or hyperglycemia; if it does develop, therapy is successful in correcting it without complications.
- The woman gives birth to a healthy newborn.

PREGNANCY-INDUCED HYPERTENSION (PIH)

Overview

Pregnancy-induced hypertension (PIH), the most common hypertensive disorder in pregnancy, is characterized by the development of hypertension, proteinuria, and edema. The definition of PIH is a blood pressure (BP) of 140/90 mm Hg during the second half of pregnancy in a previously normotensive woman. An increase in systolic blood pressure of 30 mm Hg and/or of diastolic of 15 mm Hg over baseline also defines PIH. These blood pressure changes must be noted on at least two occasions six hours or more apart for the diagnosis to be made (Sibai 1989).

Mild preeclampsia is characterized by a BP of 140/90 or +30/+15 over baseline on two occasions at least five hours apart; generalized edema of the face, hands, legs, and ankles, which is usually associated with a weight gain of more than 1 lb/week; and proteinuria of 1+ to 2+ on dipstick (less than 5 gm in 24 hours).

Severe preeclampsia is characterized by a blood pressure of 160/110 on two occasions at least six hours apart while the woman is on bed rest; proteinuria > 5 gm in 24 hours (3+ to 4+ dipstick); oliguria (urine output < 400 mL/24 hr); headache, blurred vision, scotomata (spots before the eyes), and retinal edema on funduscopy (retinas appear wet and glistening); pulmonary edema; hyperreflexia; irritability; and epigastric pain.

Eclampsia is characterized by a grand mal seizure, which may be preceded by an elevated temperature as high as 38.4°C (101°F), or the temperature may remain normal. The woman may have just one seizure or from 2 to 20 or more. Symptoms may increase in severity: BP of 180/110 or higher, 4+ proteinuria, oliguria or anuria, and increased neurologic symptoms such as decreased sensorium or coma.

Maternal risks with PIH include the following: retinal detachment, central nervous system changes including hyperreflexia and seizure, HELLP syndrome (**h**emolysis, **e**levated **l**iver enzymes, and **l**ow **p**latelet count). Women who experience HELLP, a multiple organ failure syndrome, and their offspring have high morbidity and mortality rates (Martin et al 1990).

Fetal-neonatal risks include the following: prematurity, intrauterine growth retardation, oversedation at birth because of maternal medications, and mortality rates of 10% with preeclampsia and 20% with eclampsia.

Medical Management

Mild preeclampsia (may be managed on outpatient basis in some cases):

1. **Promotion of good placental and renal perfusion.** Frequent rest periods are necessary during the day in a side-lying position. Specific guidelines regarding rest periods may be given, including the amount of time in each rest period, number of rest periods daily, and the activities during the day that are advisable or should be avoided. The more specific the guidelines, the more likely that the woman will clearly understand the information and restrictions.

2. **Dietary modifications.** Diet should be high in protein (80–100 gm/day, or 1.5 gm/kg/day). Sodium intake should be moderate, not exceeding 6 gm/day.

3. **Evaluation of fetal status.** NSTs and/or fetal biophysical profile are done on a weekly basis. Additional tests include serial ultrasounds to evaluate fetal growth, amniocentesis to determine fetal lung maturity, and a contraction stress test if nonstress test results indicate a need.

4. **Evaluation of maternal well-being.** The woman is seen every one to two weeks, is taught signs of a worsening condition, and does home blood pressure monitoring daily.

Severe Preeclampsia (hospitalization necessary):

1. **Promotion of maternal well-being.** Complete bed rest in left lateral position, which decreases pressure on vena cava, thereby increasing venous perfusion. Improved renal blood flow helps decrease angiotensin II levels, promotes diuresis, and lowers blood pressure. High protein moder-

ate sodium diet is continued. The woman is weighed daily (to detect edema), and evaluated for evidence of a change in condition through assessment of BP, TPR, deep tendon reflexes (DTRs) and clonus, edema (generalized and pitting), presence of headache, visual disturbances, and epigastric pain.

2. **Evaluation of laboratory data.** Daily hematocrit (rising value may be associated with decreasing vascular volume), daily liver enzyme testing including SGOT, SGPT, and LDH (a rise in these tests correlates with a worsening condition), daily uric acid and BUN (reflect renal status), platelet counts every two to three days if over 100,000/mm³, daily if under 100,000/mm³. (Platelet count may be included in preeclamptic or disseminated intravascular coagulation [DIC] screen, which also determines prothrombin time, partial thromboplastin time, fibrinogen and fibrin split products.) Platelet transfusion may be considered if the platelet count is below 50,000/mm³ (Scott and Worley 1990).

3. **Medication therapy.** Magnesium sulfate is the treatment of choice for preventing convulsion (see Drug Guide 6: Magnesium Sulfate). Sedation with phenobarbital 30–60 mg p.o. q6h may be indicated. (Some physicians prefer diazepam [Valium].) An antihypertensive such as hydralazine (Apresoline) 5 mg by slow IV push or a continuous infusion may be used if the diastolic pressure is over 110 mm Hg. Fluid and electrolytes are replaced as necessary based on the status of the woman.

Eclampsia

1. **Promotion of maternal well-being.** The therapies discussed previously are continued. Additional magnesium sulfate or sedation is used to stop the convulsion. The airway is maintained and the woman is monitored for pulmonary edema, which may be treated with furosemide (Lasix). Digitalis may be given for circulatory failure. The woman may be transferred to an intensive care unit.

Critical Nursing Assessments

1. Assess BP, pulse, and respirations q2–4h.
2. Assess temperature q4h unless elevated, then q2h.
3. Assess FHR when maternal vital signs (VS) are assessed or continuously with an electronic fetal monitor.

4. Assess intake and urinary output hourly or q4h. Output should be 700 mL/24 hr, or at least 30 mL/hr.
5. Assess urinary protein by dipstick of each urine specimen or a specimen from indwelling bladder catheter.
   Assessment technique: A small sample of urine is collected in a urine specimen bottle or in a syringe. A few drops of urine are placed on the treated section of the dipstick. The color of the treated urine is compared to samples on the dipstick container after a specified period of time. See dipstick container for specific instructions.
6. Assess urine specific gravity.
7. Assess for evidence of edema.
   Assessment technique: Assess for pitting edema by pressing over bony areas, usually over the shin. After pressing with one fingertip for three to five seconds, the resulting depression is evaluated. A slight depression is 1+, a pit one-inch deep is 4+.
8. Assess daily weight. Use the same scales each day, weigh at the same time each day with the woman in similar clothing.
9. Assess DTRs. Assess for clonus. (See Procedure 3: Deep Tendon Reflexes and Clonus Assessment.)
10. Assess breath sounds—rales will be heard if pulmonary edema is developing.
11. Assess laboratory results.
12. Assess woman's coping responses, level of understanding regarding her condition, and emotional status.
13. See Drug Guide 6: Magnesium Sulfate for specific nursing assessments during $MgSO_4$ therapy. **Be alert for:** Signs of worsening condition (increasing B/P, headache, scotomata, epigastric pain, pitting edema); signs of $MgSO_4$ toxicity (respirations $< 12-14$/min, diminished or absent reflexes, urine output < 100 mL in four-hour period).

Sample Nursing Diagnoses

- Fluid volume deficit related to fluid shift from intravascular to extravascular space secondary to vasospasm.
- High risk for injury related to possibility of convulsion secondary to cerebral vasospasm or edema.
- Knowledge deficit related to PIH and its implications for the woman and her unborn child.

Critical Nursing Interventions

If the woman is managed at home:

1. Teach the woman and her support person how to assess BP. Include positioning and specifics of the procedure. Assist them in developing a chart to record the findings. Instruct them about findings that should be reported to the physician.

2. Provide teaching about the rest period regimen. Explain the purpose of the side-lying position.

If the woman is hospitalized:

1. Monitor maternal BP, pulse and respirations, DTRs and clonus, and FHR q2–4h. Monitor oral temperature q4h unless elevated, then q2h.

2. Monitor intake and output; monitor urine for proteinuria and specific gravity with each voiding or hourly if an indwelling catheter is in place. Output should be at least 30 mL/hr. Specific gravity of readings > 1.040 indicate oliguria.

3. Monitor for signs of worsening condition including headache, visual disturbances, epigastric pain, and change in level of consciousness at least q4h.

4. Maintain woman in a side-lying position.

5. Provide emotional support and teaching regarding condition and treatment plan.

6. Administer $MgSO_4$ and other medications as ordered. Monitor for evidence of effectiveness or toxicity.

7. Provide a quiet, restful environment with limited visitors.

8. Pad side rails and take seizure precautions.

9. Review the following aspects of the care you have provided:

   - What is the woman's response to the medications? Am I seeing any potential side effects?

   - Is there a change in her ability to talk? Does she seem more irritable? Confused?

   - Is she complaining of headache or other symptoms that indicate a worsening condition?

   - Is the baby moving as much? Is FHR in normal range (120–160 beats/min)?

   - Positioning on which side produces the best results in fetal heart rate? Urine output? What can I do to help her maintain that position? A back rub? Pillows?

- Have I taken necessary safety precautions, including padded side rails, quiet environment, calcium gluconate (magnesium sulfate antagonist) available?

Sample Nurse's Charting

4:00 PM BP stable at 142/96, P 88, R 18, T 98.4F. FHR 138. Lungs clear to auscultation. DTRs, patellar and brachial, 2+ with no clonus. 1+ pitting edema in legs, some swelling of fingers—rings snug. Slight periorbital edema evident. Urine S.G. 1.034; hourly output 40 mL/hr through Foley. 2+ proteinuria. $MgSO_4$ maintenance dose running @ 2 gm/hr per infusion pump. No edema, redness, or c/o discomfort at infusion site. Continuous EFM with FHR baseline 140–146, LTV average, STV present. Accelerations of 20 bpm for 20 sec noted with fetal movement. No decelerations noted. Pt. alert, responsive, oriented. States she has a slight headache but denies epigastric pain or visual changes. Resting quietly on her L side. Side rails padded and up. A. Smythe, RN

Evaluation

- The woman is able to explain PIH, its implications for her pregnancy, the treatment regimen, and possible complications.
- The woman does not have any eclamptic convulsions.
- The woman and her care givers detect any evidence of increasing severity of the PIH or possible complications early so that appropriate treatment measures can be instituted.
- The woman gives birth to a healthy newborn.

PRETERM LABOR

Overview

Labor that occurs between 20 and 37 completed weeks of gestation is referred to as preterm labor. It may result from maternal factors such as cardiovascular or renal disease, PIH, diabetes, abdominal surgery during pregnancy, a blow to the abdomen, uterine anomalies, cervical incompetence, DES exposure, history of cone biopsy, and maternal infection. Fetal factors include multiple pregnancy, hydramnios, and fetal infection, and placental factors include placenta previa and placenta abruptio.

The major maternal risks involve psychologic stress related to the woman's concern for her unborn child and physiologic side effects of the drugs used to stop labor. Fetal-neonatal risks are those related to the effects of prematurity.

Medical Management

1. **Confirmation of diagnosis.** A diagnosis of preterm labor is made if the gestation is between 20 and 37 weeks, if there are documented uterine contractions (four in 20 minutes or eight in 60 minutes), and ruptured membranes. If the membranes are not ruptured one of the following must be present: 80% cervical effacement, documented cervical changes, or 2 cm dilatation (Creasy and Resnik 1989).

2. **Initial treatment.** Any medical conditions that may contribute to preterm labor should be treated. Mild symptoms may be treated with bed rest and hydration per infusion. If labor continues or if symptoms are severe, tocolysis (use of medication to stop labor) is begun.

3. **Tocolysis.** Tocolytics currently used to arrest preterm labor include β-adrenergic agents and magnesium sulfate. The β-adrenergics used include ritodrine (Yutopar), which is FDA approved, and terbutaline (Brethine), which is not FDA approved for use in preterm labor, but has become increasingly popular because it is effective and less expensive than ritodrine. (See Drug Guide 13: Ritodrine [Yutopar].) If uterine contractions are mild, 0.25 mg of terbutaline is administered subcutaneously q30min to a maximum of 1.0 mg in four hours (Anderson and Merkatz 1990). With more pronounced contractions (or if subcutaneous terbutaline is not effective) ritodrine or terbutaline is administered intravenously until uterine activity ceases. The medication is then administered orally for long-term maintenance. Some facilities are also using a subcutaneous terbutaline pump for long-term tocolysis.

   Magnesium sulfate is also effective and has fewer side effects than the β-adrenergics. Four to six gm are administered IV over 20–30 min. The dose may be increased by 0.5 gm/hr every 30 min until contractions cease or a dose of 3.0 gm/hr is reached. Maternal serum level of 5–8 mg/dL is the effective range for tocolysis (Creasy and Resnick 1989). (See Drug Guide 6: Magnesium Sulfate.) Long-term oral therapy may be accomplished with magnesium chloride, magnesium oxide, or magnesium gluconate at a dose of 250–450 mg q3hr.

4. Women who are at risk for preterm labor may benefit from participating in an at home preterm birth prevention program. Examples of major risk factors include a history of preterm labor, multiple gestation, uterine anomaly, DES exposure, hydramnios, two or more second trimester abortions, and uterine irritability (Creasy and Resnik 1989).

Critical Nursing Assessments

1. Assess carefully for evidence of complications or side effects from tocolysis. These include tachycardia, palpitations, nervousness, nausea and vomiting, headache, hypotension. Table 2–2 identifies critical nursing assessments during ritodrine therapy.

Table 2–2 Critical Nursing Assessments During Ritodrine Therapy

Time Interval	Assessment
During Initial IV Therapy and Increases in Infusion Rate	
Every 10 or 15 minutes	FHR and maternal BP, pulse, and respirations. Auscultate lung sounds for rales and rhonchi. Be alert for complaints of dyspnea, chest tightness Uterine activity
Every hour	Assess output (should be over 30 cc/hr or match intake) Assess intake (should not exceed 90–100 mL/hr
During Maintenance IV Therapy	
Every 30 minutes	Maternal BP, pulse, and respirations; FHR; lung sounds; uterine activity
Every 4 hours	Intake and output
During PO Therapy	
Before each dose	Maternal BP, pulse, and respirations; FHR; lung sounds
Every 4–8 hours	Intake and output

Whenever lab work results are available, evaluate K^+ (for hypokalemia), hemoglobin, and hematocrit (for signs of hemodilution, which, together with hypokalemia, may be associated with pulmonary edema).

Be alert for: evidence of pulmonary edema, the most serious complication. Signs include shortness of breath, chest tightness, dyspnea, rales and rhonchi.

2. Assess for symptoms of magnesium toxicity in women receiving magnesium sulfate, including respirations $< 12–14$/min, diminished or absent DTRs, urine output < 100 mL in four-hour period.

Sample Nursing Diagnoses

* Knowledge deficit related to causes, identification, and treatment of preterm labor.
* Fear related to the risks of early labor and birth.

Critical Nursing Interventions

Home care

1. Instruct women at risk about the signs and symptoms of preterm labor, which include the following:

    * Uterine contractions occurring q10min or less
    * Mild menstrual-like cramps felt low in the abdomen or abdominal cramping with or without diarrhea
    * Feelings of pelvic pressure that may feel like the baby pressing down. The pressure may be constant or intermittent
    * Constant or intermittent low backache
    * A sudden increase in vaginal discharge (an increase in amount, or a change to more clear and watery, or a pinkish tinge)

2. Instruct woman that on a home monitoring program she uses a home uterine activity monitor to record and transmit uterine contractile activity via the phone once or twice daily to a nurse specially trained in assessing the signs and symptoms of preterm labor. The nurse uses the data received and the woman's reports of symptoms to evaluate the risk of preterm labor on a daily basis.

3. Teach at-risk woman who is **not** on a preterm home monitoring program to evaluate contraction activity once or twice daily. Instruct her to lie on her side and place her fingertips on the fundus of the uterus. She checks for contractions (hardening of the fundus) for about one hour. Oc-

casional contractions are probably normal Braxton Hicks contractions.

4. If the woman experiences contractions every ten minutes or any of the previously identified signs of labor she should be instructed to do the following:

- Empty her bladder and lie down, preferably on her left side.
- Drink three to four 8-oz cups of fluid.
- Palpate for uterine contractions.
- Rest for 30 minutes after symptoms have subsided and gradually resume activity.
- Call her health care provider if symptoms persist, even if uterine contractions are not palpable (Herron 1988).

Hospital care

1. Promote bed rest in a side-lying position as much as possible.
2. Monitor BP, pulse, and respirations as ordered, especially when on tocolytic therapy (see Table 2–2).
3. Maintain continuous electronic monitoring of FHR and uterine contractions if ordered (See Chapter 3) and evaluate results.
4. Monitor intake and output.
5. Keep vaginal exams to a minimum.
6. Explain procedures to the woman and her partner; answer questions and provide emotional support.
7. Review the following critical aspects of the care you have provided:

- What is the woman's response to the tocolysis? Is she showing any side effects of the medication?
- Is she still having contractions? Have they increased or lessened? Is she showing other signs of labor?
- What is the fetus's response?
- What position is most effective? Are there nursing measures I can use to help her tolerate the side-lying position and the effects of tocolysis?
- How is she coping emotionally? Have I spent enough time helping her to cope with the stress of the situation?

Sample Nurse's Charting for Woman Receiving Subcutaneous Terbutaline

10:00 AM BP stable at 108/70, P 104 and regular, R 18, T 98.0. FHR baseline 148–152, STV present, LTV average. No decelerations noted. No contractions for past 4 hr. Receiving subq terbutaline. Lungs clear to auscultation. c/o mild headache, relieved with Tylenol. IV infusing (see IV sheet). Voided 250 mL clear urine. Resting on L side. A. Smythe, RN

Evaluation

- The woman understands the cause, identification, and treatment of preterm labor.
- The woman understands self-care measures and can identify characteristics that should be reported to her care giver.
- The woman and her baby have a safe labor and birth.

PLACENTA PREVIA

Overview

In placenta previa the placenta is implanted in the lower uterine segment instead of the upper portion of the uterus. As the lower uterine segment contracts and dilates in the later weeks of pregnancy, the villi are torn from the uterine wall and bleeding results. If the placenta previa is complete, the placenta totally covers the internal cervical os. In partial placenta previa, a portion of the os is covered. Maternal risks are related to the possibility of hemorrhage and to psychologic stress resulting from concern about fetal well-being. Fetal-neonatal risks are related to the extent of the placenta previa. If a severe bleeding episode occurs the fetus often suffers fetal distress. Fetal demise is also a possibility if the condition is not diagnosed in a timely manner.

Medical Management

1. **Diagnosis.** Diagnosis is made based on a history of painless, bright red vaginal bleeding, especially in the third trimester. The initial bleeding episode may be light but is

often followed by more severe bleeding. Diagnosis is confirmed with ultrasound to localize the placenta.

2. **Expectant management.** If < 37 weeks' gestation, expectant management is used to delay birth to allow the fetus to mature. This includes bed rest, no rectal or vaginal exams, monitoring of bleeding, ongoing assessment of fetal status with external monitor, monitoring of vital signs, laboratory evaluation (hemoglobin, hematocrit, Rh factor, urinalysis). Two units of cross-matched blood are kept available for transfusion. If the previa is partial or if the placenta is simply low-lying, vaginal birth may be attempted.

3. **Emergency management.** If severe bleeding occurs or evidence of fetal distress develops, a cesarean is performed.

Critical Nursing Assessments

1. Assess woman regularly for evidence of vaginal bleeding. If bleeding present, note amount, character.

2. Assess for signs of shock if bleeding present (decreased blood pressure, increased pulse, cool clammy skin, pallor, decreased hematocrit, urine output < 30 mL/hr).

3. Assess for uterine contractility and signs of labor. **Word of caution:** Vaginal exams may trigger a major bleeding episode and are **contraindicated.**

4. Assess woman's understanding of her condition, its implications, and treatment options.

5. Assess fetal status: During bleeding episode, continuous electronic fetal monitoring is used; when no bleeding is present, an electronic fetal monitoring strip is run, usually q4h (timing may vary according to agency policy).

Sample Nursing Diagnosis

- Altered tissue perfusion (placental) related to blood loss.
- Fear related to concern for own personal well-being and that of baby.

Critical Nursing Interventions

1. Carry out ongoing monitoring of maternal and fetal status including VS, evidence of bleeding, urinary output, electronic monitor tracing, signs of labor.

2. Explain procedures to woman and her family.
3. Administer IV fluids or blood products as ordered.
4. Review the following critical aspects of care you have provided:

   - Have I questioned the woman about bleeding? If bleeding is present, have I assessed quantity carefully?
   - Have I carefully monitored fetal status? Any signs of tachycardia? Decelerations?
   - Have I been alert for any changes in the woman's status? Any signs of labor? Any changes she has noted?
   - Have I implemented measures to help the woman be comfortable on bed rest—back rubs, positioning with pillows, diversionary activities?

Evaluation

- The woman's condition remains stable or, if bleeding occurs, it is detected promptly and therapy is begun.
- The woman and her baby have a safe labor and birth.

ADDITIONAL COMPLICATIONS

Table 2–3 describes additional complications that the nurse may encounter.

REFERENCES

Anderson HF, Merkatz IR: Preterm labor. In: *Danforth's Obstetrics and Gynecology*, 6th ed. Scott JR, et al (editors). Philadelphia: Lippincott, 1990.

Creasy RK, Resnik R: *Maternal-Fetal Medicine: Principles and Practices*. Philadelphia: Saunders, 1989.

Cunningham FG et al: *Williams' Obstetrics*, 18th ed. Norwalk, CT: Appleton & Lange, 1989.

Gabbe SG: Diabetes mellitus: Ways of individualizing care. *Contemp OB/GYN* July 1990; 35(7):68.

Garcia PM, Gall SA: Multiple pregnancy. In: *Danforth's Obstetrics and Gynecology*, 6th ed. Scott JR et al (editors). Philadelphia: Lippincott, 1990.

Ghiloni SZ: Home management. In: *Diabetes Complicating Pregnancy*. Hare JW (editor). New York: Alan R. Liss, 1989.

Table 2–3 Selected Complications During Pregnancy

Condition/Overview	Signs/Symptoms/Risk	Medical Therapy	Nursing Interventions
Acquired Immunodeficiency Syndrome (AIDS) AIDS, caused by the human immunodeficiency virus, is a multisystem disorder that enters the body through blood, blood products, and bodily fluids such as semen, vaginal fluid, and urine. HIV affects T-cells, thereby depressing the body's immune response. Persons at highest risk are homosexual or bisexual men, heterosexual partners of persons with AIDS, IV drug users, hemophiliacs, and fetuses of women at risk or HIV positive. Persons generally test positive for HIV within 2–12 weeks of exposure but may remain	The following women are considered at risk for HIV: prostitutes; women with a history of sexually transmitted infection; IV drug users; partners (currently or previously) of IV drug users, bisexual men, hemophiliacs, or those who test positive for HIV. Women with AIDS may have any of the following: malaise, weight loss, lymph-adenopathy, diarrhea, fever, neurologic dysfunction, immunodeficiency, or Kaposi's sarcoma. Maternal risks: Progression of symptoms in HIV-positive, asymptomatic	Currently there is no definitive therapy for AIDS although a variety of experimental drugs are being tested. Current goal is to detect women at risk and educate the public about the spread of AIDS. Women at risk who are pregnant or planning a pregnancy should be offered HIV antibody testing. Women who test positive should be counseled about the implications for herself and her fetus/newborn. They may be offered a therapeutic abortion. Women who continue pregnancy need excellent pre-	1. Assess history for risk factors. 2. Provide clear information about AIDS and the implications for the woman, her partner, and a child should the woman become pregnant. 3. Monitor asymptomatic pregnant woman for nonspecific symptoms such as fever, weight loss, persistent candidiasis (vaginal yeast infection or thrush in mouth), diarrhea, cough, skin lesions. 4. Implement universal precautions including use of

asymptomatic for five to seven years or more.
In the U.S. the vast majority of pediatric AIDS cases have resulted from perinatal transmission from mother to child.

women may be accelerated by pregnancy.
Fetal-neonatal risks: Risk of transmission from HIV-positive mother to fetus is about 40% to 50% (McMahon 1988). Infant often asymptomatic at birth; onset of symptoms usually occurs between 9 and 18 months.

natal care with attention to psychosocial and teaching needs.

disposable latex gloves when in contact with non-intact skin, mucous membranes, or bodily fluids (e.g. changing chux, diapers, peripads, starting IV, drawing blood); use of protective covering such as plastic apron and glasses or eye shield when contamination from splashing may occur (vaginal exam, vaginal or cesarean birth, suctioning, care of newborn before initial bath). (Consult unit procedure manual for further specifics.)

5. Provide emotional support and nonjudgmental attitude; preserve confidentiality.

Continued

Table 2–3 continued

Condition/Overview	Signs/Symptoms/Risk	Medical Therapy	Nursing Interventions
Chlamydia Sexually transmitted infection caused by *Chlamydia trachomatis*, often found in association with gonorrhea.	Women are often asymptomatic. Symptoms may include thin or purulent vaginal discharge, frequency and burning with urination, or lower abdominal pain. Infant of woman with untreated chlamydia is at risk for newborn conjunctivitis, chlamydial pneumonia, preterm birth, or fetal demise.	Nonpregnant women treated with tetracycline. Since this may permanently discolor fetal teeth, pregnant women are treated with erythromycin ethyl succinate. Erythromycin eye ointment (but not silver nitrate) can prevent conjunctivitis in the newborn.	1. Review signs and symptoms, explain importance of taking entire dose of medication.
Gonorrhea Sexually transmitted infection caused by *Neisseria gonorrhoeae*.	Majority of women are asymptomatic; disease often diagnosed during routine prenatal cervical culture. If symptoms are present, they include purulent vaginal discharge, dysuria, urinary frequency, inflammation and swelling of vulva. Cervix may appear eroded.	Pregnant women are treated with ceftriaxone plus erythromycin (CDC 1989). If the woman is allergic to ceftriaxone, spectinomycin is used. All sexual partners are treated.	1. Review medication purpose, side effects. 2. Explain that untreated gonorrhea may result in pelvic inflammatory disease and infertility. 3. Discuss safe sexual practices.

Infection at time of birth may cause ophthalmia neonatorum in the newborn.

Syphilis

Sexually transmitted infection caused by the spirochete *Treponema pallidum.*

Primary stage: chancre, slight fever, malaise. Chancre lasts about four weeks, then disappears.
Secondary stage: occurs six weeks to six months after infection. Skin eruptions (condyloma lata); also symptoms of acute arthritis, iritis, liver enlargement, chronic sore throat with hoarseness.
Diagnosed by blood tests such as VDRL, RPR, FTA-ABS. Dark field exam for spirochetes may be done.
May be passed transplacentally to fetus. If untreated, one of the following can occur: second trimester abortion, stillborn infant at term, congenitally infected infant, uninfected live infant.

For syphilis less than one year in duration: 2.4 million U benzathine penicillin G IM. For syphilis of more than one year's duration: 2.4 million U benzathine penicillin G once a week for three weeks. Sexual partners should also be screened and treated.

1. Explain the risk factors and long-term effects if syphilis is not treated.
2. Explain implications for fetus/neonate.
3. Stress importance of receiving all three doses if syphilis is greater than one year in duration.

Continued

Table 2–3 continued

Condition/Overview	Signs/Symptoms/Risk	Medical Therapy	Nursing Interventions
TORCH			
The TORCH group of infectious diseases may cause serious harm to fetus. They include toxoplasmosis (TO), rubella (R), cytomegalic inclusion disease (C), and herpes genitalis (H). Some sources identify the "O" as "other infections." Exposure of the woman during the first 12 weeks of pregnancy may cause developmental anomalies. **Toxoplasmosis** is caused by a protozoan and transmitted by eating raw or poorly cooked meat or by exposure to feces of infected cats. Innocuous in adults. **Rubella** or German measles is caused by a virus.	**Toxoplasmosis** results in a mild infection in adults but is associated with an increased risk of spontaneous abortion, prematurity, stillbirth, neonatal death, and disorders including microcephaly, hydrocephalus, convulsions, blindness, deafness, and mental retardation. **Rubella** exposure in the first trimester is associated with spontaneous abortion, congenital heart disease, intrauterine growth retardation, cataracts, mental retardation, and cerebral palsy. Infection in the second trimester is most often associated with permanent hearing impairment in the newborn.	**Toxoplasmosis:** Goal is to identify women at risk. Diagnosis made using serologic testing, physical findings, and history. Treatment includes sulfadiazine, pyrimethamine, and spiramycin. If toxoplasmosis is diagnosed before 20 weeks' gestation, therapeutic abortion may be offered because damage to the fetus tends to be more severe than if the disease is diagnosed later in pregnancy. **Rubella:** Best therapy is prevention by vaccination. Women of childbearing age should be tested for immunity and vaccinated if susceptible. HAI titer of 1:16 or greater indicates immunity. Pregnant	**Toxoplasmosis:** Explain methods of prevention to childbearing woman. She should avoid poorly cooked or raw meat, especially pork, beef, and lamb. Fruits and vegetables should be washed. Litter box should be cleaned frequently by someone else, and woman should wear gloves when gardening. **Rubella:** Assess for signs of rubella infection (maculo-papular rash, lymphadenopathy, muscular achiness, joint pain). Provide emotional support and objective information for couples contemplating therapeutic abortion. **CID:** Provide emotional support and objective information.

Cytomegalic inclusion disease (CID), caused by the cytomegalovirus (CMV), is the most prevalent infection of the TORCH group. Chronic persistent infection with viral shedding for years. Usually is asymptomatic in adults and children.

Herpes genitalis, caused by herpes simplex virus type 2 (HSV-2), is a chronic, recurring infection that causes painful lesions in the genital area and is transmitted by sexual contact.

CID may cause fetal death; in neonates it is associated with microcephaly, cerebral palsy, mental retardation, etc. Subclinical infections may cause neurologic and hearing problems that may go unrecognized for months or years.

Herpes genitalis may cause spontaneous abortion if active HSV-2 infection occurs in first trimester. Highest risk of infection for newborn who is born vaginally when mother has active HSV-2 in her vagina. Risk of neonatal death, permanent brain damage, characteristic skin lesions.

women are not vaccinated but will be offered vaccination postpartum. If infection occurs in first trimester, woman will be offered a therapeutic abortion.

CID: Diagnosis is confirmed by serologic tests to detect CMV antibodies. No effective treatment is available at this time.

Herpes genitalis: Treatment is aimed at relieving woman's pain and may include sitz baths QID, followed by drying with a hair dryer; oral acyclovir reduces healing time but is not recommended during pregnancy. A cesarean birth is recommended for pregnant women with visible HSV-2 lesions; if no lesions are visible, vaginal birth is attempted. Cultures every three to five days are recommended for women with visible lesions at or near term but before the onset of labor (Landers and Sweet 1990).

Herpes genitalis: Provide information about the disease and its spread. Advise woman to inform future health care providers of her infection. A possible association exists between herpes and cervical cancer. Thus women should understand importance of yearly Pap smears.
Provide emotional support and nonjudgmental attitude.

Continued

Table 2–3 continued

Condition/Overview	Signs/Symptoms/Risk	Medical Therapy	Nursing Interventions
Substance Abuse Indiscriminate use of alcohol or drugs such as cocaine, PCP, opiates, and methadone may affect the woman and her fetus/neonate. Alcohol abuse has been associated with fetal alcohol syndrome. Use of addicting drugs may cause the infant to be born addicted or to have serious and permanent problems.	Signs of addiction in the pregnant woman may include dilated or constricted pupils, inflamed nasal mucosa, abscesses, edema or track marks on arms and legs, inappropriate or disoriented behavior, or excessive fatigue. Risks to the fetus include the following (varies somewhat according to substance abused): neurologic changes including marked irritability, poor interactive behavior, poor consolability, seizures, and so forth.	Following diagnosis, management involves a team approach to provide care for woman and fetus/neonate. Hospitalization may be necessary to achieve detoxification. "Cold turkey" withdrawal is not advised because of risk to fetus. Urine screening may be done regularly throughout the pregnancy for women who are known or suspected substance abusers.	1. Be alert for signs of substance abuse. If it is suspected, ask direct questions, beginning with less threatening questions about use of tobacco, caffeine, and alcohol consumption. Then progress to questions about illicit drugs. 2. Provide information about the possible effects of substance abuse on the fetus.
Multiple Gestation Morbidity and mortality rates increase significantly in pregnancies with multiple fetuses. Dizygotic, or fraternal twins (resulting from two ova), are more common and are influ-	Fetal risk is significantly higher. The perinatal mortality rate is higher and there is an increased risk of preterm labor with the problems associated with prematurity.	Early diagnosis based on history, greater than anticipated uterine size, and ultrasound is crucial. Women are seen every two weeks until 28 weeks' gestation and then	1. Counsel on importance of good nutrition including adequate calories (40–45 kcal/kg/day), calcium (1800–2000 mg/day, and protein (more than 1.5 g/kg)

enced by heredity, race, maternal age and parity, and fertility drugs. Monozygotic or identical twins (resulting from one ovum) are not as common and are not influenced by external factors other than infertility therapy. Higher numbers of fetuses (triplets or quadruplets, for example) may result from either process or a combination (Cunningham et al 1989).

The incidence of intrauterine growth retardation, congenital anomalies, and abnormal presentations is all increased. For the mother, a multiple gestation may contribute to more physical discomfort during pregnancy, such as shortness of breath, backaches, and pedal edema, as well as an increased incidence of PIH, anemia, and placenta previa. Prolonged hospitalization may be necessary, especially with three or more fetuses.

weekly. Serial ultrasounds are done every three to four weeks to assess for IUGR. NST and fetal biophysical profile are done at least weekly beginning at 28–30 weeks. Bed rest in the lateral position is begun as early as 23–26 weeks to prevent preterm labor. Maternal blood pressure is monitored closely. Preterm labor is managed in the same way as it is for single pregnancy (see earlier discussion in this chapter).

(Garcia and Gall 1990).

2. Discuss importance of sufficient rest if at home (usually bed rest with BRP) or at least two hours in the morning, afternoon, and evening.

3. If woman is hospitalized, explain importance of complete bed rest (or bed rest with BRP if ordered).

4. Monitor fetal status. This involves isolating each FHR as well as running an electronic fetal monitor strip on each fetus at least q4–8h (depending on agency policy). If possible the strips will be run at the same time using two (or three) monitors. This becomes more difficult with quadruplets.

5. Monitor for signs of complications such as PIH or preterm labor.

From CDC: 1989 Sexually transmitted disease treatment guidelines. *Mortality and Morbidity Weekly Reports.* Sept. 1, 1989; 38 (5-8): 1.

Herron MA: One approach to preventing preterm birth. *J Perinatol Neonatal Nurs* 1988; 2:1.

Landers DV, Sweet RL: Perinatal infections. In: *Danforth's Obstetrics and Gynecology*, 6th ed. Scott JR et al (editors). Philadelphia: Lippincott, 1990.

Martin JN et al: Pregnancy complicated by preeclampsia-eclampsia with the syndrome of hemolysis, elevated liver enzymes, and low platelet count: How rapid is postpartum recovery? *Obstet Gynecol* November 1990; 76:737.

McMahon KM: The integration of HIV testing and counseling into nursing practice. *Nurs Clin North Am* 1988; 23(4):803.

Scott JR, Worley RJ: Hypertensive disorders of pregnancy. In: *Danforth's Obstetrics and Gynecology*, 6th ed. Scott JR et (editors). Philadelphia: Lippincott, 1990.

Sibai BM: Preeclampsia-eclampsia. In: *Gynecology and Obstetrics*. Vol. 2. Sciarra JJ (editor). Philadelphia: Lippincott, 1989.

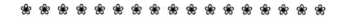

CHAPTER 3

The Intrapartal Client

OVERVIEW

Labor and birth progresses through four stages. A first time laboring woman (nullipara) will **average** twelve hours (11 hours in first stage and one hour of pushing in second stage). A multipara, **averages** about eight hours (7¼ hours in first stage and ½ hour pushing in second stage). See Table 3–1 for definitions of each stage of labor and Table 3–2 for contraction and labor progress characteristics.

NURSING CARE DURING ADMISSION

Critical Nursing Assessments

Name: _____ Age: _____

   Maternal vital signs:

   BP _____ T _____ Radial pulse _____ R _____

   Gravida _____ Para _____ Term _____

   Preterm _____ Ab _____ Living _____

   EDB _____ Weeks gestation now _____

   Risk factors present _____ Medications being taken _____

   Allergies: Medications _____ Foods _____ Substances _____

Labor status

1. **Uterine contractions.** Ask mother and support person what the contraction pattern has been prior to admission. Assess uterine contractions by palpation on admission. Information regarding uterine contractions will be needed to determine labor status, fetal status, and the need for further nursing interventions.

Table 3–1   Stages of Labor and Birth

Stage	Begins	Ends
First	Beginning of cervical dilatation	Complete dilatation
Second	Complete dilatation	Birth of the baby
Third	Birth of the baby	Birth of the placenta
Fourth	Birth of the placenta	1–4 hours past birth

Table 3–2   Contraction and Labor Progress Characteristics

Contraction Characteristics

Latent phase:	Every 10–20 min × 15–20 seconds; mild, progressing to Every 5–7 min × 30–40 seconds; moderate
Active phase:	Every 2–3 min × 60 seconds; moderate to strong
Transition phase:	Every 2 min × 60–90 seconds; strong

Labor Progress Characteristics

Primipara:	1.2 cm/hr dilatation 1 cm/hr descent <2 hr in second stage
Multipara:	1.5 cm/hr dilatation 2 cm/hr descent <1 hr in second stage

Assessment Technique: With the woman's gown over her abdomen, but blankets pulled aside, place palmar surface of fingers on fundus of uterus (upper portion, above the umbilicus). During your assessment and evaluation you will determine contraction frequency, duration, and intensity. When uterine tightening begins, note the time (use second hand on a clock or watch), continue to assess the tightening, and when it has completely relaxed, once again note the time. (This provides information regarding duration of that contraction.) Continue to watch the time and note the beginning of the next contraction. This will establish frequency (from the beginning of one contraction to the beginning of the next contraction). While feeling the tightening, slightly push your fingertips against the uterus.

If the tissue indents easily, the intensity is mild; if it indents a small amount, it is moderate intensity; if it indents a very small amount, it is strong intensity. (See Figure 3–1.) Contraction frequency and duration may also be assessed and evaluated by using external electronic monitoring. Contraction intensity may be measured more precisely by use of an intrauterine uterine pressure device that attaches to the electronic monitor.

2. **Cervical dilatation and effacement.** Cervical dilatation progresses from 0 to 10 cm and effacement progresses from 0% to 100%.
   Assessment technique: See Procedure 18: Sterile Vaginal Exam, and Figure 3–2.

3. **Amniotic fluid membrane status.** Amniotic membranes are either intact or ruptured. If ruptured, the time of rupture needs to be noted and the fluid is observed for amount (usually described as small, moderate, or large) (remember, there is about 600–800 cc of fluid at 40 weeks' gestation), color (should be colorless), odor (should be nonfoul), and consistency (should be clear; cloudy fluid may indicate infection and meconium may be associated with fetal stress).

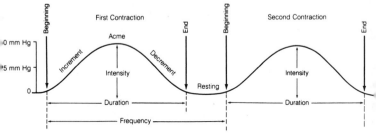

Figure 3–1   Characteristics of uterine contractions.

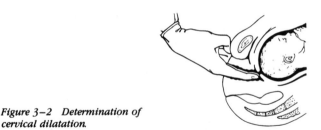

Figure 3–2   Determination of cervical dilatation.

Assessment technique: See Procedure 18: Sterile Vaginal Exam and Procedure 2: Assessment for Amniotic Fluid.

4. **Fetal status.**

  a. **Fetal heart rate (FHR).** When auscultating the FHR, the nurse determines rate, regularity, and whether slowing is heard during or just after uterine contractions. Assess FHR with the woman in high Fowler's (back of the bed is almost completely upright), in semi-Fowler's (back of bed is at approximately 45 degrees), or in side-lying position (to maximize blood flow to the fetus). When assessing the FHR by electronic fetal monitor (EFM), the nurse gathers data regarding baseline fetal heart rate, variability (short-term and long-term), and periodic changes (accelerations and decelerations). Once these data are known, the nurse can evaluate the tracing as reassuring (a normal pattern), or nonreassuring (a pattern that may be associated with fetal distress of some type).

  Assessment technique—auscultation: The FHR may be auscultated with a fetoscope or a hand-held ultrasound device. See Procedure 7: Fetal Heart Rate Auscultation.

  Assessment technique—electronic fetal monitoring: See Procedure 8: Fetal Monitoring: Electronic. A sample of a tracing is illustrated in Figure 3–3. Note that time is assessed by counting the squares or the darker vertical lines.

  Terms related to fetal heart rate monitoring include the following:

  Baseline rate: Refers to the range of FHR observed between contractions during a ten-minute period of monitoring. The range does not include the rate present during decelerations.

  Baseline changes: Defined in terms of ten-minute periods of time. Changes include: tachycardia, bradycardia, and variability of heart rate.

  Tachycardia: FHR 160 beats per minute (bpm) or more for more than ten minutes; moderate (160–179 bpm), severe (180 or more).

  Bradycardia: FHR less than 120 bpm for more than ten minutes; mild (100–119 bpm), moderate (less than 100 bpm), severe (less than 70 bpm). Other characteristics of EFM tracings are presented in Table 3–3.

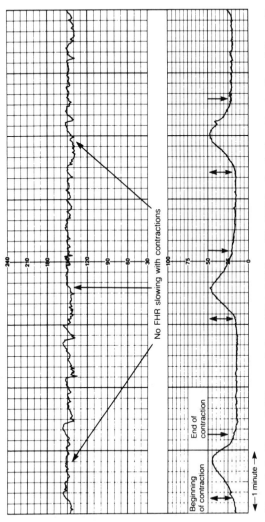

Figure 3–3   Normal FHR range is from 120 to 160 bpm. The FHR tracing in the upper portion of the graph indicates FHR range of 140–155 bpm. The lower portion is a tracing of the uterine contraction pattern (or frequency).

Table 3–3 Characteristics of FHR Tracings

Example	Characteristic	Nursing Intervention
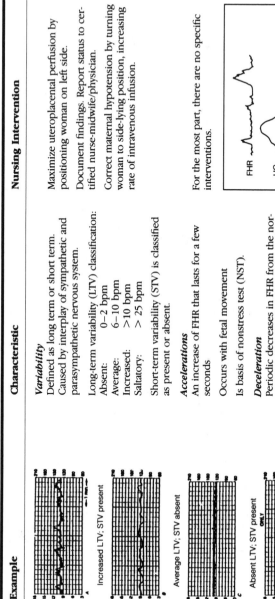Increased LTV; STV present	***Variability*** Defined as long term or short term. Caused by interplay of sympathetic and parasympathetic nervous system. Long-term variability (LTV) classification: Absent: 0–2 bpm Average: 6–10 bpm Increased: >10 bpm Saltatory: > 25 bpm Short-term variability (STV) is classified as present or absent.	Maximize uteroplacental perfusion by positioning woman on left side. Document findings. Report status to certified nurse-midwife/physician. Correct maternal hypotension by turning woman to side-lying position, increasing rate of intravenous infusion.
Average LTV; STV absent	***Accelerations*** An increase of FHR that lasts for a few seconds Occurs with fetal movement Is basis of nonstress test (NST).	For the most part, there are no specific interventions. 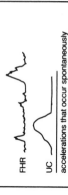
Absent LTV; STV present ONLY	***Deceleration*** Periodic decreases in FHR from the normal baseline Classified as early, late, or variable.	
Absent LTV; STV absent		

Early deceleration

Due to pressure on the fetal head as it progresses down the birth canal.

Characteristics:
Resembles upside down shape of uterine contraction.

Occurs at or just before the beginning of contraction and ends as contraction ends.

Nadir (lowest point) occurs at peak of contraction, and is within normal FHR range.

Is considered a normal variation.

No specific intervention needed.

Monitor for changes in FHR pattern.

Evaluate for possible cephalopelvic disproportion (CPD) if occurs in early labor.

Late deceleration

Due to uteroplacental insufficiency as the result of decreased blood flow and oxygen transfer to the fetus during contractions.

Characteristics:
Smooth, uniform shape that inversely mirrors contraction.

Begin at or within seconds after the peak of the contraction.

Last past end of contraction.

Turn woman to left side-lying position.

Report findings to physician/CNM and document findings.

Provide explanation to woman and partner.

Monitor for further FHR changes.

Maintain good hydration with IV fluids.

Discontinue oxytocin if it is being administered.

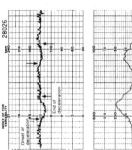

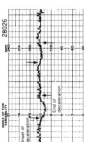

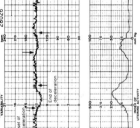

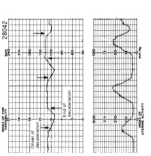

Continued

Table 3–3 continued

Example	Characteristic	Nursing Intervention
	Tend to occur with every contraction; they are persistent and consistent.	Administer oxygen by face mask at 7–10 L/min.
	Usually occur within normal FHR range.	Monitor maternal BP, P for signs of hypotension.
	In some situations, changing maternal position, providing IV hydration, and de-creasing contraction frequency decreases late decelerations.	Assist with preparation for cesarean birth if required.
	Variable deceleration	Document findings.
	Due to umbilical cord compression, which decreases the amount of blood flow (therefore oxygen supply) to the fetus.	Report status to certified nurse-midwife/physician.
	Characteristics: Vary in onset, occurrence, and waveform.	Change maternal position to one in which FHR pattern is most improved.
	Usually fall outside the normal FHR range.	Correct maternal hypotension.
	Are acute in onset.	Assist with preparation for cesarean birth if required.
		Provide explanation to woman and partner.

Discontinue oxytocin if it is being administered and there are severe variables. Oxytocin may be continued if mild or moderate decelerations are present.

Perform vaginal examination to assess for prolapsed cord or change in labor progress.

Monitor FHR continuously to assess current status and for further changes in FHR pattern.

b. **Evaluation of fetal heart rate tracings.** Although it seems an awkward way to begin, evaluation of the electronic monitor tracing begins by looking at the uterine contraction pattern. To evaluate the contraction pattern the nurse should:

1. Determine the uterine resting tone.
2. Assess the contractions:
   What is the frequency?
   What is the duration?
   What is the intensity (if internal monitoring)?

The next step is to evaluate the fetal heart rate tracing.

1. Determine the baseline:
   Is the baseline within normal range?
   Is there evidence of tachycardia?
   Is there evidence of bradycardia?
2. Determine FHR variability:
   Is short-term variability present or absent?
   Is long-term variability average? Minimal to absent? Moderate to marked?
3. Is a sinusoidal pattern present?
4. Are there periodic changes?
   Are accelerations present?
   Do they meet the criteria for a reactive nonstress test (NST)?
   Are decelerations present?
   Are they uniform in shape? If so, determine if they are early or late decelerations.
   Are they nonuniform in shape? If so, determine if they are variable decelerations.

c. **Classifying the FHR tracing as reassuring or non-reassuring.** After evaluating the FHR tracing for the factors just listed, the nurse may further classify the tracing as reassuring or nonreassuring. Reassuring patterns contain normal parameters and do not require additional treatment or intervention. Nonreassuring patterns may require continuous monitoring and more involved treatment and intervention.

5. **Fetal presentation and position.** Fetal position refers to the relationship of the fetal presenting part (the part of the fetus that enters the maternal pelvis first) to the maternal pelvis, for example: right occiput anterior (ROA) or left occiput anterior (LOA). Fetal presentation may be cephalic,

breech, or transverse. Cephalic presentation is the most common and occurs in 97% of births. Breech presentation occurs just under 3% of the time.

Assessment technique: Fetal presentation and position are determined by vaginal examination. See Procedure 18: Sterile Vaginal Exam and Figure 3–4.

6. **Information, comfort, and coping level.** Assessment of the woman's physical and emotional state and her coping methods will provide useful information for the admission process and later in the labor.

    Assessment technique: In a conversational interview format, determine the type of prenatal education program the woman has completed. What hopes and plans does she have for this birth? Has she completed a birth plan or made a formalized list of special requests during the labor and birth? What plans has she made with the certified nurse-midwife/physician? Does she verbalize the need for information or does she have questions? Does she have a resource/support person with her?

7. **Assessment findings that require immediate intervention.** See Table 3–4.

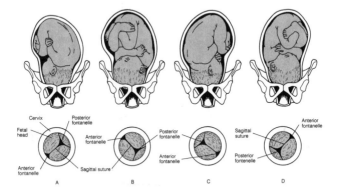

Figure 3–4 Assessment of fetal position. A, left occiput anterior (LOA). The posterior fontanelle (triangle-shaped) is in the upper left quadrant of the maternal pelvis. B, Left occiput posterior (LOP). The posterior fontanelle is in the lower left quadrant of the maternal pelvis. C, Right occiput anterior (ROA). The posterior fontanelle is in the upper right quadrant of the maternal pelvis. D, Right occiput posterior (ROP). The posterior fontanelle is in the lower right quadrant of the maternal pelvis.

Table 3–4 Deviations from Normal Labor Process Requiring Immediate Intervention

Finding	Immediate Action	Finding	Immediate Action
Woman admitted with unusual vaginal bleeding or history of painless vaginal bleeding	1. Do not perform vaginal examination. 2. Assess FHR. 3. Evaluate amount of blood loss. 4. Evaluate labor pattern. 5. Notify physician/CNM immediately.	Prolapse of umbilical cord	1. Relieve pressure on cord manually. 2. Continuously monitor FHR; watch for changes in FHR pattern. 3. Notify physician/CNM. 4. Assist woman into knee-chest position. 5. Administer oxygen. 6. Direct another person to prepare for immediate cesarean section.
Presence of greenish or brownish amniotic fluid	1. Continuously monitor FHR. 2. Evaluate dilatation status of cervix and determine whether umbilical cord is prolapsed. 3. Evaluate presentation (vertex or breech). 4. Maintain woman on complete bed rest on left side. 5. Notify physician/CNM immediately. 6. Note color and consistency of amniotic fluid.		

Absence of FHR and fetal movement	Woman admitted in advanced labor; birth imminent

1. Notify physician/CNM.
2. Provide truthful information and emotional support to laboring couple.
3. Remain with the couple.
4. Prepare for diagnostic ultrasound exam.
	1. Prepare for immediate birth.
	2. Obtain critical information:
	  a. EDB
	  b. History of bleeding problems
	  c. History of medical or obstetrical problems
	  d. Past and or present use/abuse of prescription/OTC/illicit drugs
	  e. Problems with this pregnancy
	  f. FHR and maternal vital signs if possible
	  g. Whether membranes are ruptured and how long since rupture
	  h. Blood type and Rh
	3. Direct another person to contact CNM/physician. Do not leave woman alone.
	4. Provide support to couple.
	5. Put on gloves.

Sample admission nursing note Grav I Para 0 EDB
1-13-92 40 wks gest admitted ambulatory to BR1 in labor. Contractions q3 X 50 of mod qual. Memb intact. Cervix 5 cm, 80%
effaced, small amount blood-tinged mucus present. Vertex presentation at 0 station. FHR 140 by auscultation, regular rhythm.
No increase or decrease in FHR noted during or following
UC. Maternal temp 98.6, pulse 78, resp 18, BP 120/74. Adm UA
obtained and to lab. Support person with pt and to remain
through birth. P. Gomez, RNC

NURSING CARE DURING LABOR

Critical Nursing Assessments

Additional assessments of maternal and fetal status and labor
progress are presented in Table 3–5.

Critical Nursing Interventions

1. During labor, the nursing support measures will vary depending on the progress of labor and the wishes of the
   laboring woman or couple. Table 3–6 summarizes the
   major characteristics of labor and birth and presents nursing interventions that may be used in each stage of labor.
2. Teach a visualization method. If the woman is in early labor, or is awaiting an induction, there is time to teach her a
   visualization technique that can be used during labor. Direct a visualization by saying something like the following:
   "Think about a place you have been that has pleasant mem-
   ories and feelings around it. A place that was relaxing,
   where all your stress disappeared. As you think about this,
   take in a breath and remember the smells around the
   place. If it was outside, feel the warmth of the sun or the
   way the breeze felt on your face. In your mind, sit in that
   place again. Let all your tension and tiredness leave your
   body as you feel the warmth and breezes."

   Give the woman a few moments to think about her special place. Ask if she would like to share information about
   the setting. If the woman chooses to do this add the information to help her with the visualization (for example,
   "think about the mountain cabin and the warmth of the sun
   on your face as you sit in the rocking chair on the front
   porch," etc).

Table 3–5 Nursing Assessments During Labor and Birth

Stage	Maternal Assessments	Fetal Assessments
First Stage Latent phase	Blood pressure, pulse, respirations q1hr if in normal range. Temperature q4hr unless over 37.5°C (99.6°F) or membranes ruptured, then q1hr. Uterine contractions q30min.	FHR q60min for low-risk women and q30min for high-risk women, if normal characteristics present (average variability, baseline in the 120–160 bpm range, without late or variable decelerations [NAACOG 1990]). Note fetal activity. If EFM in place, assess for reactive NST.
Active phase	BP, P, R, q1hr if in normal range. Uterine contractions q30min.	FHR q30min for low-risk women and q15min for high-risk women, if normal characteristics are present (NAACOG 1990).
Transition	BP, P, R q30min.	FHR q30min for low-risk women and every 15 min for high-risk women.
Second Stage	BP, P, R q5–15min. Uterine contractions palpated with each contraction or continuously.	FHR q15min for low-risk women and q5min for high-risk women (NAACOG 1990).

NAACOG 1990.

Table 3–6 Normal Progress, Psychologic Characteristics, and Nursing Support During First and Second Stages of Labor

Stage/ Phase	Cervical Dilatation	Uterine Contractions	Woman's Response	Nursing Support Measures
Stage 1 Latent phase:	1–4 cm	Every 15–30 min, 15–30 sec duration Mild intensity	Usually happy, talkative, and eager to be in labor Exhibits need for independence by taking care of own bodily needs and seeking information	Establish rapport on admission and continue to build during care. Assess information base and learning needs. Be available to consult regarding breathing technique if needed; teach breathing technique if needed and in early labor. Orient family to room, equipment, monitors, and procedures. Encourage woman and partner to participate in care as desired. Provide needed information. Assist woman into position of comfort (nonsupine position); encourage frequent change of position; and encourage ambulation during early labor. Offer fluids/ice chips. Keep

Active phase:	4–7 cm	Every 3–5 min, 30–60 sec duration Moderate intensity	May experience feelings of helplessness; exhibits increased fatigue and may begin to feel restless and anxious as contractions become stronger; expresses fear of abandonment. Becomes more dependent as she is less able to meet her needs	couple informed of progress. Encourage woman to void every one to two hours. Assess need for and interest in using visualization to enhance relaxation and teach if appropriate. Observe response to contractions. Encourage woman to maintain breathing patterns; provide quiet environment to reduce external stimuli. Provide reassurance, encouragement, support; keep couple informed of progress. Promote comfort by giving backrubs, sacral pressure, cool cloth on forehead, assistance with position changes, support with pillows, effleurage. Provide ice chips, ointment for dry mouth and lips. Encourage to void every one to two hours. Offer shower/Jacuzzi/warm bath if available.

Continued

Table 3–6 continued

Stage/Phase	Cervical Dilatation	Uterine Contractions	Woman's Response	Nursing Support Measures
Transition:	8–10 cm	Every 2–3 min, 45–90 sec duration Strong intensity	Tires and may exhibit increased restlessness and irritability; may feel she cannot keep up with labor process and is out of control Physical discomforts Fear of being left alone May fear tearing open or splitting apart with contractions	Encourage woman to rest between contractions; if she sleeps between contractions, wake her at beginning of contraction so she can begin breathing pattern (increases feeling of control). Provide support, encouragement, and praise for efforts. Keep couple informed of progress; encourage continued participation of support persons. Promote comfort as listed above but recognize many women do not want to be touched when in transition. Provide privacy. Provide ice chips, ointment for lips. Encourage to void every one to two hours.

			If she has difficulty focusing, cup her face in your hands and place your face close to hers. Talk her through the contraction. Have her breathe with you.
Stage 2	Complete	Every 1½–2 minutes	May feel out of control, help-less, panicky, exhausted, exhilarated	Assist woman in pushing efforts. Encourage woman to assume position of comfort. She may be most comfortable in a sitting position on a toilet, leaning over a birthing bar, on hands and knees, or perhaps on her side. Some women like to sit in high Fowler's, to have support behind their shoulders, and to have someone hold their legs up and flexed while they push. Provide encouragement and praise for efforts. Keep couple informed of progress. Provide ice chips and cool cloth for forehead. Maintain privacy as woman desires.

After the woman has a visualization set up, suggest thinking about it during contractions as a means of increasing relaxation and focusing concentration. You could say: "As each contraction begins, think about this special place for a moment and let your body relax. Keep a picture of your place in your mind as you breathe with the contraction. When the contraction is over, let your body stay relaxed. Feel the comfort of this room and support of those around you."

3. Teach a progressive relaxation sequence. If the woman is just beginning labor, you may have an opportunity to teach a relaxation exercise. Instruct her as follows:

    a. Assume a comfortable position (mid-Fowler's with arms supported by pillows, or side-lying with pillow between knees and pillows to support arms, or in a reclining or rocking chair).

    b. Breathe slowly and easily. Close your eyes and let your body sink into the bed (or chair). Adjust your position so that each part of your body is supported and comfortable.

    c. Maintain your breathing and try to keep your mind clear. To help focus, think of the number 1 as you inhale, and the number 2 as you exhale. Each time your mind begins to drift away, quietly think about the numbers.

    d. Tighten your face, hold it a few seconds, and then release all the tightness. Let it flow out with your breath. **Note:** After doing this exercise the first time, the woman may want to do the progressive relaxation exercise by herself, or may want her support person to talk through it with her.

    e. Tighten, hold, and then release the neck and shoulders . . . the right arm and hand . . . the left arm and hand . . . the chest and upper back . . . the abdomen . . . the right thigh . . . the right lower leg, ankle, and foot . . . the left thigh . . . the left lower leg, ankle, and foot. **Note:** A variation of this exercise is to have the woman tighten the body part, hold for a few seconds, and then release it as the coach lightly strokes that body part. Later in labor, gentle stroking of the woman's arms or back will enhance relaxation.

4. Teach paced breathing. Determine which breathing method the woman (couple) has learned. Provide encouragement as needed in maintaining breathing pattern. Provide support to the labor coach and assist as needed.

Lamaze breathing pattern cues

First-level breathing   Pattern begins and ends with a
cleansing breath (in through the nose and out through
pursed lips as if cooling a spoonful of hot food). While inhaling through the nose and exhaling through pursed lips,
slow breaths are taken moving only the chest. The rate
should be approximately 6–9/minute or two breaths/15
seconds. The coach or nurse may assist by reminding the
woman to take a cleansing breath and then the breaths
could be counted out if needed to maintain pacing. The
woman inhales as someone counts "one one thousand,
two one thousand, three one thousand, four one thousand."
Exhalation begins and continues through the same count.

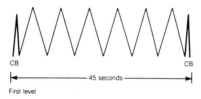

First level

Second-level breathing   Pattern begins and ends with
a cleansing breath. Breaths are then taken in and out si-
lently through the mouth at approximately four breaths/5
seconds. The jaw and entire body needs to be relaxed. The
rate can be accelerated to 2–2½ breaths/second. The
rhythm for the breaths can be counted out as "one and two
and one and two and . . ." with the woman exhaling on the
numbers and inhaling on *and*.

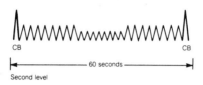

Second level

Third-level breathing   Pattern begins and ends with
a cleansing breath. All breaths are rhythmical, in and out
through the mouth. Exhalations are accompanied by a
"Hee" or "Hoo" sound in a varying pattern, which begins
as 3:1 (Hee Hee Hee Hoo) and can change to 2:1 (Hee
Hee Hoo) or 1:1 (Hee Hoo) as the intensity of the contraction changes. The rate should not be more rapid than

2–2½/second. The rhythm of the breaths would match a "one and two and . . ." count.

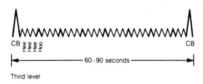

Third level

Abdominal breathing pattern cues

The abdomen moves outward during inhalation and downward during exhalation. The rate remains slow with approximately 6–9 breaths/minute.

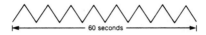

Quick method

When the woman has not learned a particular method and is in active phase of labor, the nurse may teach her a combination of two patterns. Abdominal breathing may be used until labor is more advanced. Then a more rapid pattern can be used consisting of two short blows from the mouth followed by a longer blow. (This pattern is called "pant pant blow" even though all exhalations are a blowing motion.)

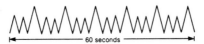

5. Administer analgesic agents as needed. The guidelines for administration are as follows:

   • Assess woman and her record for history of allergies.

   • Assess baseline FHR and maternal vital signs prior to administration of analgesic in order to have a comparison if hypotension develops. Record findings on the chart and on EFM strip (if running).

   • Encourage woman to empty her bladder prior to administration to enhance the rest and relaxation from the drug.

   • Raise side rails to provide safety and explain this precaution to client.

- Monitor maternal vital signs and FHR to assure they remain in a normal range.
- Chart analgesic administration and maternal-fetal status on client record and on EFM tracing. **Note:** Analgesics are not given if the maternal vital signs are unstable, if the woman is hypotensive, if severe hemorrhage is present, or if the baby is preterm.

6. Provide nursing support during regional blocks. See Table 3–7, which highlights nursing actions during regional blocks.

NURSING CARE AT THE TIME OF BIRTH

Critical Nursing Assessments

1. Assessments are outlined in Table 3–5.

Critical Nursing Interventions

- Prepare the birthing area as the time of birth approaches.
- The certified nurse-midwife/physician is summoned if not already present.
- Maternal-fetal assessments are continued as outlined in Table 3–5.
- The nurse and support person assist the woman in her pushing efforts.
- An instrument table and other equipment are prepared.
- Oxygen and suction equipment is readied if needed for both mother and newborn.
- Identification bracelets are prepared.
- Just prior to the birth, the nurse dons sterile gloves and cleanses the perineum.

NURSING CARE IMMEDIATELY AFTER THE BIRTH OF THE BABY

Critical Nursing Assessments

- Assess the Apgar score for the newborn at one and five minutes of age (see Table 3–8).

Table 3–7 Summary of Commonly Used Regional Blocks

Type of Block	Area Affected	Use During Labor and Birth	Nursing Actions
Lumbar epidural	Vagina and perineum	Given in first stage and second stage of labor	Assess woman's knowledge regarding the block. Act as advocate to help her obtain further information if needed. Monitor maternal blood pressure to detect the major side effect, which is hypotension. Provide support and comfort.
Pudendal	Perineum and lower vagina	Given in the second stage just prior to birth to provide anesthesia for episiotomy or for low forceps delivery	Assess woman's knowledge regarding the block. Act as advocate to help her obtain further information if needed.
Local infiltration	Perineum	Administered just before birth to provide anesthesia for episiotomy	Assess woman's knowledge regarding the block. Provide information as needed. Provide comfort and support. Observe perineum for bruising or other discoloration in the recovery period.

Table 3–8 The Apgar Scoring System*

Sign	1	2	3
		Score	
Heart rate	Absent	Slow—below 100	Above 100
Respiratory effort	Absent	Slow—irregular	Good crying
Muscle tone	Flaccid	Some flexion of extremities	Active motion
Reflex irritability	None	Grimace	Vigorous cry
Color	Pale blue	Body pink, blue extremities	Completely pink

*From Apgar V: The newborn (Apgar) scoring system: reflections and advice. *Pediatr Clin North Am* 1966; 13 (August): 645.

- Complete an initial physical assessment of the newborn (see Table 3–9).

Critical Nursing Interventions

- Don disposable gloves when handling the newborn.
- Provide warmth for the newborn by drying with warmed soft blankets, placing under a radiant warmer, or by placing the newborn skin to skin with the mother.
- Maintain a clear airway in the newborn by suctioning with the bulb syringe or by using nasopharyngeal suctioning if needed (see Procedure 19: Suctioning of the Newborn).
- Prevent infection in the newborn by washing hands thoroughly prior to the birth, maintaining asepsis in placing the umbilical cord clamp, and maintaining asepsis if eye prophylaxis is administered in the birthing area.
- Assure correct identification of the newborn by placing identification bracelets on the mother and newborn at birth (in some institutions, an identification band is also placed on the support person), and obtaining newborn's footprints and maternal finger print on birth record.
- Continue to provide support to the woman and her partner.
- Maintain birth record for the client chart.

Table 3–9 Initial Newborn Evaluation

Assess	Normal Findings
Respirations	Rate 30–60 irregular No retractions, no grunting
Apical pulse	Rate 120–160 and somewhat irregular
Temperature	Skin temp above 97.8F (36.5C)
Skin color	Body pink with bluish extremities
Umbilical cord	Two arteries and one vein
Gestational age	Should be 38–42 weeks to remain with parents for extended time
Sole creases	Sole creases that involve the heel

In general expect: scant amount of vernix on upper back, axilla, groin; lanugo only on upper back; ears with incurving of upper ⅔ of pinnae and thin cartilage that springs back from folding; male genitalia—testes palpated in upper or lower scrotum; female genitalia—labia majora larger; clitoris nearly covered.

In the following situations, newborns should generally be stabilized rather than remaining with parents in the birth area for an extended period of time:

Apgar is less than 8 at one minute and less than 9 at five minutes, or a baby requires resuscitation measures (other than whiffs of oxygen). Respirations are below 30 or above 60, with retractions and/or grunting.
Apical pulse is below 120 or above 160 with marked irregularities.
Skin temperature is below 97.8°F (36.5°C).
Skin color is pale blue, or there is circumoral pallor.
Baby is less than 38 or more than 42 weeks' gestation.
Baby is very small or very large for gestational age.
There are congenital anomalies involving open areas in the skin (meningomyelocele).

- Monitor maternal blood pressure (BP) and pulse (P).
- Administer oxytocin as ordered by physician/certified nurse-midwife (see Drug Guide: Oxytocin [Pitocin]). The pitocin may be added to the IV solution if one has already been started, or may be given IM (frequently the ventrogluteal or vastas lateralis site is used).

NURSING CARE IN THE IMMEDIATE
RECOVERY PERIOD (FOURTH STAGE)

Critical Nursing Assessments

Complete maternal assessments q15 X 4, q30 X 2, q1–2hr X two. Maternal BP and pulse are obtained first, then the uterine fundus is assessed (see Figure 3–5). After removing the peripad or chux, the perineum is observed for swelling, bruising, or lacerations. The amount of lochia is also assessed (see Procedure 5: Evaluation of Lochia After Birth). During the assessment the nurse may anticipate the findings indicated in Table 3–10.

The frequent assessments of the immediate recovery cease when:

- Blood pressure and pulse are stable.
- Uterus is firm, in the midline, and below the umbilicus.
- Lochia is rubra, moderate in amount, without clots.
- Perineum is free from bruising or excessive edema.

Critical Nursing Interventions

Support parental attachment by providing private time for the parents and the newborn. Encourage the mother to hold the infant as she desires. Facilitate eye contact by turning down the

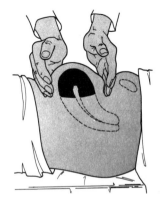

Figure 3–5   Suggested method of palpating the fundus of the uterus during the fourth stage. The left hand is placed just above the symphysis pubis, and gentle downward pressure is exerted. The right hand is cupped around the uterine fundus.

Table 3–10 Maternal Adaptations Following Birth

Characteristic	Normal Findings
Blood pressure	Should return to prelabor level
Pulse	Slightly lower than in labor
Uterine fundus	In the midline at the umbilicus or 1–2 finger-breadths below the umbilicus
Lochia	Red (rubra), small to moderate amount (from spotting on pads to ¼–½ of pad covered in 15 minutes). Should not exceed saturation of one pad in first hour
Bladder	Nonpalpable
Perineum	Smooth, pink, without bruising or edema
Emotional state	Wide variation, including excited, exhilarated, smiling, crying, fatigued, verbal, quiet, pensive, and sleepy

lights in the recovery area. If this is the first baby, some parents enjoy looking the baby over with the nurse explaining some of the newborn characteristics. Monitor newborn status (temperature, skin color, respiratory and heart rate, and need for oral suctioning).

❀ ❀ ❀ ❀ ❀ ❀ ❀ ❀ ❀ ❀ ❀ ❀ ❀ ❀ ❀ ❀ ❀ ❀ ❀

CHAPTER 4

The At-risk Intrapartal Client

FAILURE TO PROGRESS IN LABOR

Overview

Failure to progress in labor is defined as no progress in cervical dilatation or descent of the presenting part during active labor. Failure to progress may be associated with malpresentation (breech, transverse, face or brow), malposition (occiput posterior), or cephalopelvic disproportion (CPD). When such conditions are recognized and treated aggressively, 50% of women will have vaginal birth, while the other 50% will require cesarean birth (Lipshitz 1990).

Maternal risks include infection secondary to increased number of vaginal examinations to determine status, dehydration secondary to inadequate fluid intake, and exhaustion associated with lengthening of the labor. Fetal risks include stress from maternal dehydration and subsequent hypotension and from prolonged labor.

Medical Management

1. **Fluid therapy.** Intravenous fluids may be ordered to rehydrate the laboring woman.
2. **Rule out CPD.** An x-ray pelvimetry may be needed to evaluate the maternal pelvis and the fetus.
3. **Stimulation of labor.** If CPD is ruled out and uterine contractions are less than normal in frequency and quality, an oxytocin infusion may be started to augment the labor pattern.

4. **Method of birth.** If CPD is present, cesarean birth is advised.

Critical Nursing Assessments

1. Assess fetal vertex for engagement into the maternal pelvis. If engaged, the fetal head is at the level of the ischial spines on vaginal examination.

2. Assess uterine contractions. Normal contractions occur every two to three minutes, lasting 50–60 seconds, and are of moderate to strong intensity. If when palpated contraction intensity is less than expected (for this point in labor) and the amount of pain the woman experiences seems out of proportion (feels pain before contraction begins, intense discomfort during contraction, and feels pain after the contraction is gone), consider the possibility of occiput posterior position (Lipshitz 1990).

3. Assess cervical dilatation and effacement. Cervical dilatation usually progresses at 1.5 cm/hr for multiparas and 1.2 cm/hr for primigravidas. Effacement changes from 0% to 100% during the labor progress. If the cervix becomes edematous and thicker during labor, CPD may be present.

4. Assess fetal position, presentation, and descent. A vaginal examination may identify problems such as breech, transverse brow or face presentation, or occiput posterior.

5. Assess for presence of caput (edema of subcutaneous tissues in the top of the fetal head). An enlarging caput may confuse the examiner because it feels like further descent of the fetal head.

6. Assess descent of the fetal head by determining station. **Be alert for:** the presence of a caput because as the caput enlarges and extends down into the birth canal, it may be mistaken for fetal descent.

7. Assess laboring woman for hydration status, comfort/coping level.

Nursing Diagnoses

- Pain, actual, related to inability to relax secondary to labor pattern
- Ineffective individual coping related to ineffectiveness of breathing techniques to relieve discomfort

Critical Nursing Interventions

1. Assess labor status by continuous electronic monitoring and monitor labor progress, maternal and fetal status. Compare assessment findings to expected norms.
2. Provide support and comfort measures (see Chapter 3).
3. Monitor oxytocin infusion if ordered by physician (see discussion later in this chapter).
4. Maintain comprehensive charting on maternal-fetal status. Document maternal contraction status (frequency, duration and intensity of contractions), fetal status (fetal heart rate [FHR] baseline, variability, periodic changes such as accelerations or decelerations), maternal coping and comfort measures used, hydration status, and voiding patterns.
5. Prepare for cesarean birth if indicated.
6. Keep the woman and her partner informed of assessment findings and progress.
7. Review the following critical aspects of the care you have provided.

   - What position does the woman tend to seek? Would any of the following positions work: standing beside the bed and resting on the headrest? sitting on the toilet? using a kneeling or birthing bar? squatting with someone to support her? supported knee to chest? Would ambulation, a shower, or a warm bath help?
   - Have I given support to relaxation and breathing efforts?
   - Are there any other comfort measures available?

Sample Nurse's Charting

Contraction every 2½ minutes, 60 sec duration and of strong intensity. FHR BL 140–148 with two accelerations of 15 bpm with fetal movement in the last 20 minutes. STV present, LTV average. No decelerations present. Voided 200 cc clear amber urine without difficulty. Taking ice chips at will. Skin turgor and mucous membranes indicate adequate hydration. Breathing with contractions but beginning to cry out at the acme. Dozes between contractions but quickly rouses. Asking "Why is it taking so long? Why am I not making progress?" Partner and family asking to speak with physician regarding treatment plan. Call placed to physician and physician to be here in 5 minutes to see patient. P. Gomez, RNC

Evaluation

- The woman will experience a more effective labor pattern.
- The woman has increased comfort and decreased anxiety.

PRECIPITOUS BIRTH

Overview

Precipitous birth is an extremely rapid labor that lasts less than three hours from start to finish. Risks for the mother include lacerations of the cervix, vagina, and/or perineum and postpartal hemorrhage. Fetal/neonatal risks include increased pressure on and in the fetal head and possible cerebral trauma.

Medical Therapy

Close medical monitoring. Obtain previous obstetrical history to identify rapid labor.

Critical Nursing Assessments

1. Assess previous labor history if the woman is a multipara.
2. Assess contraction status. **Be alert for:** contractions that are more frequent than every two minutes and dilatation that progresses faster than normal (more than 1.5 cm per hour).
3. Assess fetal status.

Nursing Diagnoses

- Pain, actual: related to accelerated labor pattern
- Ineffective individual coping; high risk: related to ineffectiveness of breathing techniques to relieve discomfort

Critical Nursing Interventions

1. Monitor labor pattern carefully if oxytocin infusion is being used (induction or augmentation).
2. Evaluate fetal response to labor pattern.
3. Provide support and comfort measures for the woman.

4. Assist with the birth of the baby if the physician/certified nurse-midwife is not present.

- Instruct woman to pant with contractions if fetal head is crowning.
- Apply gentle pressure against the fetal head to maintain flexion and prevent it from popping out quickly. Support the perineum with the other hand and support the descending head between contractions.
- Insert two fingers along the back of the fetal neck to check for a nuchal cord. If present, bend the fingers like a fish hook, grasp the cord, and pull it over the baby's head. If the cord cannot be slipped over the head, place two clamps on it and cut between the clamps. Unwind the cord from around the neck.
- Suction the fetal nares and mouth with a bulb syringe.
- While requesting the woman to push gently, exert gentle downward pressure on the head and neck to assist in the birth of the anterior shoulder. Then exert gentle upward pressure to assist with the posterior shoulder. Support the rest of the baby's body as it is born.
- Place newborn on maternal abdomen and dry the baby with soft warm blankets.
- Check firmness of the uterus. Observe for excessive maternal bleeding.
- Complete patient records. (For detailed description of assisting at birth see Olds SB, London ML, Ladewig PW: *Maternal-Newborn Nursing: A Family Centered Approach*, 4th ed. Benjamin/Cummings, 1992.)

Evaluation

- The woman and her baby are closely monitored during labor and a safe birth occurs.
- The woman feels support and enhanced comfort during labor and birth.

GESTATIONAL AGE-RELATED PROBLEMS

See Table 4–1: Babies with Special Needs in Labor and Birth.

Table 4-1 Babies with Special Needs in Labor and Birth

Type	Implication for Labor	Treatment	Immediate Nursing Support for Newborn
Postdate	More likely to have decreased amount of amniotic fluid, so variable decelerations are more likely. Meconium may be present in amniotic fluid.	Fetal biophysical profile (FBPP) to assess fetal status. Induction if FBPP score decreases, if amniotic fluid volume decreases, or pregnancy reaches 43 wks.	Continuous EFM during labor. At birth, assist physician/CNM with visualization of cord and nasopharyngeal suctioning if fluid is meconium stained.
Preterm	Stress of labor is difficult for baby. Parents are very concerned about baby. Analgesia may be withheld to avoid depressing the fetus/newborn.	Tocolytic therapy to suppress labor. If not successful, forceps may be used to protect fetal head, or cesarean birth is performed.	Have pediatrician and nursing support available. Provide respiratory support, temperature stabilization, and rapid assessment of newborn.
Multiple gestation	Vertex-vertex presentation is most common, followed by vertex-breech. Increased risk of prolapsed cord and cord entanglement.	Vaginal birth of vertex-vertex presentation may be possible. Other presentations may be possible with guided ultrasound. Continuous EFM of both babies during labor.	If vaginal birth anticipated, double numbers of personnel. Provide respiratory support, temperature stabilization.
Macrosomia (Weight >4000 grams)	CPD is more likely. Dysfunctional labor due to overstretching of uterine muscle fibers.	If CPD present, then cesarean birth performed.	Baby is more likely to develop hypoglycemia. If shoulder dystocia, assess for shoulder movement, and crepitus over clavicle.

LABOR COMPLICATED BY MALPRESENTATION OR MALPOSITION

See Table 4–2: Impact of Fetal Malpresentation/Position on Birth. (See Figure 4–1 for selected types of fetal malpresentations.)

PROLAPSED UMBILICAL CORD

Overview

Prolapsed cord occurs when the umbilical cord precedes the fetus down the birth canal. Conditions associated with prolapsed cord include breech presentation, transverse lie, contracted pelvic inlet, small fetus, extra long cord, low-lying placenta, hydramnios, and twin gestations. Fetal/neonatal risks include decreased oxygenation and circulation from the compressed umbilical cord and possible fetal distress.

Medical Therapy

Early recognition. Once prolapsed cord is identified, an emergency cesarean birth is usually indicated.

Critical Nursing Assessments

1. Assess woman's present pregnancy for conditions associated with prolapsed cord.
2. Assess FHR. Since cord compression is associated with variable decelerations (decelerations that vary in timing with the contractions), the best method of assessing is by electronic fetal monitoring (EFM). Periodic auscultation may or may not identify a variable deceleration.
3. Assess for presence of cord prolapse.
   Be alert for: the presence of a pulsating, slick cord. (See Figure 4–2.)

Nursing Diagnoses

- Impaired gas exchange in the fetus; high risk: related to decreased blood flow secondary to compression of the umbilical cord
- Fear related to unknown outcome

Table 4–2 Impact of Fetal Malpresentation/Position on Birth

Fetal Position	Implication for Labor	Treatment Needed or Anticipated	Nursing Interventions	Impact on Newborn
Occiput posterior	Labor may be longer. Severe back pain may be present.	Forceps or manual rotation at birth may be needed.	Apply sacral pressure. Monitor labor, maternal-fetal status. Assist mother into hands and knees position and instruct her to do pelvic rock. Alternative position would be to put weight on knees and lean over raised head of bed, change position from side to side, squat, and/or sit on a toilet.	If labor is longer, fetus more likely to experience stress. Head is molded.
Brow presentation (See Figure 4.1.)	Labor may be longer.	If CPD is suspected or present, and labor is arrested, then cesarean birth is appropriate.	Monitor labor, maternal-fetal status. Provide support measures. Assist with cesarean birth if indicated.	

Face presentation (See Figure 4.1.)	Risks of CPD and prolonged labor are increased.	If no CPD present and chin (mentum) is anterior, vaginal birth may be possible. If chin is posterior a cesarean birth is necessary.	Monitor labor, maternal-fetal status. Provide support measures. Assist with cesarean birth if indicated.	May develop facial edema during labor. May have edema of throat that compromises breathing.
Breech (See Figure 4.1.)	Labor may be prolonged. Meconium may be expelled in amniotic fluid.	External version may be done at 37–38 weeks and then vaginal birth. If version unsuccessful, cesarean birth is scheduled. Some obstetricians may consider vaginal birth for frank breech.	Monitor labor, maternal-fetal status. Monitor for prolapsed cord.	Newborn has increased risk of mortality, intracranial hemorrhage from traumatic birth of head during vaginal birth. Brachial plexus palsy may occur with vaginal birth.

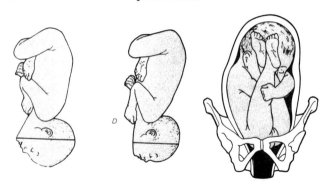

Figure 4–1   Types of malpresentation. A, Brow presentation: The largest anterior-posterior diameter presents to the maternal pelvis. B, Face presentation: Vaginal birth may be possible if the fetal chin is toward the maternal symphysis pubis. C, Breech presentation.

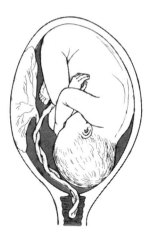

Figure 4–2   Prolapse of the umbilical cord.

Critical Nursing Interventions

1. Complete a vaginal examination to check for prolapse of the cord when variable decelerations are noted on EFM tracing.

2. Relieve pressure of the fetal presenting part by leaving the

gloved fingers in the vagina and lifting the fetal head off the cord (push fetus up toward the body of the uterus). If possible, place woman in knee-chest or Trendelenburg's position. Maintain the maternal position and pressure on the fetal presenting part until the physician arrives and/or a cesarean birth is accomplished.

3. Administer oxygen to the mother by face mask at 7–10 L/min.

4. Call for assistance. Other nurses can assist in the preparation of the woman for emergency cesarean birth.

5. Provide information and support to the laboring couple.

6. Review the following critical aspects of the care you have provided.

- What is the response of the fetal heart rate to the intervention? Has the rate returned to 120–160 range? Is there evidence of variable decelerations on the EFM tracing?

- Are the variable decelerations lessening in depth? in number?

- Is the position that I have asked the woman to assume working? Is FHR improving? (See above questions.) Can this position be maintained until a cesarean birth can be accomplished?

- Is the baby moving much? Are accelerations present?

- What do I need to protect myself from the woman's bodily fluids? Could a colleague tie a plastic apron around me?

Sample Nurse's Charting

Sterile vaginal exam done to assess dilatation status. Prolapse of the umbilical cord through the cervix and into the vagina. Immediate pressure placed on the fetal vertex. EFM monitor indicates FHR maintained BL of 144–150 from beginning of exam throughout intervention. STV present, LTV average, accelerations of 20 bpm with fetal movement and palpation of fetus. Immediate call placed to Dr. _____ to advise of status. IV of 1000 mL lactated Ringer's started in R wrist after one attempt. Running at 125 mL/hr. Indwelling Foley catheter inserted. To surgery for emergency cesarean section. Permit signed by husband. P. Gomez, RNC

AMNIOTIC FLUID-RELATED COMPLICATIONS: HYDRAMNIOS

Overview

Hydramnios occurs when there is over 2000 mL of amniotic fluid in the amniotic sac. The exact cause of hydramnios is unknown; however, it often occurs in cases of major congenital anomalies. Maternal risks include shortness of breath and edema in the lower extremities from compression of the vena cava. The fetus/neonate has an increased risk of mortality because of associated fetal malformations (more prevalent with hydramnios) and increased incidence of preterm birth. Malpresentation is more likely, as is prolapse of the cord.

Medical Therapy

1. **Provide supportive therapy.** Assess fundal size and monitor growth throughout pregnancy. Complete ultrasound examinations to determine presence of anomalies.
2. **Decrease amount of amniotic fluid.** In some instances, an amniocentesis may be done to remove fluid in order to reduce the risk of preterm labor.

Critical Nursing Assessments

1. Assess woman's history for other associated problems such as diabetes, Rh sensitization, fetal malformations, or multiple gestation.
2. Assess FHR. It may be more difficult to auscultate the FHR because of the increased amount of fluid. Placement of the EFM may also be more difficult because of the size of the maternal abdomen. **Be alert for:** the presence of variable decelerations that may indicate prolapse of the cord.
3. Assess maternal blood pressure (BP) and respiratory rate (weight of the uterus can compromise maternal circulation). If compression of the vena cava occurs, hypotension, rapid pulse, pallor, and dyspnea may be noted.
4. Assess for fetal malpresentation-malposition by sterile vaginal examination to determine fetal presenting part.

Nursing Diagnoses

- Alteration in gas exchange; high risk related to pressure on the diaphragm secondary to hydramnios
- Fear related to unknown outcome of the pregnancy

Critical Nursing Interventions

1. Position woman on left or right side.
2. Monitor maternal and fetal status frequently. Follow NAACOG recommended guidelines for labor (see Table 3–5). Because of increased incidence of fetal problems, continuous EFM may be warranted.
3. Monitor amount of amniotic fluid lost, and characteristics of fluid. **Be alert for:** presence of meconium in the fluid (may be associated with fetal stress/distress).

Evaluation

- Maternal and fetal status remains stable with BP, pulse, respirations, and FHR in normal range.
- Woman's questions and fears are addressed.

AMNIOTIC FLUID-RELATED COMPLICATION: OLIGOHYDRAMNIOS

Overview

In oligohydramnios, the amount of amniotic fluid is severely reduced and concentrated. The exact cause is unknown; however, it is found in cases of postmaturity, with intrauterine growth retardation (IUGR) secondary to placental insufficiency, and in fetal conditions associated with renal and urinary malfunction.

Since the amount of amniotic fluid is reduced the umbilical cord has less fluid to float in. The umbilical cord is more likely to be compressed (can be indicated by variable decelerations) and the blood flow to the fetus is reduced. Maternal risks include dysfunctional labor. Fetal risks may include fetal hypoxia associated with umbilical cord compression. If oligohydramnios has been present throughout the gestation, the fetus may have pulmonary hypoplasia.

Medical Therapy

1. **Identify presence of oligohydramnios.** Oligohydramnios is usually identified by serial ultrasound examinations during pregnancy. During labor, an amnioinfusion (infusion of warmed saline solution) may be done to decrease the incidence of cord compression.

2. **Monitor fetal status.** Monitor fetus with fetal biophysical profiles.

Critical Nursing Assessments

1. Assess results of any prenatal testing that indicate decreased amniotic fluid volume (ultrasound exam with notations of decreased volume, or fetal biophysical profile (FBPP) score that is decreased due to diminished amniotic fluid volume.

2. Assess FHR. **Be alert for:** variable decelerations.

3. If membranes rupture, note color and amount of fluid (will be assessed as scant, small, moderate, or large amount), and assess for the presence of meconium.

Nursing Diagnoses

- Alteration in gas exchange; high risk; related to pressure on the umbilical cord secondary to decreased amniotic fluid

- Fear related to unknown outcome of pregnancy

Critical Nursing Interventions

1. Monitor maternal and fetal status on a frequent basis. Watch for maternal hypotension, anxiety, or tension (may be associated with decreased placental-fetal perfusion).

2. Be alert for presence of variable decelerations and decreased variability.

3. Encourage woman to maintain side-lying position while in bed.

4. Assist with amnioinfusion if done.

Evaluation

- The woman and her partner understand the condition, need for monitoring, and possible associated problems.

• The woman and her baby are monitored closely throughout the labor and birth.

AMNIOTIC FLUID EMBOLISM

Overview

An amniotic fluid embolism is a catastrophic event that occurs when a small amount of amniotic fluid enters the maternal blood stream. The bolus of amniotic fluid moves through the maternal circulation, through the right atrium and ventricle, and then into the pulmonary circulation. The sequence of events is thought to include transient pulmonary arterial spasm producing hypoxia with left ventricular and pulmonary capillary injury. This is followed by left ventricular failure and the acute development of adult respiratory distress syndrome (ARDS). The etiology of the coagulopathy that also occurs is unknown (Niswander and Evans 1990).

Maternal mortality rate is 80% (Niswander and Evans 1990). Fetal hypoxia/anoxia occurs as the mother experiences respiratory difficulty or respiratory arrest.

Medical Therapy

Emergency support measures. Immediate, intensive care to support circulatory and respiratory systems is required. Oxygen is administered by mask or positive pressure. The mother may need to be intubated, and numerous IV lines are placed. Central hemodynamic monitoring lines are necessary to monitor pressures and make treatment decisions. IV fluids are given for hypotension and dopamine may be required to maintain maternal blood pressure. Coagulation studies are completed to monitor the development of consumption coagulopathy (DIC) and to monitor treatment. Continuous EFM is necessary to monitor fetal status (Niswander and Evans 1991).

Critical Nursing Assessments

1. Assess for associated factors such as multiparity, hydramnios, tumultuous labor (contractions with frequency of less

than two minutes and strong intensity. This type of labor
may occur naturally or be associated with intravenous oxytocin administration).

2. Assess maternal vital signs. **Be alert for:** signs of respiratory distress or any statement from the mother that she is
experiencing difficulty breathing. The amount of difficulty
seems to be dependent on the amount of amniotic fluid in
the bolus. A large bolus will cause immediate, overwhelm-
ing respiratory problems.

3. Assess FHR. Evaluate FHR rate, variability, and presence of
decelerations.

4. Assess labor progress and identify hypertonic labor patterns
(contractions more frequent than every two minutes and/or
duration greater than 90 seconds with strong intensity).

Nursing Diagnoses

* Alteration of gas exchange; high risk; related to cardio-
pulmonary collapse
* Fear related to unknown outcome of the complication

Critical Nursing Interventions

1. Continue to monitor and evaluate maternal-fetal status.

2. If respiratory difficulties occur, quickly assess, provide oxygen, call for emergency assistance, and provide respiratory
and cardiac support until assistance arrives. Start one or
two peripheral IV lines and assist with emergency measures. Have one nurse note the type and administration
time of all medications. Monitor fetal status at all times.

3. Complete patient records. Nurses' notes need to reflect the
time symptoms began and what the signs and symptoms
were, the actions taken and response of the patient. Continuing assessments are also documented.

4. Prepare for emergency cesarean birth.

Evaluation

* The mother and baby are monitored carefully.
* Emergency measures are instituted immediately.

ABRUPTIO PLACENTA
IN THE INTRAPARTAL AREA

Overview

When a woman is admitted to the intrapartal area and she is bleeding, it is important to quickly complete assessments and to differentiate between many possible causes of the bleeding. Knowledge of the type of bleeding and the presence or absence of pain may assist in this differentiation (see Table 4–3). Maternal mortality is approximately six percent. Other complications include hemorrhage and development of DIC. Fetal/neonatal risks include anemia and hypoxia.

Medical Therapy

1. **Mild abruption** (Vaginal bleeding absent or external bleeding of less than 100 mL). The labor can continue and vaginal birth is anticipated.
2. **Moderate abruption** (vaginal bleeding absent or from 100–500 mL) and **Severe abruption** (vaginal bleeding absent or greater than 500 mL) require continuous monitoring of the mother and fetus, monitoring and treatment of

Table 4–3 Characteristics of Placenta Previa and Abruptio Placenta

Placenta Previa	Abruptio Placenta
Bright red bleeding	May be bright red or dark red in color or no bleeding may be apparent if abruption is concealed
No pain	May have no pain if abruption was on margin of placenta and has now resolved
May have history of painless, bright red bleeding	May have pain if abruption is central (behind placenta). If contractions are present, may have increased tonus of uterus and poor uterine relaxation between contractions. Uterus may be "boardlike"

shock, possibly an amniotomy and oxytocin infusion to augment labor or begin labor, evaluation of coagulation, blood replacement, and possible cesarean section.

3. **Method of birth.** Cesarean birth is indicated when: 1) fetal distress develops and a vaginal birth is not imminent, 2) the fetus is alive and a severe abruption occurs, 3) hemorrhage becomes severe and threatens the life of the mother, and 4) labor is not progressing.

Critical Nursing Assessments

1. Assess maternal history for associated factors (pregnancy-induced hypertension [PIH], high multiparity, trauma, use of illicit drugs such as cocaine or crack).

2. Assess type and amount of bleeding. Pads may be weighed to more accurately assess blood loss (1 gram equals 1 mL). Hemorrhage of 500 mL or more increases chance of fetal death. Vaginal bleeding is present in 80% of abruptions, is absent (concealed) in other 20% (Niswander and Evans 1990).

3. Assess whether pain is present. Is pain associated with uterine contractions? Is there pain between contractions (feels as if the uterus stays tight and does not relax). Are there tender areas over the uterus? Pain is present in most women with abruptio placenta. The pain is usually of sudden onset, is constant, and is localized to the uterus or the lower back (Niswander and Evans 1991).

4. Assess uterine contractions. What is frequency, duration, intensity, and what is resting tone between contractions? (Abruptio is associated with a rising uterine tone baseline.)

5. Assess size of uterus. If bleeding is concealed, the uterus may be filling with blood and the fundus will rise.

6. Assess labor progress (vaginal examination for cervical dilatation, effacement, and fetal station). Abruption may be associated with precipitous birth.

7. Assess maternal vital signs (BP, pulse, respirations) and fetal status (by EFM).

8. Assess laboratory studies (hemoglobin, hematocrit, DIC screen).

Nursing Diagnoses

See Nursing Care Plan 7: Hemorrhage in Third Trimester and at Birth.

Critical Nursing Interventions

1. Monitor maternal status. Be alert for beginning signs of shock (decreased BP, increased pulse, increased respirations).

2. Monitor fetal status. Be alert for FHR baseline changes and late decelerations with decreased variability.

3. Monitor amount of blood loss. Measure blood loss. Wear disposable gloves when handling blood-soaked items or while cleansing blood from woman.

4. Carefully monitor labor status. Be alert for increased uterine tonus, which may be exhibited by increased frequency of contractions (< two minutes), increased intensity, incomplete uterine relaxation between contractions, tenderness of the uterine fundus, and a rising baseline of EFM monitor strip.

5. Monitor urine output. Urine output is reflective of circulatory status. Urine output needs to be at least 30 mL/hr. An indwelling bladder catheter will assist in monitoring urine output accurately. Amount of output is measured every one to four hours, depending on severity of bleeding.

6. Monitor size of abdomen. Measurement of abdominal girth may be ordered. If it is, place measuring tape under woman, bring around to the front and over the umbilicus. Use either the upper or lower edge of the umbilicus and, for consistency, consider making marks on the maternal abdomen with felt-tip pen to assure consistent placement of the tape in each measurement.

7. Monitor oxytocin if it is being administered. See discussion of induction of labor later in this chapter.

8. Monitor laboratory studies. Be alert for development of consumption coagulopathy (DIC) as evidenced by decreasing platelets and fibrinogen and increased fibrin split products. (See Table 4–4.)

9. Monitor oxygen status by pulse oximetry (pulse oximetry needs to be 90 or above). If reading is below 90, administer oxygen by face mask at 7–10 L/min.

10. Monitor fluid and blood replacement.

11. Monitor for signs of decreased platelet count such as purpura, petechiae, bruising, hematemesis, rectal bleeding.

12. Prepare for cesarean if birth not imminent.
    Note: for additional information, see Nursing Care Plan 7: Hemorrhage in Third Trimester and at Birth.

Table 4–4 Laboratory Findings Associated with DIC

Lab Test	Normal Value	Value in DIC
Partial thromboplastin	60–70 sec	Prolonged
Platelets	150,000–400,000 μL	Decreased
Fibrinogen	200–400 mg/dL	Decreased
Fibrin degradation products (also called fibrin split products or fibrin)	2–10 μg/mL	Increased

13. Follow body substance isolation and CDC precautions at all times of exposure to bodily fluids.
14. Review the following critical aspects of the care you have provided.

- Are the woman's vital signs stable? Are they responding in an anticipated way to the medical therapy? What does the woman say about her condition? Is she anxious?
- Is the amount of bleeding increasing? What are the measured amounts of blood loss? Is there bleeding from any other site?
- Is the uterus becoming more tender, more sensitive?
- Is there a rising uterine resting tone?
- Is there a better position to place the woman in to maximize circulation and comfort?
- What other information can I provide?
- Has there been a change in her consciousness level? **Note:** for further information see Nursing Care Plan 7: Hemorrhage in Third Trimester and at Birth.

Sample Nurse's Charting

Uterine contractions every 3 min, 60 sec duration and strong intensity. Uterus relaxes between contractions. Patient reports slight tenderness in the upper uterine fundus on the right when palpated. FHR 140–146, STV diminished, LTV decreased, no accelerations with fetal movement. Deceleration of 15 bpm lasting 15 sec begins just after acme of each contraction. O_2 per face mask at 8 L/min. Patient lying on left side. BP stable at 112/70. Admitting BP 114/72. Pulse 80 and regular. 100 cc dark red vaginal bleeding present on chux in last hour. Patient breathing with contractions and relaxing well with encouragement. Partner provides continuous, ongoing support. P. Gomez, RNC

Evaluation

See Nursing Care Plan 7: Hemorrhage in Third Trimester and at Birth.

PLACENTA PREVIA IN THE INTRAPARTAL PERIOD

Overview

Placenta previa may occur as a low placental implantation, a partial or marginal previa, or a complete previa. Maternal risks include hemorrhage and possible complications of emergency cesarean birth. Fetal/neonatal risks include anemia, and hypoxia if bleeding occurs.

Medical Therapy

Management. Obtain diagnosis from ultrasound examination. If complete previa, gestation >37 weeks, and documented fetal maturity, schedule cesarean birth. If marginal placenta previa, labor and vaginal birth may be possible.

Critical Nursing Assessments

1. Assess type and amount of bleeding (as in abruption section just discussed).
2. Assess maternal vital signs and fetal status.
3. Assess labor progress (uterine contraction frequency, duration, and intensity; fetal descent).
4. Assess laboratory findings.

Nursing Diagnoses

See Nursing Care Plan 7: Hemorrhage in Third Trimester and at Birth.

Critical Nursing Interventions

1. Monitor bleeding. Weigh all absorbent pads to determine amount of blood loss.
2. Monitor maternal vital signs for signs of shock.
3. Monitor FHR for evidence of normality (baseline stable, short-term variability (STV) present and average long-term variability (LTV), no periodic decelerations or early decelerations). Note signs of possible fetal problems such as rising or falling baseline, decreased variability, late and/or variable decelerations.
4. Monitor laboratory studies. **Be alert for:** evidence of decreasing hemoglobin and hematocrit.
   Note: Coagulation problems are not as common with previa.
5. Administer and monitor IV fluids and blood replacement.
6. Monitor oxygen status. If vital signs unstable or questionable, monitor pulse oximetry. If pulse oximetry is below 90, administer oxygen by face mask at 7–10 L/min. Continue to monitor pulse oximetry.
   Note: See Nursing Care Plan 7: Hemorrhage in Third Trimester and at Birth for additional information.

Evaluation

See Nursing Care Plan 7: Hemorrhage in Third Trimester and at Birth.

DIABETES MELLITUS IN THE INTRAPARTAL PERIOD

Overview

Diabetes affects the labor process in a variety of ways. Insulin/glucose balance is affected by the expenditure of energy during labor. The method of birth will be influenced by assessment of the fetal size. A large fetus (> 4500 grams or a fetus larger than the maternal pelvis) will be born by cesarean.

Effect of Diabetes	**Medical Therapy**	**Nursing Interventions**
Alteration of insulin/ glucose balance	Schedule cesarean in early AM. Advise patient to have her usual evening insulin dose, evening meal, and snack.	Monitor blood glucose by finger-stick at evening meal and at bedtime.
		Be watchful for signs and symptoms of hypo- or hyperglycemia.
		Expect precipitous drop in insulin requirements after birth.
	If patient is laboring monitor blood glucose by hourly fingersticks and administration of insulin and IV fluids. Maintain glucose control at < 100 mg/dL.	Assist with finger-sticks. Adjust IV fluids per physician order. Administer insulin per physician order.
Increased incidence of large fetus	Estimate fetal size.	Maintain mother in side-lying position.
		Monitor FHR by EFM.
		Evaluate labor progress carefully to watch for failure to progress or evidence of CPD.
		Evaluate EFM tracing for late deceleration and/or decreased variability.
Increased incidence of congenital anomalies		Assess newborn for signs of congenital problems.
Acceleration of fetal lung maturity	Determine fetal lung maturity prior to labor.	Have resuscitation equipment and personnel available at birth.

PREGNANCY-INDUCED HYPERTENSION IN THE INTRAPARTAL PERIOD

Overview

The woman with pregnancy-induced hypertension needs to be watched closely in the intrapartal area. Her blood pressure may increase with the stress of labor. Hyperirritability of the central nervous system (CNS) may affect the woman's ability to cope with the labor process.

Effect of Labor	Medical Therapy	Nursing Interventions
Possible increase of blood pressure	IV magnesium sulfate therapy	Start and monitor IV magnesium sulfate therapy by infusion pump.
		Check BP, pulse, respirations, patellar and brachial reflexes, and urine output at least hourly (more often if maternal condition requires).
		Remember therapeutic magnesium sulfate level is from 4 to 7 mEq/L.
		Loss of patellar reflex is the earliest sign of magnesium toxicity; this occurs at about 7–10 mEq/L.
		Respiratory and cardiac arrest may occur if magnesium levels rise further. See Drug Guide 6: Magnesium Sulfate (Mg SO$_4$).
Stress of labor on fetus	Evaluate fetal status.	Maintain continuous EFM. Assess tracing frequently for late decelerations or decreased variability.

INDUCTION OF LABOR

Overview

Labor may be induced when diabetes, PIH, premature rupture of membranes (PROM), postterm pregnancy, intrauterine growth retardation (IUGR), and intrauterine fetal death (IUFD) are present. The most frequent methods of induction are amniotomy, intravenous oxytocin, or both. Prostaglandin E_2 is currently being used for labor priming (softening of the cervix) at term but is not used to induce labor at that time.

Cervical readiness for induction can be assessed by determining a Bishop's score. A score of at least 9 is usually associated with a successful induction (see Table 4–5).

For oxytocin induction 1000 mL of solution (such as lactated Ringer's) is started IV by a large-bore plastic IV catheter (18 or 20 gauge). Ten units of pitocin are added to a second 1000-mL bottle of IV fluid (second bottle needs to match the other primary IV). The IV containing the pitocin is the secondary bottle and this bottle is administered via an infusion pump. (See Drug Guide 10: Oxytocin [Pitocin] for further information.)

Maternal risks include water intoxication; rapid labor and birth; cervical, vaginal, and/or perineal lacerations. Fetal/neonatal risks include rapid intracranial pressure changes if rapid labor and birth occur, possible decreased placental-fetal circulation if labor pattern is overstimulated.

Critical Nursing Assessments

See Nursing Care Plan 8: Induction of Labor.

Nursing Diagnoses

See Nursing Care Plan 8: Induction of Labor.

Critical Nursing Interventions

See Nursing Care Plan 8: Induction of Labor.

Evaluation

See Nursing Care Plan 8: Induction of Labor.

Table 4–5 Prelabor Status Evaluation Scoring System*

Factor	Assigned Value			
	0	1	2	3
Cervical dilatation	Closed	1–2 cm	3–4 cm	5 cm or more
Cervical effacement	0%–30%	40%–50%	60%–70%	80% or more
Fetal station	–3	–2	–1, 0	+1, or lower
Cervical consistency	Firm	Moderate	Soft	
Cervical position	Posterior	Midposition	Anterior	

*Modified from Bishop EH: Pelvic scoring for elective induction. *Obstet Gynecol* 1964; 24:266.

OBSTETRIC PROCEDURE: EXTERNAL VERSION

Procedure Overview

Version is done to change the fetal position from breech to cephalic. It is usually scheduled in the 38th week of pregnancy, but may be done in the 39th or 40th.

Critical Nursing Assessments

1. Assess the mother for presence of contraindications (nonreactive nonstress test [NST], evidence of CPD, multiple gestation, oligohydramnios, and placenta previa).
2. Assess maternal BP, pulse and respirations, and fetal heart rate (establish presence of reassuring characteristics: FHR baseline between 120–160, presence of short-term variability and average long-term variability, absence of late or variable decelerations).

Nursing Diagnoses

- Knowledge deficit related to procedure and possible complications

Critical Nursing Interventions

1. Monitor maternal BP and pulse prior to the version and every five minutes during the procedure.
2. Monitor fetal heart rate continuously during the version.
3. Provide support to the woman and her partner.
4. Provide information regarding the version.
5. Determine woman's Rh status. If she is Rh negative, obstetrician will probably order mini-dose of RhoGam.

Evaluation

- The version is accomplished successfully and no complications have occurred.
- The woman is knowledgeable regarding possible complications.

OBSTETRIC PROCEDURE: FORCEPS-ASSISTED BIRTH

Procedure Overview

Forceps may be used for rotation of the fetus when there is a persistent posterior position or transverse arrest (anterior-posterior diameters of the fetal head remain transverse in the maternal pelvis), and for traction to assist birth. Maternal risks include laceration of the cervix, vagina, or perineum; or hematoma. Fetal/neonatal risks include possible stress, facial edema, and/or bruising.

Critical Nursing Assessments

1. Assess maternal ability to relax perineal muscles during forceps application and use.
2. Assess maternal and fetal status (vital signs) and contraction pattern.

Nursing Diagnoses

- Knowledge deficit related to procedure and possible complications
- Ineffective coping related to unexpected labor progress and use of procedure

Critical Nursing Interventions

1. Monitor woman's comfort/coping level.
2. Monitor uterine contractions and inform physician of presence of contractions.
3. Monitor FHR after each contraction or continuously by EFM.
4. Provide information and support to the woman.

Evaluation

- Mother and baby have experienced no complications.
- Mother and partner understand procedure and possible complications.

OBSTETRIC PROCEDURE: VACUUM EXTRACTION

Procedure Overview

The vacuum extractor is composed of a suction cup attached to a suction device (bottle). The suction cup is placed against the fetal occiput and traction can be applied by the obstetrician to assist the birth. The maternal risks are similar to those in the use of forceps. Fetal/neonatal risks are similar except that facial edema or bruising does not occur; instead, a caput (called a chignon) forms under the suction cup.

Nursing assessments, diagnoses, interventions, and evaluation are similar to those in forceps-assisted birth.

REFERENCES

Lipshitz J: Failure to progress in labor. In: Rivlin ME, Morrison JC, Bates GW (editor): *Manual of Clinical Problems in Obstetrics and Gynecology*. Boston: Little, Brown, 1990.

Niswander KR, Evans A: *Manual of Obstetrics*. Boston: Little, Brown, 1991.

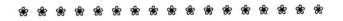

CHAPTER 5

The Normal Newborn

At the moment of birth, numerous physiologic adaptations begin to take place in the newborn's body. Because of these dramatic changes, the newborn requires close observation to determine how smoothly she or he is making the transition to extrauterine life. The newborn also requires care that enhances her or his chances of making the transition successfully.

Two broad goals of nursing care during this period are to promote the physical well-being of the newborn and to promote the establishment of a well-functioning family unit. The first goal is met by providing comprehensive care to the newborn while he or she is in the nursery. The second goal is met by teaching parents how to care for their new baby and by supporting their parenting efforts so that they feel confident and competent.

TRANSITIONAL PERIOD

The transitional period involves three periods, called the first period of reactivity, sleep phase, and second period of reactivity. The characteristics of each period demonstrate the newborn's progression to independent functioning.

First Period of Reactivity

This period lasts from birth to 30–60 minutes after birth.

Characteristics

1. The newborn's vital signs are as follows: apical pulse rate between 120–150 bpm (but may be as high as 180 bpm) and irregular in rhythm. Respiratory rate between 30 and

60 breaths/minute, irregular, and some may be labored, with nasal flaring, expiratory grunting, and retractions.

2. Color fluctuates from pale pink to cyanotic.

3. Bowel sounds are absent and the baby usually does not void or stool during this period.

4. The newborn has minimal amounts of mucus at this time, a rigorous cry, and strong suck reflex. Special tip: During this period of time, the newborn's eyes are open more than they will be again for days. It is an excellent time for the attachment process to begin as the newborn is able to maintain eye contact for long periods of time.

Care needs specific to first period of reactivity

1. Assess and monitor heart rate and respirations q30 min for the first four hours after birth.

2. Keep baby warm (axillary or skin probe temperature between 36.5° C to 37° C [97.7° F–98.6° F]) with warmed blankets or overhead warming lights.

e. Couple mom and baby together skin to skin to facilitate attachment.

4. Delay instillation of eye prophylactic for first hour to promote newborn-parent interaction.

Sleep Phase

The sleep phase lasts from 30–60 minutes after birth to four to six hours after birth.

Characteristics

1. As the baby moves into the sleep phase, the heart rate may remain irregular until sleep occurs. While asleep, the respiratory rate increases and the apical pulse rate ranges from 120–140 bpm.

2. Skin color stabilizes and may show some acrocyanosis.

Care needs specific to sleep phase   The baby doesn't respond to external stimuli. Mother and father can still enjoy holding and cuddling their baby.

Second Period of Reactivity

The second period of reactivity lasts from four to six hours of age to 8–12 hours of age.

Characteristics

1. Baby has intense sensitivity to internal and environmental stimuli. Apical pulse ranges from 120–160 bpm and can vary from this range from bradycardia (< 120 bpm) to tachycardia (> 160 bpm). Respiratory rate (RR) is 30–60 breaths/minute with periods of more rapid respirations, but they remain unlabored (no nasal flaring or retractions).

2. Skin color fluctuates from pink or ruddy to cyanotic with periods of mottling.

3. Baby often voids and passes meconium during this period.

4. Mucus secretions increase and the baby may gag on secretions. Sucking reflex is again strong and baby may be very active.

Care needs specific to second period of reactivity

1. Close observation of newborn for possible choking on the excessive mucus normally present. Use bulb syringe to remove mucus and teach parents how to use the bulb syringe.

2. Observe for any episode of apnea and initiate methods of stimulation if needed (stroke baby's back, turn baby to side, etc).

3. Assess baby's interest in and ability to feed (no choking or gagging during feeding, no vomiting of feeding in unchanged form).

Additional Assessments and Interventions in the Transitional Period

In these first few hours of life, the nurse will accomplish the following:

1. Monitor newborn vital signs. See Table 5–1 for summary of normal findings.

2. Weigh the newborn, and measure length, head, and chest circumference (see Table 5–2 and Figure 5–1). To determine length, place the newborn flat on her/his back with legs extended as much as possible. Hold the head still at the top of the measuring tape and gently stretch the legs downward toward the bottom of the tape (see Figure 5–2). To measure head circumference place the tape over the

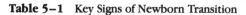

Table 5-1 Key Signs of Newborn Transition

Pulse: 120–150 beats/min
   During sleep as low as 100 beats/min; if crying, up to 180 beats/min

Respirations: 30–60 respirations/min
   Predominantly diaphragmatic but synchronous with abdominal movements

Temperature: Axillary: 36.5° C–37° C (97.7° F–98.6° F)
   Skin: 36° C–36.5° C (96.8° F–97.7° F)

Dextrostix: greater than 45 mg %

Hematocrit: less than 65%–70% central venous sample

Blood pressure: 90–60/45–40 mm Hg

Table 5-2 Newborn Weight and Measurements

Weight
Average: 3405 grams (7 lb, 8 oz)
Range: 2500–4000 grams (5 lb, 8 oz to 8 lb, 13 oz)
Weight is influenced by racial origin and maternal age and size

Length
Average: 50 cm (20 in)
Range: 45–55 cm (18–22 in)

Head Circumference
Average: 32–37 cm (12½–14½ in)
Approximately 2 cm (about 1 inch) larger than chest circumference

most prominent part of the occiput and bring it around above the eyebrows (see Figure 5–3). The circumference of the head is approximately 2 cm greater than the circumference of the chest at birth. To obtain chest circumference, place the tape measure at the lower edge of the scapulas and bring it around anteriorly over the nipple line.

3. Complete gestational age assessment of the newborn. The nurse needs to complete this assessment during the first four hours of life so that age-related problems can be identified. Clinical gestational age assessment tools have two components: external physical characteristics and neuromuscular status.

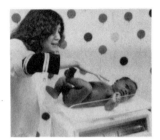

Figure 5–1 Weighing of newborns. The scale is balanced before each weight, with the protective pad in place. The care giver's hand is poised above the infant as a safety measure. (From Swearingen P: The Addison-Wesley Photo Atlas of Nursing Procedures. Menlo Park, CA: Addison-Wesley, 1984.)

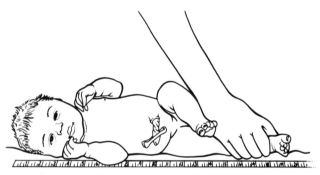

Figure 5–2 Measuring the length of a newborn.

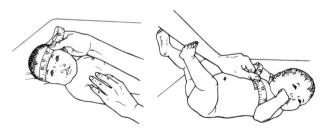

Figure 5–3 Obtaining newborn measurements. A, Measuring the head circumference of the newborn. The tape is placed on the occiput and then brought around and placed just above the eyebrows. B, Measuring the chest circumference of the newborn. The tape is placed over the lower edge of the scapula and brought around to the front and placed over the nipple line.

Physical characteristics can be assessed (with the exception of sole creases) over the first 24 hours. Neuromuscular development may be influenced by the newborn's unstable nervous system or labor and birth events. It can be assessed in the first 24 hours; however, if the findings drastically differ from the gestational age determined by looking at physical characteristics, the assessment may be repeated after 24 hours (see Table 5–3).

Method of assessment Use Estimation of Gestational Age by Maturity Rating (Figure 5–4). Assess each of the factors listed and assign a score of 0 to 4 for each one. It is helpful to circle the results for each assessment.

Physical characteristics

a. **Skin** in the preterm neonate appears thin and transparent, with veins prominent over the abdomen early in gestation. As term approaches, the skin appears opaque because of increased subcutaneous tissue. Disappearance of the protective vernix caseosa promotes skin desquamation (peeling).

b. **Lanugo**, a fine hair covering, decreases as gestational age increases. The amount of lanugo is greatest at 28–30 weeks and then disappears, first from the face, then from the trunk and extremities.

c. **Sole (plantar creases)** needs to be assessed within 12

Table 5–3 Characteristics of Gestational Age Assessment

Physical Characteristics	Neuromuscular Characteristics
Characteristics of skin	Posture
Amount of lanugo	Square window (wrist)
Sole creases	Arm recoil
Amount of breast tissue	Popliteal angle
Cartilaginous development of the ear	Scarf sign
Male: testicular descent and rugae on scrotum OR	Heel to ear
Female: labial development	

**Estimation of Gestational Age
by Maturity Rating**
Symbols: X=First exam   O=Second exam

Neuromuscular Maturity

	0	1	2	3	4	5
Posture						
Square window (wrist)	90°	60°	45°	30°	0°	
Arm recoil	180°		100°-180°	90°-100°	<90°	
Popliteal angle	180°	160°	130°	110°	90°	<90°
Scarf sign						
Heel to ear						

Gestation by dates _____ wks.

Birth date _____ Hour _____ am / pm

APGAR _____ 1 min _____ 5 min

Score	Wks
5	26
10	28
15	30
20	32
25	34
30	36
35	38
40	40
45	42
50	44

Physical Maturity

	0	1	2	3	4	5
Skin	gelatinous red, transparent	smooth pink, visible veins	superficial peeling and/or rash, few veins	cracking pale area, rare veins,	parchment, deep cracking, no vessels	leathery, cracked, wrinkled
Lanugo	none	abundant	thinning	bald areas	mostly bald	
Plantar creases	no crease	faint red marks	anterior transverse crease only	creases anter. 2/3	creases cover entire sole	
Breast	barely perceptible	flat areola, no bud	stippled areola, 1-2 mm bud	raised areola, 3-4 mm bud	full areola, 5-10 mm bud	
Ear	pinna flat, stays folded	sl. curved pinna, soft with slow recoil	well-curv. pinna, soft but ready recoil	formed and firm with instant recoil	thick cartilage, ear stiff	
Genitals (male)	scrotum empty, no rugae		testes decending, few rugae	testes down, good rugae	testes pendulous, deep rugae	
Genitals (female)	prominent clitoris and labia minora		majora and minora equally prominent	majora large, minora small	clitoris and minora completely covered	

Figure 5–4   Newborn maturity rating and classification. (From Ballard JL, et al: A simplified assessment of gestational age. Classification of the low-birth-weight infant. In: Klaus MH, Pediatr Res *1977; 11:374. Figure adapted from Sweet AY, Fanaroff AA:* Care of the High-Risk Infant. *Philadelphia: Saunders, 1977, p 47.)*

hours of birth because after this the skin of the foot begins drying and superficial creases disappear. Development of sole creases begins at the top of the sole and proceeds downward toward the heel.

d. **Areola** is inspected and the breast bud tissue is gently palpated to determine the size. It is important to place your index and middle finger over this tissue and roll over the breast bud to estimate the size, rather than pinching the tissue. Another method of measuring involves placing a ruler just above the breast bud tissue for more accurate measurement. Most experienced nurses have completed the assessment often enough that they can estimate the size very accurately.

e. **Ear form and cartilage** change throughout gestation. By 36 weeks some cartilage and slight incurving of upper pinna are present, and the pinna springs back slowly when folded. To assess, observe ear form and then fold pinna of the ear forward against the side of the head, release it, and observe the results.

f. **Genitals** change in appearance during gestation because of the amount of subcutaneous fat present. **Female genitals** at 30–32 weeks have a prominent clitoris and the labia majora are small and widely separated. At 36–40 weeks the labia nearly cover the clitoris, and at 40-plus weeks, the labia majora completely cover the clitoris. The nurse completes the assessment by observation. **Male genitals** are evaluated for size of the scrotal sac, presence of rugae, and the descent of the testes. The nurse observes the size of the scrotal sac and whether rugae are present. The scrotal sac can be gently palpated to determine descent of the testes.

Neuromuscular characteristics

a. **Resting posture** should be assessed as the baby lies undisturbed on a flat surface such as his or her bed.

b. **Square window (wrist)** is elicited by flexing the baby's hand toward the ventral forearm. The angle formed at the wrist is measured (by estimation and matching it against the angles on the scoring tool) (see Figure 5–5).

c. **Arm recoil** is a test of flexion development. It is best evaluated after the first hour of life when the baby has had time to recover from the stress of birth. To assess, place the newborn in a supine position (lying on his/ her back), completely flex both elbows (by holding the newborn's hands and placing the hands up against the forearms), hold them in this position for about five seconds, and then release them. On release, the elbows of a full-term newborn form an angle of less than 90° and rapidly recoil back to flexed position. The arms of a preterm have slower recoil time and form greater than a 90° angle.

d. **Popliteal angle** is determined with the newborn supine and flat. The thigh is flexed on the abdomen/chest, and the nurse places the index finger of the other hand behind the newborn's ankle to extend the lower leg until resistance is met. The angle formed is then measured. Results vary from no resistance in the very immature infant to an 80° angle in the term infant.

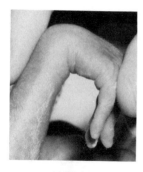

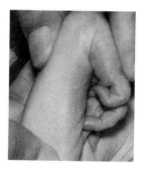

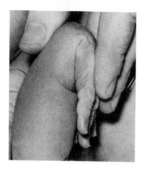

Figure 5–5   Square window sign. A, *This angle is 90° and suggests an immature newborn of 28 to 32 weeks' gestation.* B, *A 30° angle is commonly found from 38–40 weeks' gestation.* C, *A 0° angle occurs from 40–42 weeks. (From Dubowitz L, Dubowitz V:* Gestational Age of the Newborn. *Menlo Park: CA, Addison-Wesley, 1977.)*

   e. **Scarf sign** is elicited by placing the neonate supine and drawing an arm across the chest toward the infant's opposite shoulder. The arm is pulled until resistance is met. (The newborn needs to remain lying on his/her back. The location of the elbow is then noted in relation to the midline of the chest) (see Figure 5–6).
   f. **Heel to ear** is performed by placing the baby in a supine position and, while stabilizing the hip on the bed, gently drawing the foot toward the ear on the same side until resistance is felt. Both the popliteal angle and the proximity of the foot to the ear are assessed. In a very preterm newborn, the leg will remain straight and the foot will go to the ear or beyond. If the newborn was in a breech presentation, this assessment should be delayed until the legs are positioned more normally.

Scoring   All individual scores are added and the total number is compared to the score on the Estimation of Gesta-

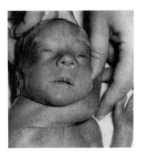

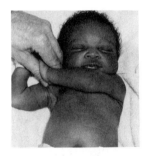

Figure 5–6 Scarf sign. A, No resistance is noted until after 30 weeks' gestation. The elbow can be readily moved past the midline. B, The elbow is at midline at 36–40 weeks' gestation. C, Beyond 40 weeks' gestation, the elbow will not reach the midline. (From Dubowitz L, Dubowitz V: Gestational Age of the Newborn. *Menlo Park, CA, Addison-Wesley, 1977.)*

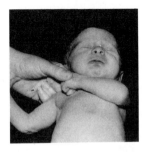

tional Age by Maturity Rating tool. A score of 35 equals 38 weeks, a score of 37 equals 39 weeks, and a score of 40 equals 40 weeks.

The estimated gestational age is plotted on a tool that classifies newborns by birth weight and gestational age (see Figure 5–7). Most newborns are appropriate for gestational age (AGA). A baby that is large for gestational age (LGA) or small for gestational age (SGA) may require additional assessment and intervention (for further discussion see Chapter 6).

4. Administer Ilotycin ointment (or silver nitrate drops) into the newborn's eyes. This is a legally required prophylactic eye treatment for *Neisseria gonorrhoea*. which may have infected the newborn during the birth process. Ilotycin has the advantage of being useful for both gonorrhea and chlamydia; it is also less irritating to the newborn's eyes, which results in decreased incidence of swelling and discharge.

5. Administer prophylactic dose of vitamin K. The vitamin K is given to prevent hemorrhage, which can occur due to low prothrombin levels in the first few days of life (see Figure 5–8 for injection sites).

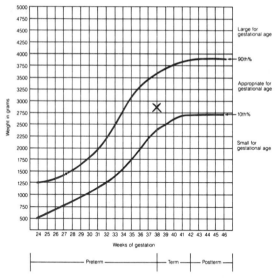

Figure 5–7 Classification of newborns by birth weight and gestational age. The newborn's birth weight and gestational age are plotted on the graph. The newborn is then classified as large for gestational age (LGA), appropriate for gestational age (AGA), or small for gestational age (SGA). For example, a baby who is 38 weeks' gestation and weighs 2875 gm is considered AGA (see X). (From Battaglia FC, Lubchenco LO: A practical classification of newborn infants by weight and gestational age. J. Pediatr 1967; 71:161.)

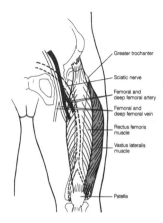

Figure 5–8 Newborn injection sites. The middle third of the vastus lateralis muscle is the preferred site for intramuscular injection in the newborn.

6. Assess glucose level. A drop of blood is obtained by heel stick and blood glucose is determined (see Figure 5–9). The glucose strip should read > 45 mg/dL; a value < 45 mg/dL needs to be followed up by drawing a central blood sample (drawn from a vein in the hand or antecubital space) for further laboratory evaluation. Treatment is begun if needed (see Chapter 6 for discussion of hypoglycemia). **Be alert for:** Hypoglycemia in high-risk babies such as SGA, infant of diabetic mother (IDM), AGA preterm, and any newborn that was stressed during labor and at birth. Outward signs of hypoglycemia may include lethargy, jitteriness, poor feeding, vomiting, pallor, apnea, irregular respirations, and/or tremors.

7. Maintain temperature through use of a controlled radiant warmer. A probe is placed on the newborn's abdomen just under the ribs or over the area of the liver. The probe indicates the newborn's temperature and the radiant heater responds by becoming warmer or cooler. **Be alert for:** Newborns at risk for hypothermia (temperature < 97.7° F), including preterms, SGA, and any baby that was stressed at birth.

    If the newborn's temperature is 97.7° F or below (axillary or skin probe temperature), rewarming is needed. The baby is placed under a radiant warmer, undressed so that the skin can be warmed, and the warmer set for 98.6° F. When the skin probe indicates that the desired temperature has been reached, recheck axillary temperature. The baby may be removed from the warmer; however, axillary temperature should be rechecked about every 30 minutes for an hour or so to make sure the baby is maintaining a normal temperature.

    Successful transition to extrauterine existence is documented by stabilization of vital signs and establishment of awake/sleep cycles and feeding, stooling, and voiding patterns.

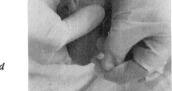

Figure 5–9   Blood is obtained by a heel stick for a glucose (Chemstrip) test.

POST-TRANSITIONAL NURSING CARE

Overview

Once the newborn has passed through the transitional period, he/she is transferred to a normal newborn area. Normal newborn care usually includes assessment of vital signs (axillary temperature, apical pulse, and respirations) every four hours, a physical assessment every eight hours, application of a drying agent to the umbilical stump every eight hours, feeding every three to four hours, diapering as needed, and weighing once every 24 hours.

Physical Assessment

It is usually easier to proceed from head to toe; however, you need to assess axillary temperature, apical pulse, and respirations while the baby is quiet. Completing the assessment in the mother's room provides a wonderful opportunity for teaching, sharing, and role modeling for first-time mothers.

1. **Head.** Palpate and observe fontanelles. The anterior fontanelle is the largest and is diamond shaped. The posterior fontanelle is triangular in shape. The sagittal suture (located on the top of the head, from front to back) is smooth and without ridges.
    Common variations: bulging of fontanelle (increased intracranial pressure), depressed fontanelle (dehydration), overriding of sagittal suture (molding), caput succedaneum (edema in tissues from trauma), cephalhematoma (bleeding into the periosteal space).
    Be alert for: Premature closing of both anterior and posterior sutures and overriding of sutures may indicate craniosynostosis and requires further assessment.

2. **Eyes.** Inspect eyes and lids. Eyes should be clear, without drainage, and no swelling of eyelids. Subconjunctival hemorrhage may be present.
    Common variations: swelling of eyelid (birth trauma, reaction to eye prophylaxis).
    Be alert for: Purulent drainage is an indication for further assessment and treatment.

3. **Ears.** Inspect outer ear. A full-term baby has incurving of the top two-thirds of the pinna. The top of the ear should be above an imaginary line drawn from the inner canthus

to the outer canthus of the eye and extended around toward the ear. Rotation of the ear should be in the midline, and not tipped forward or backward.

Be alert for: Low-set ears may be associated with a variety of congenital problems.

4. **Nose.** Inspect. Nares should be clear and without mucus. (Remember, newborn is an obligatory nose breather, so a stuffy nose has much greater implications for a newborn baby.)

Common variations: none.

Be alert for: Assess for presence of nasal flaring. If present, assess respiratory rate, retractions and grunting, and skin color. A pulse-oximeter determination may provide further information (reading should be above 90%).

5. **Mouth.** Inspect inside of mouth and palpate hard palate. Hard and soft palate should be intact (may visualize while the baby is crying or may palpate with a gloved finger). (An opening indicates cleft palate.) Inspect gums for supernumerary teeth (these teeth usually will not cause a problem, but may loosen and fall out unexpectedly).

Common variations: supernumerary teeth and Epstein's pearls.

Be alert for: An opening in the palate (cleft palate) needs to be evaluated quickly. Presence of white patches on the mucus membranes that appear as milk deposits but cannot be wiped away with a 4 × 4 may indicate thrush (*Candida*). Excessive mucus may be associated with atresia.

6. **Chest.** Inspect. Chest should be symmetric. Breasts may be flat or slightly enlarged due to the effects of maternal estrogen (this may last about one week). Count respiratory rate over one minute (uncover baby and look at movement of chest or abdomen).

Common variations: Supernumerary nipple.

Be alert for: If retractions (intercostal or sternal) are present, assess respiratory rate and determine baby's need for oxygen.

7. **Heart.** Auscultate. Apical pulse ranges from 120 to 160 bpm. May be as low as 100 with sleep. Palpate brachial, radial, femoral, and pedal pulses.

Common variations: A transitory murmur may be heard for the first few hours of life.

Be alert for: Bradycardia (< 100 bpm) or tachycardia (> 160 bpm) need further evaluation.

8. **Abdomen.** Inspect, auscultate, palpate. Abdomen should be flat (without distention) and bowel sounds should be heard in all quadrants. Umbilical stump should be drying and have no redness, discharge, or bleeding.
   Common variations: none.
   Be alert for: Bleeding and/or purulent drainage from cord require further assessment and treatment.

9. **Genitalia.** Inspect. Genitalia should be clearly differentiated. Both testes should be palpable in scrotum.
   Common variations: pseudomenstruation (small amount vaginal bleeding) in female infants due to maternal estrogen exposure. Clear mucus from the vagina, vaginal skin tag.
   Be alert for: Urinary meatus on the underside of the penis (hypospadias).

10. **Back.** Inspect. Back should be smooth with no tufts of hair present over the lower back.
    Common variations: mongolian spot over lower back.

11. **Hips.** Inspect and perform Ortolani maneuver to detect subluxation or congenital dislocation of hips. Legs should be of equal length, skin folds on both right and left posterior thighs should be symmetrical (see Figure 5–10). To do Ortolani maneuver, place newborn on her/his back. Place the palm of your right hand on the newborn's left knee and extend your index and middle finger toward the hip. Your fingertips should be on the top of the greater trochanter. Place your left hand in the same manner. Put downward pressure on the knees and rotate the knees outward. Feel for a "click" under your fingertips. If a click is felt, notify baby's care provider. The baby will most likely be triple diapered to keep the hip abducted.

12. **Extremities.** Inspect. All extremities should be symmetrical and move equally. Count digits on hands and feet; inspect palmar creases. Note any webbing (syndactyly).
    Common variations: none.
    Be alert for: Asymmetrical movement or no movement of an extremity needs to be reported and assessed further.

13. **Skin color.** Inspect. Skin color appropriate for ethnic grouping. Any evidence of acrocyanosis usually should have abated. Observe closely for signs of jaundice. Jaundice is first detectable on the face, the mucous membranes of the mouth, and the sclera. It is evaluated by blanching the tip of the nose or the forehead. If jaundice is present,

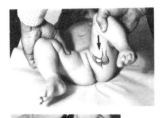

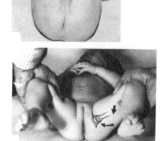

Figure 5–10 Congenital dislocation of the right hip. A, *Ortolani's maneuver puts downward pressure on the hip and then inward rotation. If the hip is dislocated, this will force the femoral head over the acetabular rim with a noticeable "clunk."* B, *Dislocated right hip in a young infant as seen on gross inspection. (From Smith DW:* Recognizable Patterns of Human Deformation. *Philadelphia: Saunders, 1981.)*

the area will appear yellowish immediately after blanching. Laboratory testing will verify the total bilirubin level.
Common variations: Milia may be present over the nose. A variety of markings may be present on the skin (see Table 5–4).
Be alert for: Cyanosis requires immediate reassessment and treatment. Jaundice requires additional assessment, evaluation, and then treatment as needed. Pallor may be associated with anemia, and ruddiness may indicate an elevated hematocrit (> 65%).

Newborns with levels above 10–11 mg/dL may be placed under phototherapy. A newborn under phototherapy needs to be blindfolded (to protect eyes from the lights), undressed (to allow ultraviolet light to shine on skin), rotated every 30–60 minutes (for even exposure), fed adequate amounts of breast milk and/or water (to stimulate intestinal movement of absorbed bilirubin), and soothed frequently (being undressed and unwrapped can make the baby feel uncomfortable).

14. **Elimination.** Note newborn record. Newborn should

Table 5–4   Birthmarks

Type	Characteristics	Parent Teaching
Telangiectatic nevi (stork bites)	Pale pink or red flat dilated capillaries over eyelids, nose, and nape of neck	Seen more with crying Blanch easily, fade during infancy, gone by 2 years of age
Mongolian spots	Bluish-black macular areas over dorsal area and buttocks	Common in dark-skinned races Gradually fade in 1st–2nd year of life
Nevus flammeus (Port-wine stain)	Nonelevated, sharply outlined, red-purple dense area of capillaries, primarily on face In black infants appears jet black	Doesn't fade with time nor blanch as a rule. Can cover with opaque cosmetic cream. Suggestive of Sturge-Weber syndrome (involving 5th cranial nerve)

void and stool within 24 hours after birth. After that, most babies have six to eight wet diapers a day and may stool at least once a day. Breast-fed babies tend to have more frequent stools.

Common variations: none.

Be alert for: If baby does not void within 24 hours, assess amount of fluid taken in, assess urethral opening. If no stool, assess abdomen for distention and bowel sounds. In some areas, a rectal thermometer coated with a lubricant is inserted (about ½ inch) into the rectum in order to stimulate the stool. Check on agency policy before attempting. Diarrhea stools can be very serious for the newborn. Observe stool characteristics closely, and test the stool for occult blood (Hematest) and sugar loss (Clinitest or other glucose testing).

15. **Behavioral.** Observe. Baby quiets to soothing, cuddling, or wrapping. Moves through all sleep-awake states.

    Common variations: none.

    Be alert for: Excessive crying, fretfulness, and inability to quiet self may be associated with drug withdrawal in the neonate.

Tip: Completing the assessment in the mother's room provides a wonderful opportunity for teaching, sharing, and role modeling for first-time mothers.

Assessment of Reflexes

At some point during the time you spend with this newborn, assess normal newborn reflexes.

1. **Moro.** Elicited by startling the newborn with a loud noise, or sudden movement. Newborn straightens arms and hands out while flexing knees. The arms then return to the chest as in an embrace. The fingers spread, forming a C, and the infant may cry.
2. **Grasp.** Elicited by stimulating the newborn's palm with a finger or object. The newborn will grasp and hold the object or finger firmly enough to be lifted momentarily from the crib.
3. **Rooting.** Elicited when the side of the newborn's mouth or cheek is touched. In response, the newborn turns toward that side and opens the lips to suck.

Documenting Assessment Findings and Care

Assessment findings may be recorded on computer charting systems, neonatal flow sheets, or in narrative notes. A narrative note might be recorded as follows:

Anterior fontanelle soft and flat, posterior fontanelle palpated closed at this time, some molding present with overriding of sagittal suture, caput succedaneum over posterior aspect of head. Eyes clear and without discharge or swelling. Nares clear without flaring or discharge. Mouth clear, and palate palpated intact. Chest movements symmetrical without retractions, apical pulse 134, regular, and no murmurs auscultated. Abdomen soft and nondistended. Baby has had a meconium and transitional stool, bowel sounds × 4. Umbilical stump drying and is without redness or discharge. Alcohol applied. No redness or discharge noted on genitalia. Perineal area cleansed and A and D ointment applied. Back clear. Moves all extremities equally. No hip click. Palmar creases normal. Skin color appropriate to ethnic group and without cyanosis. Soothes with cuddling and rocking. M. Chin, RNC

Additional Aspects of Daily Care

1. **Suctioning.** Achieved by compressing the bulb syringe, in-serting it into the side of the mouth, and then releasing the bulb. The bulb should be withdrawn, the contents expelled onto a paper towel or cloth. The bulb is then recompressed and placed back into the mouth if needed. It is best to have the bulb available at all times for the newborn. It is impor-tant to teach the parents the use of the bulb at their first contact with the baby. Some parents are frightened of the bulb, and it helps for them to actually hold it and compress it. When choking occurs, the baby may be picked up, held with her/his head slightly down and the mouth to the side to facilitate the drainage of mucus. It can be frightening to deal with a choking baby.

2. **Positioning.** Place the baby on his/her right side follow-ing feedings with a rolled blanket at the back to hold him/her in this position. The baby can be placed on the tummy after the cord (and circumcision if done) heals. A newborn should never be placed on her/his back because of the risk of choking.

3. **Wrapping.** The newborn seems to be comforted by being wrapped snugly in blankets (see Figure 5–11).

4. **Holding.** To pick up the newborn, take hold of the feet with one hand, and slide the other hand up under the baby until you reach the back of the shoulders and neck. The baby can now be picked up and placed up over your shoul-der, or cradled in the crook of your arm. (Sometimes it is easier to place the baby against your shoulder first, get settled, and then change the baby to the crook of your arm. If you are right handed, you will tend to be most comfort-able cradling the baby in your left arm. Remember to teach

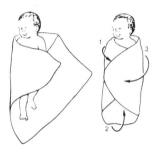

Figure 5–11 Steps used for wrapping a baby.

new parents this technique.) The baby may also be held in a football hold.

5. **Circumcision care.** Some parents choose to have their male newborn circumcised. Prior to the procedure, the parents need to validate that they understand the procedure and sign an informed consent. After the circumcision, the penis needs to be assessed for bleeding. If a Gomco clamp is used, A and D ointment is applied at each diaper change to provide protection to the skin and keep the penis from sticking to the diaper. If a Plastibell is used, the remaining plastic ring protects the penis. Other than cleansing by letting warm water softly rinse over the penis to clear away urine, no other care is required. The Plastibell usually falls off by itself in about three to four days. If it is still in place in seven days, the parents need to contact their care provider.

   Comfort measures immediately after the circumcision may include wrapping the baby in soft blankets and rocking, walking with the baby, using a pacifier, feeding after initial crying has abated, singing, gently rubbing the back, talking to the baby, and using therapeutic touch (use short, light, feathery strokes for a short period of time).

6. **Testing for phenylketonuria (PKU).** Prior to the newborn's discharge, blood needs to be obtained by heel stick for PKU testing. A second test will be done in 7–14 days and it is important to stress the need for the second test with the parents. It is usually done on an outpatient basis.

Parent Education

Provide information as needed on the following topics:

1. **Axillary temperature.** To use a glass thermometer, you must first shake the mercury down below the numbers, and then place the thermometer in the baby's right or left axilla. The thermometer needs to have contact with skin on all sides (see Figure 5–12). Hold the thermometer in place for three minutes. It is important to keep your hand on the thermometer at all times to assure correct placement and prevent an accident. After reading the temperature, cleanse the thermometer by rinsing in cool water and wiping with a soft towel. Review normal range of temperature (axillary: 97.8 to 99° F). **Teaching Tip:** Make a thermometer out of poster board. The mercury can be simulated with alumi-

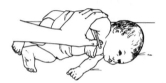

Figure 5–12   The axillary temperature should be taken for three minutes. The newborn's arm should be tightly but gently pressed against the thermometer and the newborn's side as illustrated.

num foil. Or, warm a thermometer between your fingers (if this is the first time you have taught the class it probably won't work because your fingers will be very cold!). You may find it helpful to tell the parents what the temperature is before passing the thermometer around, as many parents may feel uncomfortable telling you they cannot read a thermometer. Tell parents to let you know at the end of class if they would like any assistance or a review.

2. **Bathing the newborn.** Collect supplies (see Table 5–5). For the first few baths, schedule uninterrupted time if at all possible. Wash baby's face using a washcloth that has been moistened in warm water but does not contain soap. The eyes are done first (while the washcloth is the most clean). Using a corner of the washcloth around your finger, wipe the right eye from the inner canthus to the outer canthus, in one stroke. If another swipe is needed, use another corner of the washcloth. The left eye is washed in the same manner. Then the face is washed, as well as under the chin, and then dried. You may choose to wash the baby's hair at this point or at the end of the bath. (Those most interested in organization and saving steps would say to shampoo the hair now; others would say it needs to be done at the end of the bath to better maintain the newborn's temperature.) The chest and abdomen are then washed, rinsed, and dried. You can either use your hands or a washcloth. Umbilical care is completed by cleansing around the umbilical stump with a cotton ball that has a small amount of alcohol applied. Be sure that alcohol does not run from the cotton ball (that is too wet). The diaper is removed. If bathing a male baby, be sure to keep a diaper or rag at hand in case of another voiding (since a male infant is able to spray the urine on you). Carefully and gently clean from the area of the symphysis (pubic bone) down toward the anus. Use a separate portion of the washcloth for each motion. The baby's back and buttocks may be washed, rinsed, and dried. If the hair has not yet been washed, carefully wrap the baby in a dry blanket. Use a football hold to allow you to support the baby safely, and yet have one hand free for the sham-

---

Table 5–5 Bath Time Supplies

A plastic tub	Vitamin A and D ointment (for dry skin)
Two bath towels or baby blankets	70% isopropyl alcohol
Two washcloths	Cotton balls or Q-tips™ for alcohol application
Mild soap (unperfumed is best because it is not as drying to the baby's skin)	

---

poo. Wet the baby's hair and apply a mild shampoo. Suds, rinse thoroughly, and dry. You may want to make a hood over the baby's wet hair until the baby is completely dressed and rewarmed from the bath. Brushing the baby's hair provides stimulation to the scalp and also removes dead skin cells and prevents cradle cap.

3. **Nails.** The nails may be trimmed with special baby-sized cuticle/nail scissors. Clippers may not provide sufficient visibility.

4. **Diapering with reusable cloth diapers.** Many diaper-folding methods are available, as well as diaper wraps that allow the diaper to be placed inside a Velcro™-fastened wrapper (see Figure 5–13).

5. **Diapering with single-use paper diapers.** The baby is placed on the diaper, the front is pulled up toward the navel, and the sides are brought forward and attached by a sticky tab to the front of the diaper. Care needs to be followed to fold the diaper below the level of the umbilicus for the first seven to ten days. In addition, soiled diapers should not be left in open waste containers.

6. **Highlights of parent teaching for newborn care.**

Cord care	Complete cord care two to four times/day. Cord falls off in seven to ten days.
Perineal care	Wash and dry diaper area with each diaper change.
Circumcision care	If Gomco clamp was used, apply A and D ointment with each diaper change. If Plastibell was used, do NOT apply ointment. Plastibell falls off in three to four days. Contact care provider if it has not fallen off in seven days. Cleanse penis

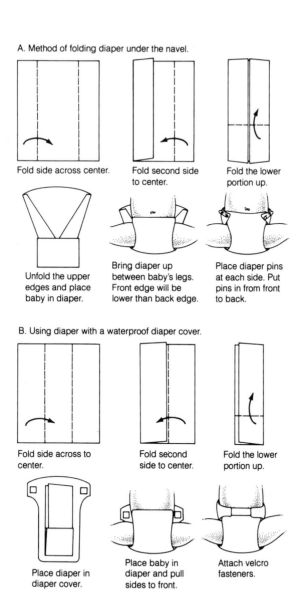

A. Method of folding diaper under the navel.

Fold side across center.

Fold second side to center.

Fold the lower portion up.

Unfold the upper edges and place baby in diaper.

Bring diaper up between baby's legs. Front edge will be lower than back edge.

Place diaper pins at each side. Put pins in from front to back.

B. Using diaper with a waterproof diaper cover.

Fold side across to center.

Fold second side to center.

Fold the lower portion up.

Place diaper in diaper cover.

Place baby in diaper and pull sides to front.

Attach velcro fasteners.

Figure 5-13   Two methods of using cloth diapers.

by letting warm water rinse over penis after each voiding. Do NOT attempt to remove whitish area on skin.

Bath   Give sponge baths until cord has fallen off and area healed (about 10–14 days). Then tub bath may be given.
Bathe every other day (or every third day) in dry climates. Those in warm, humid climates may bathe baby every day.

Axillary temperature   Shake mercury down below numbers. Leave in place at least three minutes, positioned so skin contacts the thermometer on all sides. Normal findings are 97.8° F to 99° F.

When to call   Water-loss stools (small amount of stool surrounded by a ring of water in the diaper)
Axillary temperature of > 101° F or < 97.6° F
Any color change involving pallor or cyanosis
Refusing two feedings in a row
Vomiting, especially projectile
Failure to have at least six wet diapers each day
Crying that persists for two to three hours and the baby cannot be soothed
Lethargy or listlessness

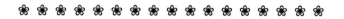

CHAPTER 6

The At-risk Newborn

HYPOGLYCEMIA

Overview

Hypoglycemia is a condition of abnormally low levels of serum glucose. It can be defined as a blood glucose level below 30 mg/dL in first 72 hours after birth or below 40 mg/dL after the first three days of life. In clinical practice, any infant with a blood glucose level less than 45 mg/dL requires intervention. Hypoglycemia can be asymptomatic or symptomatic. Presentation of symptoms and blood glucose levels vary greatly with each baby. Symptoms usually occur at < 45 mg/dL and appear between 24 and 72 hours after birth or within 6 hours after birth in severely stressed infants. A glucose level of 45 mg/dL or more by 72 hours of age is the goal regardless of weight, gestational age, or other predisposing factors. Clinical manifestations vary greatly but can include tremors or jittery movements, irritability, lethargy or hypotonia, irregular respirations, apnea, cyanosis, refusal to suck, high-pitched or weak cry, hypothermia, diaphoresis, or neonatal seizure activity. When left untreated, hypoglycemia can cause cerebral damage and mental retardation.

Medical Management

Drug therapy. Initially, 5% to 10% glucose is given with a follow-up blood glucose test. If baby can't take oral glucose, a 10% glucose intravenous infusion is ordered at a rate that gives 6–8 mg/kg/min of glucose (@90–100 mL/kg/day). For symptomatic acute hypoglycemia a bolus dose of D10W IV at rate of 1–2 mL/kg is given followed by 10% glucose infusion. Alternative treatment may be: hydrocortisone 5 mg/kg p.o. q12hrs after 6–12 hours of glucose treatment, or glucagon 0.3 mg/kg IM only as an emergency treatment. Insulin infusion drip may be preferred to glucagon administration.

Critical Nursing Assessments

1. Assess newborn and record for any risk factors.
   Be alert for: Special gestational newborns, such as premature, small for gestational age (SGA), and infant of diabetic mother (IDM) infants, and newborns with problems of asphyxia, cold stress, sepsis, or polycythemia are particularly at risk.
2. Assess dextrostix or blood glucose chemstrip on all newborns within one to two hours of birth (see Procedure 11: Glucose Chemstrip Test Using Accu-Check II Machine). For some babies a different protocol may be followed: LGA newborn—qhr X 8, then as needed; preterm appropriate for gestational age (AGA)—q4hrs for first 24 hrs, then as needed; SGA—q4hrs for first 24 hrs, then q8hrs for next 72 hrs; any symptomatic infant qhr until stable.
3. Assess all newborns for symptoms of hypoglycemia.

Sample Nursing Diagnoses

- Pain related to multiple heel sticks for glucose monitoring
- Alterations in nutrition: less than body requirements related to increased glucose use secondary to physiologic stresses
- Ineffective family coping related to fear over infant's condition

Critical Nursing Interventions

1. Based on agency glucose testing protocol, provide early feedings of breastmilk or 5% glucose for infants at risk for hypoglycemia.
2. Obtain chemstrip blood glucose per agency protocol. If < 45 mg/dL, obtain STAT blood glucose per venous stick by lab. Then provide oral glucose water (about 1 oz) to infant. Recheck chemstrip in one hour.
   Note: If initial chemstrip is < 20 mg/dL, obtain STAT blood glucose and prepare to start IV glucose therapy.

3. Monitor all babies for signs and symptoms of hypoglycemia.

4. Monitor infants with low chemstrips who have been given oral glucose water for rebound hypoglycemia in approximately three to four hours.

5. If IV therapy is ordered by the physician or indicated by your agency protocol:

   a. Start 10% dextrose and water IV on infusion pump on infants at risk for hypoglycemia or give bolus for symptomatic infants then continue glucose infusion as ordered.

   b. Administer infusion in peripheral vein of upper extremity to avoid lower extremity varicosities and potential tissue necrosis if IV infiltrates.

   c. Obtain glucose levels using chemstrip or dextrostix hourly during therapy until condition stabilizes. Obtain blood glucose levels q4–8hrs minimum.

6. Provide comfort measures to insure rest, and maintain the optimal thermal environment specific for each newborn to reduce activity and glucose consumption.

7. Assist parents to identify feelings and concerns about baby's condition. Encourage and provide maximal contact between parents and their baby.

8. Review the following critical aspects of the care you have provided:

   • Did I identify the baby's risk for hypoglycemia early in its care?

   • Have I been alert for the early signs of hypoglycemia?

   • Have I monitored the blood glucose levels carefully and instituted care per agency protocol promptly?

Sample Nurse's Charting

6:25 AM T 97.7° F, P 150, R 35 & periodic. Ant. fontanel soft & flat. Breath sounds equal bilaterally, slight substernal retractions. Abdomen soft and nondistended. Hypoactive bowel sounds. Fine tremors of arms and hands. Chemstrip 38 mg/dL. Poor suck, took 25 mL of G/W with difficulty. Lab blood glucose pending. Dr. Rich notified of glucose level. M. Chin, RN.

Evaluation

- Newborn's glucose level is stable at > 45 mg/dL, and the baby is symptom free.
- Newborn is free from further complications.

COLD STRESS

Overview

Cold stress occurs when babies are placed in less than their neutral thermal environment. When babies become chilled, they increase their oxygen consumption and use of glucose for physiologic processes. The complications that occur because of this alteration in metabolic processes are respiratory distress, respiratory and metabolic acidosis, hypoglycemia, and jaundice. Premature, SGA, hypoxic, hypoglycemic, and central nervous system (CNS) depressed newborns are at higher risk to become hypothermic and suffer the consequences.

Medical Management

Initially, medical management is directed to prevention and then to the management required by the specific complication.

Critical Nursing Assessments

1. Assess newborn temperature, using either axillary or skin probe method.
   Be alert for: A drop in skin temperature (it drops before core temperature), which may be an early indicator of cold stress. **Tip:** Axillary temperature can be misleading because of the nearness to brown fat, which can increase heat production.
2. Assess for signs of hypothermia: Shallow, irregular respirations, retractions, diminished reflexes, bradycardia, oliguria, lethargy, and temperature < 97.8° F.
3. Assess for complications such as hyperbilirubinemia, hypoglycemia (blood glucose < 45 mg/dL), and respiratory distress.

Sample Nursing Diagnoses

- Hypothermia related to exposure to cold environment, trauma, illness, or inability to shiver
- Ineffective thermoregulation related to immaturity
- Knowledge deficit related to maintenance of neutral thermal environment

Critical Nursing Interventions

1. Institute measures to prevent heat loss due to radiation, evaporation, convection, and conduction. Measures include: Dry off baby immediately and remove wet linen after birth; place baby on prewarmed bed under radiant heat source for all care and procedures, cover scales before weighing, warm stethoscope bell prior to auscultation; keep beds away from drafts and air vents, use warmed humidified oxygen, keep baby wrapped when not skin to skin or under radiant heat source with temperature probe in place; turn up thermostat in birthing area prior to birth; do not place warmer bed near windows or outside walls.

2. If chilled: Rewarm slowly to prevent apnea (see Procedure 20: Temperature Stabilization of the Newborn).

3. Monitor blood glucose levels and arterial blood gases for signs of respiratory distress.

4. Carry out care needed by newborns placed under phototherapy (see Nursing Care Plan 11: Newborn with Jaundice).

5. Instruct parents about causes of temperature fluctuation, infant's current status, heat conservation methods, and temperature stabilization methods.

6. Review the following critical aspects of the care you have provided:

   - Have I provided for sufficient warmth during all procedures and care activities? During baths? During IV starts or blood work?
   - Have I been alert for any signs of hypoglycemia, hyperbilirubinemia, or respiratory distress?

Evaluation

- Baby is maintained in a neutral thermal environment.
- Parents understand the importance of preventing heat loss and methods to prevent complications of hypothermia.

SPECIAL NEWBORNS AND THEIR ASSOCIATED CLINICAL PROBLEMS

Classification	Physical Characteristics	Clinical Problems
Small for gestational age (SGA)	Large-appearing head in proportion to chest and abdomen	1. **Perinatal asphyxia.** Chronic hypoxia in utero, which leaves little reserve to withstand the demands of labor and birth. Thus, intrauterine asphyxia occurs with its potential systemic problems.
	Loose dry skin	
	Scarcity of subcutaneous fat, with emaciated appearance	
	Long, thin appearance	
	Sunken abdomen	2. **Aspiration syndromes.** Gasping secondary to in utero hypoxia can cause aspiration of amniotic fluid into the lower airways, or can lead to relaxation of the anal sphincter with passage of meconium. This results in meconium aspiration with first breaths after birth.
	Sparse scalp hair	
	Anterior fontanelle may be depressed	
	May have vigorous cry and appears alert	
	Birth weight below tenth percentile	
		3. **Heat loss.** Decreased ability to conserve heat results from diminished subcutaneous fat (used for survival in utero), depletion of brown fat in utero, and large surface area. The surface area is diminished somewhat be-

Classification	Physical Characteristics	Clinical Problems
Small for gestational age (SGA) (*continued*)		cause of the flexed position assumed by the SGA infant. (See "Cold Stress" in this chapter for management.) 4. **Hypoglycemia.** High metabolic rate (secondary to heat loss), poor liver glycogen stores, and inhibited gluconeogenesis lead to low blood sugar levels. (See "Hypoglycemia" in this chapter for management.) 5. **Hypocalcemia.** Calcium depletion secondary to birth asphyxia. 6. **Polycythemia.** A physiologic response to in utero chronic hypoxic stress. (See this chapter for management.) 7. See Nursing Care Plan 17: Small-for-Gestational-Age Newborn.
Large for gestational age (LGA), especially infant of diabetic mother (IDM)	Appears fat and enlarged If IDM, Cushingnoid facial (round face) and neck features Overall ruddiness Has enlarged liver, spleen, and heart	1. **Hypoglycemia.** After birth the most common problem of an IDM is hypoglycemia. Even though the high maternal blood supply is lost, this

Classification	Physical Characteristics	Clinical Problems
Large for gestational age (LGA) (*continued*)	Initially lethargic then irritable and jittery	newborn continues to produce high levels of insulin, which deplete the blood glucose within hours after birth. IDMs also have less ability to release glucagon and catecholamines, which normally stimulate glucagon breakdown and glucose release. (See "Hypoglycemia" in this chapter for management.)

2. **Hypocalcemia.** Associated with prematurity and hyperphosphatemia or asphyxia.

3. **Hyperbilirubinemia.** This condition may be seen at 48 to 72 hours after birth. It may be caused by slightly decreased extracellular fluid volume, which increases the hematocrit level. Enclosed hemorrhages resulting from complicated vaginal birth may also cause hyperbilirubinemia. There may also be an increase in rate of bilirubin pro-

Classification	Physical Characteristics	Clinical Problems
Large for gestational age (LGA) (*continued*)		duction in the presence of polycythemia. (See Nursing Care Plan 11: Newborn with Jaundice.)
		4. **Polycythemia.** This condition may be caused by the decreased extracellular volume in IDMs. Current research centers on the fact that hemoglobin A_{1c} binds oxygen, which decreases the oxygen available to the fetal tissues. This tissue hypoxia stimulates increased erythropoietin production, which increases the hematocrit level. (See "Polycythemia" in this chapter for management.)
		5. **Birth injuries** such as fractures of the clavicle, facial nerve paralysis, Erb's paralysis, and diaphragmatic paralysis.
		6. **Cephalhematoma**
		7. **Respiratory distress.** This complication occurs especially in newborns of White's classes A–C dia-

Classification	Physical Characteristics	Clinical Problems
Large for gestational age (LGA) (*continued*)		betic mothers. Increasing evidence suggests that IDMs may have normal levels of the phospholipids that make up surfactant, which leads others to theorize that the composition of the lipids themselves is altered in the lungs of IDMs. (See Nursing Care Plan 12: Newborn with Respiratory Distress Syndrome.)
Preterm infant	Color—usually pink or ruddy but may be acrocyanotic; observe for cyanosis, jaundice, pallor, or plethora Skin—reddened, translucent, blood vessels readily apparent, lack of subcutaneous fat Lanugo—plentiful, widely distributed Head size—appears large in relation to body Skull—bones pliable, fontanelle smooth and flat Ears—minimal cartilage, pliable, folded over Nails—soft, short	1. **Apnea.** Cessation of breathing for more than 20 seconds. It is thought to be primarily a result of neuronal immaturity, a factor that contributes to the tendency for irregular breathing patterns in preterm infants. When cyanosis and bradycardia (heart rate less than 100 beats/min) are also present, these periods are called apneic episodes or spells. 2. **Patent ductus arteriosus.** Failure of ductus arteriosus to close

Classification	**Physical Characteristics**	**Clinical Problems**
Preterm infant (*continued*)	Genitals—small; testes may not be descended	due to decreased pulmonary arteriole musculature and hypoxemia.
	Resting position—flaccid, froglike	3. **Respiratory distress syndrome (RDS).** Respiratory distress results from inadequate surfactant production. (See Nursing Care Plan 12: Newborn with Respiratory Distress Syndrome.)
	Cry—weak, feeble	
	Reflexes—poor sucking, swallowing, and gag	
	Activity—jerky, generalized movements (seizure activity is abnormal)	4. **Intraventricular hemorrhage.** Up to 35 weeks' gestation the preterm's brain ventricles are lined by the germinal matrix, which is highly susceptible to hypoxic events. The germinal matrix is very vascular, and these blood vessels rupture in the presence of hypoxia.
		5. **Hypocalcemia.** The preterm infant lacks adequate amounts of calcium secondary to early birth and growth needs.
		6. **Hypoglycemia.** The preterm infant's decreased brown fat and

Classification	**Physical Characteristics**	**Clinical Problems**
Preterm infant (*continued*)		glycogen stores and increased metabolic needs predispose this infant to hypoglycemia. (See "Hypoglycemia" and "Cold Stress" in this chapter for management.)

7. **Necrotizing enterocolitis.** This condition occurs when blood flow to the gastrointestinal tract is decreased secondary to shock or prolonged hypoxia.

8. **Anemia.** The preterm infant is at risk for anemia because of the rapid rate of growth required, shorter red blood cell life, excessive blood sampling, decreased iron stores, and deficiency of vitamin E.

9. **Hyperbilirubinemia.** Immature hepatic enzymatic function decreases conjugation of bilirubin, resulting in increased bilirubin levels. (See Nursing Care Plan 11: Newborn with Jaundice.)

Classification	Physical Characteristics	Clinical Problems
Preterm infant (*continued*)		10. **Infection.** The preterm infant is more susceptible to infection than term infants. Most of the neonate's immunity is acquired in the last trimester. Therefore the preterm infant has decreased antibodies available for protection.
Post-term infant	Generally has normal skull, but reduced dimensions of rest of body make skull look inordinately large Dry, cracked skin (desquamating), parchmentlike at birth Nails of hard consistency extending beyond fingertips Profuse scalp hair Subcutaneous fat layers depleted, leaving skin loose and giving an "old person" appearance Long and thin body contour Absent vernix Often meconium staining (golden yellow to green) of skin, nails, and cord May have an alert, wide-eyed appear-	1. **Hypoglycemia** Nutritional deprivation and resultant depleted glycogen stores. (See "Hypoglycemia" in this chapter for management.) 2. **Meconium aspiration** Response to hypoxia in utero. 3. **Polycythemia** due to increased production of red blood cells (RBCs) in response to hypoxia. (See "Polycythemia" in this chapter for management.) 4. **Congenital anomalies of unknown cause.** 5. **Seizure** activity Because of hypoxic insult.

Classification	Physical Characteristics	Clinical Problems
Post-term infant (*continued*)	ance symptomatic of chronic intrauterine hypoxia	6. **Cold stress** Because of loss or poor development of subcutaneous fat. (See earlier discussion of cold stress management.)

HEMATOLOGICAL PROBLEMS OF THE NEWBORN

Type	Characteristics	Critical Nursing Management
Anemia Term (Hb < 13 gm/dL) Preterm (Hb < 11 gm/dL)	Pale, > 5% to 10% expected weight loss in first few days of life, slow weight gain in first months of life. Tachycardia may be present. Profound tachycardia (HR > 160) seen in hemorrhage.	**Preventive:** Term baby: Provide iron-fortified formula (2 mg/kg/day). Preterm baby: Give 25 IU of vitamin E p.o. daily with feedings until baby is two to three months of age. After two months of age switch to iron supplementation in formula. **Symptomatic newborn:** (Needs increased oxygen as do growing premature infants.) Administer packed RBCs transfusion: • Warm blood. • Give ordered amount over > 30 min. • Monitor for hypocalcemia and hypoglycemia.

Type	Characteristics	Critical Nursing Management
Anemia (*continued*)		• Don't exceed 10 mL/kg (of weight) volume per transfusion. • Recheck Hct/Hb per agency protocol.
Polycythemia Venous Hct > 65% and increased viscosity leads to impaired blood flow through blood vessels and decreased oxygen transport. LGA, IDM, SGA, and infants of pregnancy-induced hypertension (PIH) mothers are at risk.	Plethoric but cyanotic when crying. Tachypnea, tachycardia, possible murmur, congenital heart failure (CHF), respiratory distress. Feeding intolerance and necrotizing enterocolitis (NEC). Hypoglycemia, lethargy, tremors, hypotonia, poor reflexes, and possible seizures secondary to decreased cerebral perfusion. Jaundice secondary to increased RBC breakdown. Microthrombi may occur in renal and cerebral artery.	Monitor pulse, respirations. Keep urine specific gravity < 1.015. Assess color at rest and when crying. Obtain capillary blood sample for Hct (warm heel prior to heel stick; this increases blood flow and mirrors central Hct). If heel stick Hct is > 65%, obtain central Hct to verify polycythemia. **If Hct > 65% but baby is asymptomatic:** Increase fluid intake by 20–40 mL/kg/day. Recheck heel stick Hct q6hrs. **If Hct > 65% and baby is symptomatic:** Assist with partial exchange transfusion (remove some RBCs and replace with fresh frozen plasma [FFP] or 5% albumin). The goal is to lower Hct to 60% or less. Monitor newborn's response to the procedure: Take VS (**Be**

Type	Characteristics	Critical Nursing Management
Polycythemia (*continued*)		**alert for:** increased P, R, and T), signs of hypoglycemia and NEC. Obtain serial Hcts after exchange as ordered.

JAUNDICE

Overview

Hyperbilirubinemia is an above normal amount of bilirubin in the blood, which, when the level is high enough, produces jaundice. Jaundice can be seen as a visible yellowing of the skin, mucosa, sclera, and urine. Physiologic jaundice is the rise and fall in the serum bilirubin (indirect) level (4 to 12 mg/dL) by the fourth day after birth and peaking by the third to fifth day. Physiologic jaundice is common in term infants and is a result of neonatal hepatic immaturity. Pathologic jaundice is marked by yellow skin discoloration and an increase in the serum bilirubin level above 13 mg/dL within 24 hours after birth. The bilirubin level rises faster than 5 mg/dL in 24 hrs and may continue beyond a week in full-term newborns and two weeks in premature infants. Pathologic jaundice is most commonly associated with blood type or blood group incompatibility, infection, or biliary, hepatic, or metabolic abnormalities.

Medical Management

Phototherapy and exchange transfusions are the primary medical treatments for hyperbilirubinemia (see Procedure 6: Exchange Transfusion: Nursing Responsibilities). Drug therapy (albumin, phenobarbital) may also be used.

Critical Nursing Assessments

1. Assess for risk factors.
   Be alert for: Prenatal history of Rh immunization, ABO incompatability, maternal use of aspirin, sulfonamides, or antimicrobial drugs; American Indian, Japanese, Chinese, or Korean nationality (predisposed to higher bilirubin levels);

yellow amniotic fluid, which indicates significant hemolytic disease.

2. Assess color of skin, sclera, mucous membranes.
   Assessment technique: Observe in the daylight, or, using white fluorescent lights, blanch skin over bony prominence to remove capillary coloration and then assess degree of yellow discoloration. Assess oral mucosa and conjunctival sac in dark-skinned infants.
   Be alert for: In first 24 hours after birth, jaundice mandates immediate investigation. Pallor is associated with hemolytic anemia.

3. Assess laboratory results.
   Be alert for: Serum bilirubin increase of 5 mg/dL/day or more than 0.5 mg/hr, or increase in cord bilirubin to 4 mg/dL indicates severe hemolysis or pathologic process. Increased reticulocytes and decreased Hct and Hb levels are also significant.

4. Assess clinical signs and symptoms.
   Be alert for: Poor feeding, lethargy, tremors, high-pitched cry, absent Moro reflex are often first signs of bilirubin encephalopathy (kernicterus). Vomiting, irritability, rigid musculature, opisthotonos, seizures are later signs of encephalopathy and may indicate permanent damage.

Sample Nursing Diagnoses

* Fluid volume deficit related to decreased intake, loose stools and increased insensible water loss
* Alteration in parenting related to interruption in bonding between infant and parents secondary to separation. (See Nursing Care Plan 11: Newborn with Jaundice.)

Critical Nursing Interventions

While under phototherapy:

1. Place infant under phototherapy lights unclothed, except for genitalia covering, to maximize exposure to lights. Phototherapy reduces bilirubin in the skin.
   Be alert for: If surgical mask is used, remove metal nose strip to prevent burns.

2. Cover infant's eyes when under the lights. Remove eye covers at least every four hours for ten minutes with pho-

totherapy lights off. Change eye patches every 24 hours. Mark patches with time, date, and right and left eye designation (to avoid cross contamination). Inspect eyes and check under the eye dressings for pressure areas.

Be alert for: High density light may cause retinal injury and corneal burns. Irritation from patches may cause corneal abrasions and conjunctivitis.

3. Monitor vital signs every four hours. If hypo/hyperthermia occurs, check temperature every hour.

4. Monitor intake and output every eight hours. Weigh infant daily (provides more accurate determination of fluid intake and insensible water loss caused by phototherapy). Determine urine specific gravities q8hrs. Notify physician if specific gravity > 1.015, an indication of dehydration.
   Be alert for: Urine specific gravity results can be influenced by sugar, protein, blood, and urobiligen in the urine. Urine may be green because of the photodegradation of bilirubin. Stools are usually loose and green in color.

5. Provide fluid intake 25% above normal requirements to meet increase in insensible water losses and losses in the stools. Offer D5W p.o. between breast–feeding or formula intake.

6. Reposition infant at least every four hours. Monitor skin for excoriations, rash, or bronzing of the skin. Change diaper and clean area as soon after stooling to prevent skin breakdown.
   Tip: Ongoing assessment of skin must be done with the phototherapy lights off.

7. Turn phototherapy lights off when parents visit and for feedings. Coordinate care activities with parent visits so parents have maximal contact with their baby with the phototherapy lights off.

8. Monitor phototherapy lights' wave-length using bilimeter every shift.

9. Monitor bilirubin levels every eight hours for first one to two days after discontinuation of phototherapy. Bilirubin levels may rebound following phototherapy.
   If an exchange transfusion is done: See Procedure 6: Exchange Transfusion: Nursing Responsibilities.

Evaluation

See Nursing Care Plan 11: Newborn with Jaundice.

NURSING CARE NEEDS OF NEWBORNS OF SUBSTANCE-ABUSE MOTHERS

Type	Physical Characteristics	Early Neonatal Nursing Interventions
Fetal alcohol syndrome (FAS)	SGA Abnormal features: Microcephaly Craniofacial abnormalities Epicanthal folds Prenatal and postnatal growth defects Congenital heart defects Mental retardation Abnormal palmar creases *Withdrawal symptoms:* hyperactivity, tremors, lethargy, poor suck reflex Can start after birth and usually subside within first 72 hours after onset Potential for seizures	Monitor vital signs. Be alert for: apnea, cyanosis, and hypothermia. Provide heat conservation measures, ie, cap for head, double wrap; for additional management see "Cold Stress" in this chapter. Note feeding problems/patterns (offer small, frequent feedings). Measure abdominal girth. Be alert for abdominal distention. Provide oxygen via nasal cannula or mask and bulb suction as ordered for respiratory distress or aspiration. Place baby in dimly lit environment to prevent overstimulation.
Newborn of drug-dependent mother	SGA or premature Withdrawal symptoms (onset varies from birth to two weeks of age): Nasal stuffiness, sneezing, yawning, increased sucking efforts, hiccups Increased secretions, difficulty feeding,	Assess ability to feed (hyperactivity and increased secretions causes difficulty). Be alert for difficult feeder with poor suck and regurgitation/vomiting. Provide small, frequent feedings. Bulb suction newborn. Position on

Type	Physical Characteristics	Early Neonatal Nursing Interventions
Newborn of drug-dependent mother (*continued*)	drooling, gagging, vomiting, diarrhea	side with head elevated to prevent choking.
	Increased respiratory rate, shrill cry, respiratory distress	Initiate safety precautions to prevent baby self-injury during periods of hyperactivity. Observe for seizures.
	Irritability, tremors, hyperactivity, hypertonia, hyperreflexia, increased Moro reflex, disturbed sleeping pattern	
	Seizures (infrequent, but may occur in severe cases or with intrauterine asphyxia)	Decrease stimulating activities and provide quiet environment during withdrawal period. Provide gentle handling, pacifier, talk in soothing voice, play quiet music, swaddle snugly, and hold as much as baby tolerates. Encourage parent-infant attachment by explaining baby's behavior and giving comfort suggestions.
	Fever, flushing, diaphoresis	
	Dehydration	
		Administer drugs (Phenobarbital, Thorazine, Paregoric, Valium, Codeine) as ordered for relief of withdrawal symptoms. (See Nursing Care Plan 10: Newborn of a Drug-addicted Mother.)

CONGENITAL HEART DISEASE IN THE NEWBORN PERIOD

Overview

Congenital heart disease (CHD) occurs in about 8% of live births. The CHDs seen most often in the first week of life are transposition of the great vessels and hypoplastic left heart syndrome. Within the first month of life, the presenting conditions are coarctation of the aorta, ventricular septal defect, tetralogy of fallot, and patent ductus arteriosus. Initial assessment of the newborn suspected of having CHD includes: complete physical exam, blood pressure in all four extremities, electrocardiogram (ECG), chest x-ray, and evaluation of oxygenation in 100% oxygen. Now many newborns with congenital heart disease are diagnosed by fetal echocardiography and corrective management can be done during the first month of life.

Medical Management

Cardiac defects of the early newborn period include:

Congenital Heart Defect	Clinical Findings	Medical/Surgical Management
Patent ductus arteriosus (PDA): ↑ in females, maternal rubella, RDS, <1500 g preterm newborns, high-altitude births	Harsh grade 2–3 machinery murmur at upper left sternal border (LSB) just beneath clavicle ↑ difference between systolic and diastolic pulse pressure Can lead to right heart failure and pulmonary congestion ↑ left atrial (LA) and left ventricular (LV) enlargement, dilated ascending aorta ↑ pulmonary vascularity	Indomethacin—0.2 mg/kg orally (prostaglandin inhibitor) up to 3 doses Surgical ligation/resection Use of O_2 therapy and blood transfusion to improve tissue oxygenation and perfusion Fluid restriction and diuretics

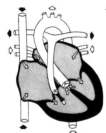

Figure 6–1(A) Patent ductus arteriosus.

Congenital Heart Defect	Clinical Findings	Medical/Surgical Management
Coarctation of aorta Can be preductal or postductal	Absent or diminished femoral pulses Increased brachial pulses Late systolic murmur in left intrascapular area Systolic BP in lower extremities Enlarged left ventricle Can present in CHF at 7–21 days of life	Surgical resection of narrowed portion of aorta Prostaglandin E_1 to maintain ductus open

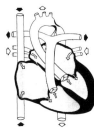

Figure 6–1(B)   Coarctation of the aorta.

Transposition of great vessels (TGA) (↑ females, IDMs, LGAs)	Cyanosis at birth or within three days Possible pulmonic stenosis murmur Right ventricular hypertrophy Polycythemia "Egg on its side" x-ray	Prostaglandin E to vasodilate ductus to keep it open Initial surgery to create opening between right and left side of heart if none exists Total surgical repair—usually the arterial switch

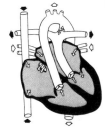

Figure 6–1(C)   Complete transposition of great vessels. (All illustrations from Congenital Heart Abnormalities. *Clinical Education Aid no. 7. Ross Laboratories, Columbus, Ohio.)*

Congenital Heart Defect	Clinical Findings	Medical/Surgical Management
Hypoplastic left heart syndrome	Normal at birth—cyanosis and shocklike congestive heart failure develop within a few hours to days	Currently no effective corrective treatment (total repair)
	Soft systolic murmur just left of the sternum	Palliative use of Prostaglandin E_1
	Diminished pulses	
	Aortic and/or mitral atresia	
	Tiny, thick-walled left ventricle	
	Large, dilated, hypertrophied right ventricle	
	X-ray: Cardiac enlargement and pulmonary venous congestion	

Critical Nursing Assessments

Nursing assessment of the following signs and symptoms assists in identifying the newborn with a cardiac problem.

1. Tachypnea: reflects increased pulmonary blood flow
2. Dyspnea: caused by increased pulmonary venous pressure and blood flow; can also cause chest retractions, wheezing
3. Color: ashen, gray, or cyanotic
4. Difficulty in feeding: requires many rest periods before finishing even 1 or 2 ounces
5. Diaphoresis: beads of perspiration over the upper lip and forehead; may accompany feeding fatigue
6. Stridor or choking spells
7. Failure to gain weight
8. Heart murmur: may not be heard in left-to-right shunting defects since the pulmonary pressure in the newborn is greater than pressure in the left side of the heart in the early newborn period

9. Hepatomegaly: in right-sided heart failure, caused by venous congestion in the liver
10. Tachycardia: pulse over 160, may be as high as 200
11. Cardiac enlargement

Sample Nursing Diagnoses

- Altered tissue perfusion related to decrease in circulating oxygen
- Ineffective breathing pattern related to fatigue
- Altered nutrition: less than body requirements related to increased energy expenditure
- Knowledge deficit of parents related to cardiac anomaly and future implications for care

Critical Nursing Interventions

1. Give small, frequent feedings (oral), or gastric tube feeding to conserve energy (see Procedure 10: Gavage Feeding).
2. Obtain daily weights and strict intake and output.
   Be alert for: Failure to gain weight, inability to take more than an ounce of formula in 30–45 min of feeding, and decrease in urine output. Also note weight gain reflected as body edema.
3. Provide oxygen to relieve respiratory distress and keep oxygen level at 30% to 40%. Oxygen will not remove cyanosis.
4. Administer digoxin per order. Dosage should be double-checked by a second RN. It is given only after listening to the apical pulse for one minute and if no irregularities or slowing are noted. **Tip:** In most agencies, if pulse is lower than 120 bpm, check with physician before giving medication.
5. Diuretics (such as Lasix) are administered; potassium levels should be monitored since diuretics cause excretion of potassium.
6. Morphine sulfate, 0.05 mg/kg of body weight per dose, may be given for irritability. It decreases peripheral and pulmonary resistance, and therefore decreases tachypnea. Place in semi-Fowler's position to ease breathing.
7. Counsel parents on home care: administration of drugs, indications of drug toxicity, and measures used to prevent fatigue and promote nutrition for growth and development.

Evaluation

- Newborn's oxygen consumption and energy expenditure are minimal while at rest and during feedings.
- Newborn is protected from additional stresses such as infection, cold stress, and dehydration.
- Parents verbalize their concerns about their baby's health maintenance and need for ongoing follow-up care.

CONGENITAL ANOMALIES: IDENTIFICATION AND CARE IN NEWBORN PERIOD

Congenital Anomaly	Nursing Assessments	Nursing Goals and Interventions
Congenital hydrocephalus (1 in 1200 live births)	Enlarged head	Assess presence of hydrocephalus: Measure and plot occipital-frontal baseline measurements, then measure head circumference once a day.
	Enlarged or full fontanelles	
	Split or widened sutures	
	"Setting sun" eyes	
	Head circumference >90% on growth chart	Check fontanelle for bulging and sutures for widening.
		Assist with head ultrasound and transillumination.
		Maintain skin integrity: Change position frequently.
		Clean skin creases after feeding or vomiting.
		Use sheepskin pillow under head.
		Postoperatively, position head off operative site.
		Watch for signs of infection.

Congenital Anomaly	Nursing Assessments	Nursing Goals and Interventions
Choanal atresia	Occlusion of posterior nares	Assess patency of nares: Listen for breath sounds while holding baby's mouth closed and alternately compressing each nostril.
	Cyanosis and retractions at rest	
	Snorting respirations	
	Difficulty breathing during feeding	Assist with passing feeding tube to confirm diagnosis.
	Obstruction by thick mucus	
		Maintain respiratory function: Assist with taping airway in mouth to prevent respiratory distress.
		Position with head elevated to improve air exchange.
Cleft lip (1 in 850–1000 live births)	Unilateral or bilateral visible defect	Provide nutrition: Feed with special nipple.
	May involve external nares, nasal cartilage, nasal septum, and alveolar process	Burp frequently (increased tendency to swallow air and reflex vomiting).
	Flattening or depression of midfacial contour	Clean cleft with sterile water (to prevent crusting on cleft prior to repair).
		Support parental coping: Assist parents with grief over loss of idealized baby.
		Encourage verbalization of their feelings about visible defect.
		Provide role model in interacting with infant. (Parents internalize others' responses to their newborn.)

Congenital Anomaly	Nursing Assessments	Nursing Goals and Interventions
Cleft palate (1 in 2500 live births)	Fissure connecting oral and nasal cavity	Prevent aspiration/infection: Place prone or in side-lying position to facilitate drainage.
	May involve uvula and soft palate	Suction nasopharyngeal cavity (to prevent aspiration or airway obstruction).
	May extend forward to nostril, involving hard palate and maxillary alveolar ridge	During neonatal period, feed in upright position with head and chest tilted slightly backward (to aid swallowing and discourage aspiration).
	Difficulty in sucking	
	Expulsion of formula through nose	Provide nutrition: Feed with special nipple that fills cleft and allows sucking. Also decreases chance of aspiration through nasal cavity.
		Clean mouth with water after feedings.
		Burp after each ounce (tend to swallow large amounts of air).
		Thicken formula to provide extra calories.
		Plot weight gain patterns to assess adequacy of diet.
		Provide parental support: Refer parents to community agencies and support groups. Encourage verbalization of frustrations as feeding process is long and frustrating.

Congenital Anomaly	Nursing Assessments	Nursing Goals and Interventions
Cleft palate (*continued*)		Praise all parental efforts.
		Encourage parents to seek prompt treatment for upper respiratory infection (URI) and teach them ways to decrease URI.
Tracheoesopha-geal fistula (type 3) (1 in 3500 live births)	History of maternal hydramnios	Maintain respiratory status and prevent aspiration: Withhold feeding until esophageal patency is determined.
	Excessive mucus secretions	
	Constant drooling	
	Abdominal distention beginning soon after birth	Quickly assess patency before putting to breast in birth area.
	Periodic choking and cyanotic episodes	Place on low intermittent suction to control saliva and mucus (to prevent aspiration pneumonia).
	Immediate regurgitation of feeding	
	Clinical symptoms of aspiration pneumonia (tachypnea, retractions, rhonchi, decreased breath sounds, cyanotic spells)	Place in warmed, humidified Isolette (liquefies secretions, facilitating removal).
		Elevate head of bed 20°–40° (to prevent reflux of gastric juices).
	Failure to pass nasogastric tube	Keep quiet (crying causes air to pass through fistula and to distend intestines, causing respiratory embarrassment).
		Maintain fluid and electrolyte balance: Give fluids to replace esophageal drainage and maintain hydration.

Congenital Anomaly	Nursing Assessments	Nursing Goals and Interventions
Tracheoesophageal fistula (type 3) (*continued*)		Provide parent education: Explain staged repair: provision of gastrostomy and ligation of fistula, then repair of atresia.

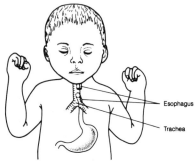

Figure 6–2   The most frequently seen type of congenital tracheoesophageal fistula and esophageal atresia.

Keep parents informed; clarify and reinforce physician's explanations regarding malformation, surgical repair, pre- and postoperative care, and prognosis (knowledge is ego strengthening).

Involve parents in care of infant and in planning for future; facilitate touch and eye contact (to dispel feelings of inadequacy, increase self-esteem and self-worth, and promote incorporation of infant into family).

Congenital Anomaly	Nursing Assessments	Nursing Goals and Interventions
Diaphragmatic hernia (1 in 4000 live births)	Difficulty initiating respirations	Maintain respiratory status: Immediately administer oxygen.
	Gasping respirations with nasal flaring and chest retraction	Initiate gastric decompression.
	Barrel chest and scaphoid abdomen	Place in high semi-Fowler's position (to use gravity to keep abdominal organ's pressure off diaphragm).
	Asymmetrical chest expansion	
	Breath sounds may be absent, usually on left side	Turn to affected side to allow unaffected lung expansion.
	Heart sounds displaced to right	

Congenital Anomaly	Nursing Assessments	Nursing Goals and Interventions
Diaphragmatic hernia (*continued*)	Spasmodic attacks of cyanosis and difficulty in feeding Bowel sounds may be heard in thoracic cavity	Carry out interventions to alleviate respiratory and metabolic acidosis. Assess for increased secretions around suction tube (denotes possible obstruction). Aspirate and irrigate tube with air or sterile water.
Omphalocele (1 in 6000–10,000 live births)	Herniation of abdominal contents into base of umbilical cord May have an enclosed transparent sac covering	Maintain hydration and temperature: Provide D_5LR and albumin for hypovolemia. Place infant in sterile bag up to above defect. Cover sac with moistened sterile gauze and place plastic wrap over dressing (to prevent rupture of sac and infection). Initiate gastric decompression by insertion of nasogastric tube attached to low suction (to prevent distention of lower bowel and impairment of blood flow). Prevent infection and trauma to defect. Position to prevent trauma to defect. Administer broad-spectrum antibiotics.

Congenital Anomaly	Nursing Assessments	Nursing Goals and Interventions
Myelomeningo-cele (0.5 in 1,000 live births)	Saclike cyst containing meninges, spinal cord, and nerve roots in thoracic and/or lumbar area	Prevent trauma and infection.
		Position on abdomen or on side and restrain (to prevent pressure and trauma to sac).
	Myelomeningocele directly connects to subarachnoid space so hydrocephalus often associated	Meticulously clean buttocks and genitals after each voiding and defecation (to prevent contamination of sac and decrease possibility of infection).
	No response or varying response to sensation below level of sac	
	May have constant dribbling of urine	May put protective covering over sac (to prevent rupture and drying).
	Incontinence or retention of stool	
	Anal opening may be flaccid	Observe sac for oozing of fluid or pus.
		Credé bladder as ordered (to prevent urinary stasis).
		Assess amount of sensation and movement below defect.
		Observe for complications: Obtain occipital-frontal circumference baseline measurements, then measure head circumference once a day (to detect hydrocephalus).
		Check fontanelle for bulging.
Congenital dislocated hip (1 in 200 live births)	Asymmetrical gluteal and anterior thigh fold	Maintain abduction position via Pavik harness, Frejka pillow splint, and plastic abduction splint.
	One leg may be shorter	

Congenital Anomaly	Nursing Assessments	Nursing Goals and Interventions
Congenital dislocated hip (*continued*)	Positive Ortolani test (clunk noted with gentle forced abduction of leg and palpable bulge of head of femur)	Provide good perineal care to prevent skin breakdown. Instruct parents on home care of appliance.
Clubfoot (1 in 1000 live births)	Abnormal turning of foot/feet either inward or outward Unable to rotate to normal position	If casted, keep casts dry, protect legs from irritation. Carry out circulatory and neurological checks. Soothe infant during and after castings. Provide parents with cast-care instructions (handling, cleaning, and signs of complications).
Imperforate anus (1 in 5000 live births)	Visible anal membrane Absence of patent anus Inability to take rectal temperature No passage of meconium Abdominal distention	Monitor passage of first stool. Take axillary temperature. Measure abdominal girth (increasing abdominal distention). Prepare parents for possible need for temporary colostomy.

PERINATALLY ACQUIRED NEWBORN INFECTIONS

Infection	Critical Nursing Assessments	Critical Nursing Interventions
Group B Streptococcus 1% to 2% colonized with one in ten developing disease	Assess for risk factors, ie: low apgars Assess for: Severe respiratory distress (grunting and cyanosis)	Closely monitor VS for signs of respiratory distress and infection.

Infection	Critical Nursing Assessments	Critical Nursing Interventions
Group B Strepto-coccus (*continued*) Early onset—usually within hours of birth or within first week Late onset—one week to three months	May become apneic or demonstrate symptoms of shock Meconium-stained amniotic fluid seen at birth	Assist with x-ray—shows aspiration pneumonia or hyaline membrane disease. Immediately obtain blood, gastric aspirate, external ear canal and nasopharynx cultures. Administer antibiotics, usually aqueous penicillin or ampicillin combined with gentamicin as soon as cultures are obtained. Initiate referral to evaluate for blindness, deafness, learning or behavioral problems.
Escherichia coli K1 (ECK1) 2nd most common cause of newborn sepsis/meningitis. Incidence 1% to 2% of live births	Assess for: seven to ten green, watery stools/day Dehydration, electrolyte imbalances, sepsis	Institute infection control measures. Isolate from other babies. Strict handwashing. Weigh at least daily. Maintain hydration by IV/PO. Administer antibiotics per order.
Gonorrhea Onset 7–14 days after birth	Assess for: Ophthalmia neonatorum (conjunctivitis) Purulent discharge and corneal ulcerations	Administer 1% silver nitrate solution or ophthalmic antibiotic ointment (see Drug Guide 5: Erythromycin [Ilotycin] ophthalmic ointment), or 1% tetracycline ointment.

Infection	Critical Nursing Assessments	Critical Nursing Interventions
Gonorrhea (*continued*)	Neonatal sepsis with temperature instability, poor feeding response, and/or hypotonia, jaundice	May give aqueous penicillin G IM as ordered if mother's culture positive. Maintain body substance isolation during procedures, educate parents regarding need for handwashing, etc. Initiate follow-up referral to evaluate any loss of vision.
Chlamydia Trachomatis Appears 5–14 days after birth	Assess for perinatal history of preterm birth Symptomatic newborns present with pneumonia—conjunctivitis (purulent yellow discharge and eyelid swelling) after three to four days Chronic follicular conjunctivitis (corneal neovascularization and conjunctival scarring)	Maintain body substance isolation. Obtain smears for cultures as ordered. Administer erythromycin p.o. and topical 10% sulfonamide drops. Wash eyes with warmed normal saline solution as needed. Initiate follow-up referral for eye complications.
Herpes Type 2	Assess for: Small cluster vesicular skin lesions over all the body Check perinatal history for active herpes genital lesions Disseminated form—DIC, pneumonia, hepatitis with jaundice, hepatosplenomegaly; and neurologic abnormalities.	Carry out careful handwashing and gown and glove isolation with linen precautions. Administer intravenous vidarabine (Vira A) or acyclovir (Zovirax). Initiate follow-up referral to evaluate potential sequelae of microcephaly, spasticity, seizures, deafness, or blindness.

Infection	Critical Nursing Assessments	Critical Nursing Interventions
Herpes Type 2 (*continued*)	Without skin lesions, see fever or subnormal temperature, respiratory congestion, tachypnea, and tachycardia.	Encourage parental rooming-in and touching of their newborn. Show parents appropriate handwashing procedures and precautions to be used at home if mother's lesions are active. Obtain throat, conjunctiva, cerebral spinal fluid (CSF), blood, urine, and lesion cultures to identify herpesvirus type 2 antibodies in serum IgM fraction. Cultures positive in 24–48 hours.
AIDS (placental transmission)	See Nursing Care Plan 9: Infant with AIDS	
Monilial infection (thrush)	Assess buccal mucosa, tongue, gums, and inside the cheeks for white plaques (seen five to seven days of age). Check diaper area for bright red, well-demarcated eruptions. Assess for thrush periodically when newborn is on long-term antibiotic therapy.	Differentiate white plaque areas from milk curds by using cotton tip applicator (if it is thrush, removal of white areas causes raw bleeding areas). Maintain cleanliness of hands, linen, clothing, diapers, and feeding apparatus. Instruct breast-feeding mothers on treating their nipples with nystatin.

Infection	Critical Nursing Assessments	Critical Nursing Interventions
Monilial infection (*continued*)		Administer gentian violet (1% to 2%) swabbed on oral lesions one hour after feeding, or nystatin instilled in baby's oral cavity and on mucosa.
		Swab skin lesions with topical nystatin.
		Discuss with parents that gentian violet stains mouth and clothing.
		Avoid placing gentian violet on normal mucosa; causes irritation.

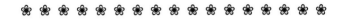

CHAPTER 7

The Postpartum Client

OVERVIEW

The period of time (approximately six weeks) following child-birth, during which the body returns to a prepregnant state, is called the puerperium. Because of current practice some women may be discharged as early as 12 hours following birth, while in most cases women are discharged within one to three days. Nursing care during this time focuses on assessment for developing complications and on client teaching. The nurse should use every opportunity to explain the normal physiologic changes to the woman so that she will be able to recognize deviations and contact her care giver if complications arise.

Table 7–1 identifies the basic assessments that the postpartum nurse should make, explains postpartum physiologic changes, and identifies basic teaching that is indicated.

NURSING INTERVENTIONS FOR POSTPARTUM DISCOMFORT

Perineal Discomfort: Episiotomy and Hemorrhoids

Suggested nursing interventions for the first few hours after birth include:

1. Ice glove or chemical ice bag on the perineal area. If glove is used, wash it first to remove powder, then wrap it in a washcloth or towel. Leave on 20 minutes, then off ten minutes.

Suggested nursing interventions after first few hours:

1. Sitz bath, usually ordered for 20 minutes TID or QID and PRN. It is soothing and cleansing, and its warmth promotes

healing. **Note:** Some research suggests that a cool sitz bath may be more effective in reducing perineal edema. Offer women a choice of temperature.

Procedure: Clean tub. Add water 102–105° F. Place a towel in the bottom and, if it is a standard sitz tub, drape a towel over the edge to cushion the woman's legs. Woman can sit in sitz tub with hospital gown draped over the edge of the tub to provide privacy and prevent chilling. Some tubs have a temperature control lever that permits the water to run with a stable temperature. In such cases leave the water running and open the drain. This creates a whirlpool effect. Warm, moist environment may make woman faint, so check on her frequently and have a call light available.

Disposable sitz tubs fit over a toilet with raised lid. At home the woman can fill a tub with 4 to 6 inches of water at a comfortable (not too hot) temperature. She should not bathe in the sitz tub because of the risk of introducing infection.

2. A perineal heat lamp provides dry heat to increase circulation, dry tissues, and promote healing. Usually used for 20 minutes TID PRN. Perineum should be cleansed first to prevent drying of secretions and to remove any ointments or sprays. Woman lies on the bed with her knees flexed and her legs spread apart. Use a 60-watt bulb and place lamp about 12 inches from perineum. The sheet can be draped over the woman's knees to provide privacy. **Never** place the lamp on the floor between uses.

3. Topical agents such as Dermoplast aerosol spray or Nupercainal ointment may be applied by the woman following a sitz bath. She should **not** use them before a heat lamp treatment because of the danger of tissue burn.

The above treatments are effective for episiotomy and hemorrhoids. In addition, suggested nursing interventions for hemorrhoids include the following:

1. Encourage side-lying position.
2. Teach woman to digitally reinsert hemorrhoids. To do this she should lie on her side, place lubricant on her finger, and apply steady gentle pressure against the hemorrhoids, pushing them inside. She should hold them in place for 1 to 2 minutes then withdraw her finger. The anal sphincter should then hold them in place. She should maintain the side-lying position for a period of time.

Table 7-1 Postpartum Assessment and Teaching

Physiologic Changes	Nursing Assessment	Client Teaching
Vital Signs		
Temperature: normal range; may increase to 100.4° F (38° C) due to exertion and mild dehydration.	Normal: 98–100.4° F (36.2–38° C) After first 24 hours temperature > 100.4° F (38° C) suggests infection.	Advise woman that following discharge, if she experiences chills, malaise, etc, she should take her temperature and report fever to her care giver.
Pulse: Puerperal bradycardia may occur for six to ten days postpartum due to decreased blood volume and cardiac strain, and increased stroke volume.	Pulse: 50–90 beats/min. Tachycardia may result from difficult labor and birth or from hemorrhage. Assess for additional signs of hemorrhage.	Explain that pulse slows normally. Advise woman to report palpitations, rapid pulse.
Respirations: unchanged	Respirations normally 16–24/min. If decreased, evaluate for medication effects; if marked tachypnea present, assess for signs of pneumonia or other respiratory disease.	Advise woman to report symptoms of complications, including difficulty breathing, cough, rapid respirations.
Blood pressure (BP): remains consistent with baseline BP. A slight decrease may indicate normal physiologic readjustment to decreased intrapelvic pressure.	BP elevated: Consider pregnancy-induced hypertension (PIH), especially if accompanied by headache (see Chapter 2). Note proteinuria, edema. BP decreased: Evaluate for additional signs of hemorrhage (rapid pulse, clammy skin).	Explain findings to woman.

Breasts

Immediately after birth, breasts are smooth, soft, and show changes in pigmentation, presence of striae, etc, characteristic of pregnancy.

Anterior pituitary secretion of prolactin promotes milk production by stimulating alveolar cells of breast. Oxytocin, produced by posterior pituitary when infant suckles, promotes milk letdown reflex and flow of milk results. At this time breasts are producing colostrum, which is creamy and high in maternal antibodies. By two to four days after birth, the breast begins producing milk. Breasts tend to become full and hard due to milk production and venous congestion. This is called engorgement.

Assess fit and support provided by bra, which should hold all the breast tissue, and, for breast-feeding women, have cotton straps that don't stretch. Nursing bras have flaps that open for breast-feeding.

Assess size and shape of breasts (one breast often larger than the other). Palpate and note whether breast is soft (initially), somewhat firm (associated with filling), firm (full of milk), or hard (engorgement). Note tenderness, palpable mass, heat, edema (suggest caked breast or mastitis). If present, assess for other signs of infection, including fever, malaise. Assess nipples for fissures, cracks, soreness, inversion.

Discuss importance of wearing a well-fitting bra 24 hours a day until breast milk is suppressed in non-nursing mother, or until breast-feeding mother stops nursing.

Discuss methods for relieving discomfort of engorgement for non-nursing and nursing mothers as indicated. (See "Breast Engorgement in the Non-nursing Mother" in this chapter, and Table 7–2.)

Review signs of infection.

Abdomen

Abdominal wall is stretched; appears loose and flabby for some time. Tone can improve in two to three months with exercise. Diastasis recti abdominis is a separation of the rectus abdominis muscle so that a portion of abdominal wall has no muscular support.

Abdomen feels soft, may have a "doughy" texture.

Palpate rectus abdominis muscle, which should be intact. If a separation is felt, determine its length and width. If difficult to determine, ask woman to elevate her head, which causes tightening of the abdominal muscle.

Discuss exercises that can be done to improve tone. (See discussion on p. 193 and Figure 7–3.)

Continued

Table 7-1 *continued*

Physiologic Changes	Nursing Assessment	Client Teaching
Uterus		
Involution: rapid reduction in size of the uterus and its return to a near prepregnant size following childbirth. Involution is enhanced by an uncomplicated birth, breast-feeding, and early ambulation. Immediately following expulsion of the placenta, uterus is contracted, about the size of a large grapefruit, located midway between symphysis and umbilicus. It gradually rises up to the level of the umbilicus as blood collects and forms clots within the uterus. It stays there for about one day, then decreases in size about one fingerbreadth/day. Within ten days to two weeks it is again a pelvic organ.	See Procedure 9: Fundal Assessment for correct technique. Fundus should be firm and in the midline. Displacement to the side may be caused by a full bladder. A fundus that is not firm is called "boggy." This may be caused by pressure from a full bladder, by the presence of clots, or because of diminished contractility in a woman who has borne several children. Massage fundus gently with the fingertips until firm; if the uterus does not contract more vigorous massage may be necessary; assess bladder for distention and have woman void if necessary; **only attempt to express clots when the uterus is firm; do not attempt to express clots from a boggy uterus.** This could cause uterine inversion. If bogginess remains or returns notify physician or nurse-midwife. Note height of uterus in relation to umbilicus and chart. For example: Uterus firm, in the midline 1 FB U.	Teach mother to evaluate her fundus herself. If it is boggy she can then massage it until it is firm and report this to the nurse. Explain the importance of voiding regularly to avoid pressure on the uterus.
Muscles stay contracted to clamp off blood vessels at placental site to prevent hemorrhage.		
Uterine ligaments are still stretched so uterus is moveable and can be displaced by a full bladder.		
Placental site takes up to six weeks to heal. Healing occurs by exfoliation so		

that no scar is formed, which would limit area available for future placental implantation.

Lochia

After birth the uterus rids itself of the debris that remains by a discharge called lochia. **Lochia rubra,** which lasts for two to three days, is dark red, like menstrual flow. **Lochia serosa** lasts from about the 3rd to 10th day. It is similar to serosanguineous drainage. **Lochia alba,** the final discharge, is a creamy brownish or yellowish discharge. When it stops the cervix is considered closed and risk of ascending infection is decreased. Lochia tends to be heavier in amount on arising (probably due to pooling in the vagina during the night). The amount may also increase with breast-feeding (oxytocin is released with suckling and it stimulates uterine contraction) and with exertion. The type, amount, and consistency of lochia indicate the degree of healing of the placental site. Persistent lochia rubra or a return to rubra from serosa may indicate subinvolution or late postpartal hemorrhage.

Assess lochia for character, amount, odor (should have a slightly musty but not offensive odor. Foul odor suggests infection), and the presence of clots. A few small clots are normal but large clots are abnormal and should be investigated. Flow should never exceed moderate amount, ie, four to eight perineal pads daily. If woman reports heavy bleeding, have woman apply clean pad and reassess in one hour. If she reports passage of clots, ask her to save all pads with clots and not flush toilet if clots are expelled with urination. If accurate assessment of blood loss is necessary, weigh pads after first balancing scale with a clean, dry pad. One gram is considered equivalent to 1 mL blood. Chart amount, followed by character. For example:

Lochia: small amount, rubra, no clots.

Instruct woman that tampons should not be used postpartum because of risk of infection. Perineal pads are generally used with a sanitary belt. (Adhesive-backed pads that are placed inside the panties move more when the woman walks and may bring contamination from the anal area forward to the episiotomy and vaginal opening.) Many young women have never worn a belt and may need assistance the first time. (Some agencies instead use a snug mesh panty that holds the pad in place.) Explain the progression of lochia from rubra to serosa to alba. Instruct the woman to save and report excessive clots, and heavily saturated pads. She should also report failure of lochia to progress from rubra to serosa or a return to rubra from serosa. Teach woman to change pads with each voiding or bowel movement and after showering or use of a sitz bath.

Continued

Table 7-1 *continued*

Physiologic Changes	Nursing Assessment	Client Teaching
Perineum		
Following birth the soft tissue of the perineum may be edematous and bruised. Episiotomy may be present. Woman may also have some hemorrhoids present as a result of pushing during labor.	Perineum should appear intact; slight edema and bruising are normal. Marked fullness, bruising, and pain may indicate hematoma and require further evaluation.	The woman may apply an ice glove or pack initially to prevent edema. Teach woman to use a perineal bottle filled with warm water or a surgigator after each voiding to wash the perineum and promote healing. Teach importance of wiping from the front (urinary meatus) to the back (anal area) to prevent contamination of the episiotomy from the anal area. Teach comfort measures for hemorrhoids.
	Inspect episiotomy. There should be no redness, **e**dema, **e**cchymosis, **d**rainage, and the edges should be well **a**pproximated (the acronym REEDA can help recall these criteria). If present, they may indicate infection.	
	If hemorrhoids are present, they should be small and nontender; full, reddened, inflamed hemorrhoids are painful and require comfort measures (see "Perineal Discomfort: Episiotomy and Hemorrhoids" in this chapter).	

Urinary Tract

Urinary output greatly increases in the early postpartum period due to diuresis. Woman may have difficulty voiding because of decreased bladder sensation, swelling and bruising of tissues around urethra, increased bladder capacity, and difficulty voiding while recumbent.

Assess voiding; woman should be voiding sufficient quantities (at least 250–300 mL) every four to six hours; ask about symptoms of urinary tract infection (UTI) (urgency, frequency, dysuria); note whether bladder is palpable; determine whether fundus is in the midline. Palpate costovertebral angle (CVA) for tenderness.

Explain the importance of adequate voiding; help woman with difficulty by providing privacy, suggesting she pour warm water over perineum, encouraging ambulation, and describing visualization techniques.

Identify symptoms of UTI; explain importance of adequate fluid intake (at least 2000 mL) daily.

Lower Extremities

Stasis of blood in legs dues to positioning, trauma to blood vessels, and use of stirrups, etc, increases risk of thrombophlebitis.

Inspect legs for redness, edema. Assess for Homans' sign (pain in calf when foot sharply dorsiflexed); palpate for tenderness, warmth.

Stress the importance of early ambulation to promote venous return. Encourage woman to avoid crossing legs or using knee-gatch position on bed.

Bowel Elimination

Bowels tend to be sluggish due to lingering effects of progesterone, decreased abdominal muscle tone, and lack of food and fluid. Woman may fear bowel movement will be painful because of episiotomy, hemorrhoids, etc.

Ask woman about bowel elimination. She should have a normal bowel movement by second or third day after birth. Stool softeners may be indicated if hemorrhoids or episiotomy increase possibility of discomfort.

Explain importance of bowel elimination. Encourage ambulation, increased fluid intake, diet high in roughage. Explain risks of constipation.

3. Witch hazel pads may be placed against the hemorrhoids and held in place by the perineal pad. They are soothing and cool.
4. Encourage actions that help prevent constipation such as increased fluid intake, roughage in diet, early ambulation, use of stool softeners as prescribed.

Afterpains

Afterpains are the result of intermittent uterine contractions and are more common in multiparas, women who had a multiple pregnancy, and women who had hydramnios. They may be intensified by breast–feeding since oxytocin is released when the baby suckles. Suggested nursing interventions:

1. Have woman lie prone with small pillow under abdomen. This places constant pressure on the uterus, causing it to remain contracted. Tell her the pain will be intensified for a few minutes but then will subside.
2. Administer analgesic as needed. For breast–feeding women, administer about one hour before scheduled feeding.

Postpartum Diaphoresis

Diaphoresis results as the body works to eliminate excess fluid and waste. Frequently occurs at night and woman awakens drenched with perspiration. Suggested nursing interventions:

1. Protect woman from chilling by changing bedding and providing a fresh gown.
2. Encourage a shower (unless cultural practices forbid it).
3. Prevent thirst by offering fluids as the woman desires.

Discomfort from Immobility

Woman may have muscular aches from pushing or from spending time in stirrups. Suggested nursing interventions:

1. Encourage early ambulation. Woman may be light-headed initially because of blood loss, fatigue, medication, etc, so nurse should assist her the first few times. This is especially important during the first shower or sitz bath, when heat may add to the problem. Stay close, have a call light and chair readily available, and check the woman frequently.

Suppression of Lactation in the Non-nursing Mother

Lactation may be suppressed through medication and mechanical inhibition.

Medications used:

1. Bromocriptine (Parlodel), see Drug Guide 2: Bromocriptine (Parlodel).
2. Estrogen-based medications such as chlorotrianisene (TACE) are seldom used because of increased risk of thromboembolism.

Mechanical suppression:

1. Have woman wear a well-fitting supportive bra continuously until lactation is suppressed (about five days). Bra is removed only for showers. Breast binder may be applied if woman prefers or if no bra is available.
2. Apply ice packs over axillary area of both breasts for 20 minutes QID.
3. Avoid any stimulation of breasts by woman, her partner, or infant.
4. Avoid warmth, which stimulates milk production; avoid letting shower water flow over breasts.

Breast Engorgement in the Non-nursing Mother

1. Interventions are the same as those for suppression.
2. Administer analgesics as necessary.

Note: In the nursing mother engorgement is handled differently. See Table 7–2.

INFANT FEEDING

Breast–feeding

The hormone prolactin, from the anterior pituitary, is initially responsible for milk production, while oxytocin, from the posterior pituitary, is responsible for the letdown reflex, which triggers the flow of milk. The letdown reflex is stimulated by infant suckling but it can also be stimulated by the newborn's presence or cry, or even thinking about the infant. It may also occur during sexual orgasm because oxytocin is released. The letdown reflex may be inhibited by a mother's lack of self-confidence, feelings of fear or embarrassment, or physical discomfort.

Milk production is based on the law of supply and demand. Repeated inhibition of the letdown reflex or failure to empty the breasts completely and frequently may decrease milk supply.

Breast–feeding technique

1. Put the newborn to breast as soon as possible.
2. Position baby so that entire body is turned toward breast. Figure 7–1 shows a variety of positions.
3. Direct nipple straight into infant's mouth with as much of the areola included as possible so that as infant sucks, his or her jaws compress the ducts under the areola, where milk is stored (see Figure 7–2).
4. To do this, the mother holds the breast with thumb placed on upper portion and remainder of her fingers cupping the breast. She then lightly strokes the infant's lips with the nipple.
5. Avoid the temptation to use a nipple shield. This confuses the baby and makes it more difficult for him/her to learn to nurse.
6. Avoid setting artificial time limits on the amount of time the baby should nurse. It may take up to three minutes for the letdown reflex to occur. Instead advise the woman to let the baby nurse at one breast as long as he/she is sucking well and positioned correctly. To avoid trauma to the breasts the mother should not let the infant sleep with the nipple in his/her mouth. When the baby has emptied the first breast she/he is burped and switched to the second breast. When the baby has completed feeding she/he is burped again.
7. The baby's suck tends to be most vigorous initially. To avoid undue trauma to the breasts the mother should alternate the breast from which she nurses first.
8. Baby's are obligatory nose breathers. To avoid blocking the nares with a full breast the mother should either lift the breast slightly or compress the breast tissue away from the baby's nose.

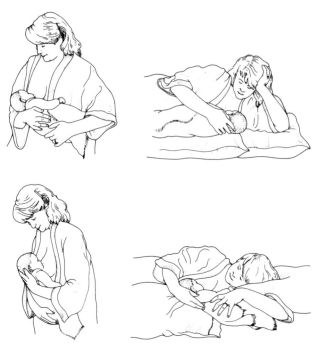

Figure 7–1 Examples of breast-feeding position changes to facilitate thorough breast emptying and prevent nipple soreness.

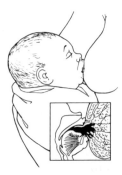

Figure 7–2 To nurse effectively, it is important that the infant's mouth cover the majority of the areola to compress the ducts below. (Courtesy of Ross Laboratories, Columbus, Ohio.)

9. To prevent trauma to the nipple the mother should break suction before removing the infant from the breast by inserting a finger into the infant's mouth next to the nipple.

10. When feeding is completed the woman should wash the nipples with warm water to prevent milk drying and should inspect them for trauma.

11. Frequent nursing helps establish a good supply of milk and prevents nipple trauma from the too vigorous suck of a ravenous infant. Thus, during the first few days the mother should nurse frequently (every 1 1/2 to 3 hours).

12. Table 7–2 cites suggested interventions for common problems.

Bottle Feeding

Bottle feeding is also a nurturing choice for infant feeding and allows both parents to share in this nurturing activity with their child. A variety of commercial formulas are available. Whole milk and skim milk should not be used for children under two years. Whole milk has too high a protein content; skim milk also has too much protein and lacks adequate calories and essential fatty acids.

Bottle feeding technique

1. Formula tends to be digested more slowly, so the bottle-fed infant may go longer between feedings.

2. Infants are usually fed "on demand," which typically is every three to five hours.

3. The mother should assume a comfortable position with adequate arm support so that she can cradle her baby in her arm close to her body .

4. The bottle should be held, not propped, with the baby's head somewhat elevated. Feeding the infant horizontally may result in positional otitis media.

5. The nipple should have a large enough hole to permit milk to flow in drops when the bottle is inverted. Too large an opening may cause overfeeding and regurgitation.

6. The nipple should be pointed directly into the mouth and on top of the tongue. The nipple should be kept full of formula to avoid ingestion of extra air.

Table 7–2   Self-care Measures for the Woman with Breast–feeding Problems

Nipple Inversion

Use Hoffman's exercises to increase protractility.

Use special breast shields such as Woolrich or Eschmann.

Use hand to shape nipple when beginning to nurse.

Apply ice for a few minutes prior to feeding to improve nipple erection.

Use electric or hand pump to cause nipple prominence, express a few drops of breast milk, then switch to regular nursing.

Inadequate Letdown

Massage breasts prior to nursing.

Feed in a quiet, private place, away from distraction.

Take a warm shower before nursing to relax and stimulate letdown.

Apply warm pack for 20 minutes before nursing.

Use relaxation techniques and focus on letdown.

Drink water, juice, or noncaffeinated beverages before and during feeding.

Avoid overfatigue by resting when the baby sleeps, feeding while lying down, and having quiet time alone.

Develop a conditioned response by establishing a routine for starting feedings.

Allow the baby sufficient time on each side to trigger the letdown reflex.

Use breast-alternating method (either use different breast for each feeding or switch breasts several times during a single feeding).

If all else fails obtain a prescription for oxytocin nasal spray from the health care provider.

Nipple Soreness

Ensure that infant is correctly positioned at the breast with the infant's ear, shoulder, and hip in straight alignment.

Rotate breast–feeding positions.

Use finger to break suction before removing infant from the breast.

Hold baby close when feeding to avoid undue pulling on nipple.

Continued

Table 7–2   *continued*

Don't allow baby to sleep with nipple in mouth.

Nurse more frequently.

Begin nursing on less sore breast.

Apply ice to nipples and areola for a few minutes prior to feeding.

Protect nipples to prevent skin breakdown.

Clean nipple gently with warm water.

Allow nipples to air dry, or dry nipples with hair dryer set to low heat, or expose nipples to sunlight initially for 30 seconds, then increase to three minutes.

If clothing rubs nipples, use ventilated shields to keep clothing away from skin.

To promote healing, apply a small amount of breast milk to nipple and areola after nursing and allow to dry.

The routine application of ointment to nipple, areola, or breast (eg, lanolin, Massé cream, Eucerin cream, or A & D ointment) should be discouraged.

Apply tea bags soaked in warm water.

Change breast pads frequently.

Nurse long enough to empty breasts completely.

Alternate breasts several times during feedings.

Cracked Nipples

Use interventions discussed under sore nipples.

Inspect nipples carefully for cracks or fissures.

Temporarily stop nursing on the affected breast and hand express milk for a day or two until cracks heal.

Maintain healthy diet. Protein and vitamin C are essential for healing.

Use a mild PO analgesic such as acetaminophen for discomfort 20–30 minutes before feedings.

Consult health care providers if signs of infection develop.

Nipple shield should be tried before nursing on a breast is permanently discontinued, but it should be used only as a last resort. Some women find it contributes to their discomfort. Consult a lactation specialist prior to use.

Continued

Table 7–2 *continued*

Breast Engorgement

Nurse frequently (every 1½ to 3 hours) around the clock.

Wear a well-fitting supportive bra at all times.

Take a warm shower or apply warm compresses to trigger letdown.

Massage breasts and then hand express some milk to soften the breast so the infant can "latch on."

Breast-feed long enough to empty breast.

Alternate starting breast.

Take a mild analgesic 20 minutes before feeding if discomfort is pronounced.

Plugged Ducts (Caked Breasts)

Nurse frequently and for long enough to empty the breasts completely.

Rotate feeding position.

Massage breasts prior to feeding, in a warm shower when possible.

Maintain good nutrition and adequate fluid intake.

---

7. The infant should be burped at regular intervals, preferably at the middle and end of the feeding, or, during the first few feedings, after about every 1/2 ounce. If the infant was crying vigorously before feeding, he/she should be burped before feeding or after taking just enough formula to calm down.

8. Burping is done by holding the infant upright on the shoulder or by holding the infant in a sitting position on the feeder's lap with the chin and chest supported by one hand. The back is then stroked or patted gently.

9. Newborns frequently regurgitate small amounts. The feeder may find it helpful to keep a "burp cloth" handy. Forceful emesis requires medical evaluation, especially if other symptoms are present.

10. Infants should be encouraged but not forced to feed. Overfeeding can lead to infant obesity.

THE Rh-NEGATIVE MOTHER

A woman who is Rh negative with an indirect Coombs' test negative, and whose infant is Rh positive with a direct Coombs' negative, is given Rh Ig G (RhoGAM) within 72 hours after childbirth. See Procedure 17: Rh Ig G Administration, and Drug Guide 12: Rh_o (D) Immune Globulin (Human).

RUBELLA VACCINE

Women who are not immune to rubella (German measles) as evidenced by a titer of less than 1:10, are usually given the rubella vaccine during the immediate postpartal period because it is known that they are not pregnant. Because the rubella vaccine is a live, attenuated vaccine, they are advised **not** to be-

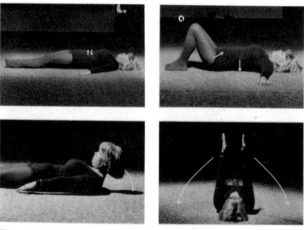

Figure 7–3   Postpartal exercises. Begin with five repetitions two or three times daily and gradually increase to ten repetitions. First day: A, Abdominal breathing. Lying supine, inhale deeply using the abdominal muscles. The abdomen should expand. Then exhale slowly through pursed lips, tightening the abdominal muscles. B, Pelvic rocking. Lying supine with arms at sides, knees bent and feet flat, tighten abdomen and buttocks and attempt to flatten back on floor. Hold for a count of ten, then arch the back, causing the pelvis to "rock." On second day add: C, Chin to chest. Lying supine with no pillows, legs straight, raise head and attempt to touch chin to chest. Slowly lower head. D, Arm raises. Lying supine, arms extended at 90° angle from body, raise arms so they are perpendicular and hands touch. Lower slowly. On fourth day add: E, Knee rolls. Lying supine with knees bent, feet flat, arms extended to the

come pregnant for at least 3 to 4 months after receiving it. See Drug Guide 14: Rubella Virus Vaccine.

POSTPARTUM EDUCATION: SELECTED TOPICS

Postpartal Exercises

The woman should be encouraged to begin simple exercises in the hospital and to continue them at home. Exercise helps to improve muscle tone, contributes to postpartum weight loss, and aids in preventing constipation. Many agencies have a booklet on appropriate exercises. Figure 7–3 identifies some commonly used exercises.

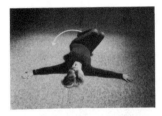
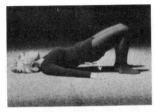
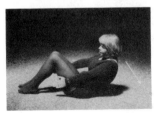
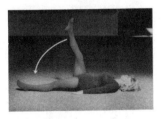

side, roll knees slowly to one side, keeping shoulders flat. Return to original position and roll to opposite side. F, Buttocks lift. Lying supine, arms at sides, knees bent, feet flat, slowly raise buttocks and arch the back. Return slowly to starting position. On sixth day add: G, Abdominal tighteners. Lying supine, knees bent, feet flat, slowly raise head toward knees. Arms should extend along either side of legs. Return slowly to original position. H, Knee to abdomen. Lying supine, arms at sides, bend one knee and thigh until foot touches buttocks. Straighten leg and lower it slowly. Repeat with other leg. After two to three weeks, more strenuous exercises such as bent knee sit-ups and side leg raises may be added as tolerated. Kegel exercises, begun antepartally, should be done many times daily during postpartum to restore vaginal and perineal tone.

Sibling Preparation

Most agencies now permit siblings to visit the postpartum area. This visit reassures the children that their mother is well and still loves them. The parents may ask for advice about dealing with the siblings when mother and baby return from the hospital. The following advice may be helpful:

- If possible, have the father carry the new baby inside so that the mother's arms are free to embrace her other children.

- Some mothers bring a doll home for the older sibling. The sibling can then care for the doll when the mother is caring for the baby.

- Involving older children in baby care helps them develop a sense of closeness with the baby. Even very young children can hold the baby with supervision.

- Each parent should spend quality time in a one-to-one experience with each of their older children. Hugs, kisses, and words of praise are also important.

- Regression is common, and a toilet-trained child may begin to wet or may request a bottle for meals.

Resumption of Sexual Activity

The couple is advised to abstain from sexual intercourse until the episiotomy is healed and the lochia has stopped, which is usually by the end of the third week.

- Because the vagina may be dry (hormone-poor), some form of water-soluble lubricant such as K-Y jelly may be necessary to prevent discomfort.

- Warn breast–feeding couples that the woman may leak milk with orgasm because of the release of oxytocin. Some couples find this pleasurable or amusing; others prefer to have the woman wear a bra. Nursing the baby prior to intercourse may help prevent this.

- The woman may experience decreased interest in sex due to hormonal changes, fatigue, dissatisfaction with her personal appearance, and lingering discomfort (often related to the episiotomy). This may be frustrating, especially for her partner, and they may find it helpful to discuss it openly.

- To avoid an unplanned pregnancy, the couple should be advised to use contraception when they resume sexual activity, even if the woman's menses have not yet returned.

CONTRACEPTION

Contraceptive information should be made available before the woman is discharged. In choosing a method, consistency of use outweighs absolute reliability of a given method. The nurse should review for the woman (or couple) the advantages and disadvantages of each method, risk factors and contraindications, and the ways of using a given method to enable the woman (or couple) to choose the best method for her and her partner. Different methods of contraception may be appropriate at different times in the couple's life. Table 7–3 identifies factors to consider in selecting a method of contraception.

Table 7–3 Factors to Consider in Choosing a Method of Contraception

Effectiveness of method in preventing pregnancy

Safety of the method:
   Are there inherent risks?
   Does it offer protection against STDs or other conditions?

Client's age and future childbearing plans

Any contraindications in client's health history

Religious or moral factors influencing choice

Personal preferences, biases, etc

Life-style:
   How frequently does client have intercourse?
   Does she have multiple partners?
   Does she have ready access to medical care in the event of complications?
   Is cost a factor?

Partner's support and willingness to cooperate

Personal motivation to use method

Methods of Contraception

Condom   A condom is a barrier contraceptive; its effectiveness is increased when it is used in combination with a spermicide.

Advantages: Small, lightweight, disposable, and inexpensive; has no side effects; requires no medical examination or supervision; offers visual evidence of effectiveness; provides some protection against sexually transmitted infections.

Disadvantages: Risk of breakage or displacement; may cause perineal or vaginal irritation, some dulling of sensation.

Method of use: Condoms are applied to the erect penis, rolled from the tip to the end of the shaft before vulvar or vaginal contact is made. A small space is left at the tip to accommodate ejaculate, thereby avoiding breakage. Condom rim should be held when penis is withdrawn from vagina to prevent spillage. Latex may be weakened by prolonged exposure to heat.

Note: Only latex condoms offer protection against AIDS. "Skin condoms" made of lamb's intestine do not.

Diaphragm   The diaphragm is a barrier contraceptive used with a spermicidal cream or jelly.

Advantages: Excellent choice for women who are unable or unwilling to take birth control pills or who have an intrauterine device (IUD). Involves no medication; contraception only used as necessary; may be inserted up to four hours before intercourse.

Disadvantages: Women who are not comfortable manipulating their genitals may find it unacceptable; some couples feel it interferes with sexual spontaneity.

Contraindications: Women with a history of toxic shock syndrome or urinary tract infections.

Method of use: A diaphragm must be fitted by a trained care giver. It is inserted into the vagina prior to intercourse with approximately 1 teaspoonful of spermicidal jelly or cream placed around the rim and in the cup. When correctly placed it covers the cervix. If more than 4 hours elapse between insertion and intercourse, additional spermicide should be inserted into the vagina (see Figure 7–4). The diaphragm is left in place for 6 to 8 hours after intercourse. Then it is removed, cleaned, and allowed to dry. It should be inspected periodically for holes or tears.

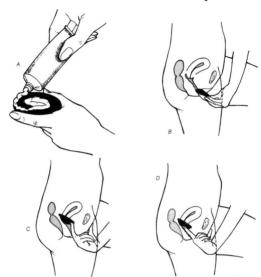

Figure 7–4 A, Diaphragm and jelly. Jelly is applied to the rim and center of the diaphragm. B, Insertion of the diaphragm. C, Rim of the diaphragm is pushed under the symphysis pubis. D, Checking the placement of the diaphragm. Cervix should be felt through the diaphragm.

Cervical cap The cervical cap is similar to the diaphragm, except it fits snugly over the cervix. It may be left in place up to 48 hours. Tends to be more difficult for women to insert and remove.

Contraceptive sponge The contraceptive sponge is a barrier contraceptive impregnated with spermicide.
Advantages: May be used for multiple acts of coitus up to 24 hours; professional fitting or prescription not required; one size fits all; may offer some protection against chlamydia and gonorrhea.
Disadvantages: Cost (approximately $1.50 per sponge); may be difficult to remove; and may cause vaginal dryness, irritation, or allergic reactions.
Contraindication: Women with a history of toxic shock syndrome.

Method of use: The sponge is moistened thoroughly with water and inserted into the vagina so that cupped end fits over cervix (see Figure 7–5). It should be left in place for six hours following intercourse, then removed and discarded.

Intrauterine Device (IUD) The IUD provides continuous contraceptive protection by producing an inflammatory reaction in the endometrium and tubes. Best suited for multiparous women in a monogamous relationship.

Types available: Copper-containing Cu380T (ParaGard) and progesterone-containing Progestasert

Advantages: High effectiveness, continuous contraceptive protection, no coitus-related activity, and relative inexpensiveness over time.

Disadvantages: Possible adverse effects including pelvic inflammatory disease (PID), severe dysmenorrhea, irregular menses, increased bleeding during menses, uterine perforation, expulsion; if IUD fails and pregnancy results, there is increased risk of ectopic pregnancy.

Contraindications: History of PID. Not recommended for women with multiple sexual partners because of the increased risk of PID.

Method of use: Requires signed consent before insertion by a physician, nurse midwife, or trained nurse practitioner. The woman should check for the presence of the string once weekly for the first month and then after each menses.

Oral contraceptives Oral contraceptives provide contraceptive protection by inhibiting release of ovum and by maintaining cervical mucus that is hostile to sperm.

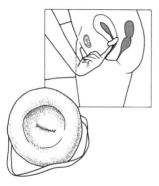

Figure 7–5   Contraceptive sponge is moistened with water and inserted into the vagina with concave portion over the cervix.

Advantages: No coitus-related activity, high effectiveness rate. Noncontraceptive benefits include the following: decreased menstrual cramps, decreased menstrual flow, increased cycle regularity, decreased incidence of functional ovarian cysts; in addition there is a substantial reduction in the incidence of ectopic pregnancy, ovarian cancer, endometrial cancer, iron deficiency anemia, and benign breast disease (Connell et al 1989).

Disadvantages: Must be taken daily; has some serious associated side effects, especially those related to thrombus formation.

Contraindications: Pregnancy, previous history of thrombophlebitis, acute or chronic liver disease, presence of estrogen-dependent carcinoma, undiagnosed uterine bleeding, heavy smoking, hypertension, diabetes, and hyperlipidemia.

Method of use: Pills are prescribed after a careful review of the woman's history and a thorough physical exam including blood pressure (BP) check and pap smear. The woman is seen yearly while on the pill. Pills are begun on the first Sunday after the beginning of the menstrual cycle and are taken daily for 21 days. The woman then stops for one week (or takes seven "blank" pills if she prefers a 28-day package.) She then resumes the pills. Low-dose pills should be taken within four hours of the same time daily. She should use a backup method such as condoms during her first cycle on the pills. If she misses a pill she should take it when she remembers and take her pill for the day at the regular time. Many women take their pills at night when they are less rushed, so they are asleep when most side effects such as nausea would occur.

Spermicides Spermicides provide contraceptive protection by destroying sperm or neutralizing vaginal secretions and thereby immobilizing sperm. They are available in a variety of forms including cream, foam, jelly, film, and suppositories. Spermicides are only minimally effective when used alone. Their effectiveness increases when used with a condom.

Advantages: Wide availability and low toxicity. Offers high degree of protection against gonorrhea and some protection against *Chlamydia, Trichomonas,* and herpes.

Disadvantages: Low reliability, some messiness.

Vasectomy A vasectomy is a male sterilization procedure in which the vas deferens are severed surgically. Relatively simple procedure that does not interfere with erectile function.

Tubal ligation Tubal ligation is a method of female sterilization in which the fallopian tubes are severed. Because it involves general anesthesia it has more associated risks than a vasectomy.

Both procedures should be considered irreversible despite some success with microsurgical techniques to reverse the operation.

Subdermal implants (Norplant) Six silastic capsules of levonorgestrel, a progestin, are implanted in the woman's arm. They act by preventing ovulation in most women and by stimulating the production of thick cervical mucus, which inhibits sperm penetration (Kaunitz 1990). Requires a minor surgical procedure for insertion.

Advantages: Provides continuous contraception that is removed from the act of coitus. Effects last up to five years.

Disadvantages: Variety of side effects (spotting or irregular bleeding, amenorrhea, weight gain, increased incidence of ovarian cysts, hirsutism, headaches, depression [Kaunitz 1990]). Implants may be visible in very slender users.

CARE OF THE WOMAN FOLLOWING CESAREAN BIRTH

The new mother who has given birth by cesarean section has postpartal needs similar to those of women who gave birth vaginally; however, she also has nursing care needs similar to those of women who have undergone major abdominal surgery. Nursing interventions include the following:

1. Encourage woman to cough, deep breathe, and use incentive spirometry every 2 to 4 hours while awake for the first day or two following birth.

2. Encourage leg exercises q2h until woman is ambulatory.

3. Monitor temperature for fever (infection), BP for decrease, and pulse for increase (hemorrhage). Elevated BP may indicate pregnancy-induced hypertension (PIH) (may occur for up to 48 hours postpartum).

4. Assess for adequate voiding after the Foley is removed. Implement nursing interventions if necessary to encourage voiding (privacy, increased fluid, warm water over perineum, ambulation).

5. Assess for evidence of abdominal distention. Note presence or absence of bowel sounds. Measures to prevent or minimize gas pains include leg exercises, abdominal tightening,

early ambulation, and avoiding the use of straws. Flatulence may be relieved by lying on the left side, using a rocking chair, and the use of antiflatulents (such as mylicon), suppositories, and enemas.

6. Measures to alleviate pain include the following:
    - Administer analgesics as needed. Patient-controlled analgesia (PCA) is available in many facilities.
    - Offer comfort through positioning, back rubs, oral care, and reduction of noxious stimuli such as noise or odors.
    - Encourage presence of significant others, including baby.
    - Encourage breathing, relaxation, and distraction techniques (such as those taught in childbirth preparation classes).

7. Encourage shower by second or third postpartal day (cover incision with plastic wrap until staples are removed, and stay close in case woman becomes faint).

8. Discharge teaching includes need for adequate rest, warning signs of infection, ways of lifting and feeding infant to avoid strain.

9. Provide opportunities for parent-infant interaction.

REFERENCES

Connell EB et al: Contraceptive advances. Part I. Hormonal methods. *Female Patient* 1989 (December); 14:29.

Kaunitz AM: Long-acting progestin contraceptives. *Contemp OB/GYN* October 15, 1990; 35(special issue):59.

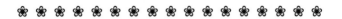

CHAPTER 8

The At-risk Postpartal Client

POSTPARTAL HEMORRHAGE

Overview

Postpartum hemorrhage is defined as a blood loss of 500 mL or more at any time after birth. The main causes of postpartal hemorrhage are uterine atony (relaxation of uterus due to hydramnios, large infant, multiple gestation, grand multiparity, use of magnesium sulfate in labor), retained placental fragments, laceration of genital tract, or hematoma development (resulting from trauma to uterus, vagina, or perineum). Postpartum hemorrhage is characterized by bright red vaginal bleeding in the presence of either a soft boggy uterus with clots or a well-contracted uterus without clots. This condition most commonly occurs within the first 24 hours after giving birth. Hematomas present as severe pressure anywhere along the genital tract and purple color to the vaginal mucosa or ecchymotic perineum. Late or delayed hemorrhage can occur up to four to six weeks postpartum and is usually caused by subinvolution.

Medical Management

1. **Uterine atony.** Oxytocic drugs are administered after separation of the placenta to prevent uterine atony (see Drug Guide 10: Oxytocin [Pitocin]). Fundal height and firmness are determined; if the uterus is not firm and well contracted after expulsion of the placenta fundal massage is initiated. If there is excessive bleeding (more than 350–500 mL), the clinician may do bimanual uterine compression. Oxygen via mask is administered at 6–10 liters per minute. Hematocrit, partial thromboplastin, prothrombin times, and fibrinogen levels are monitored.

2. **Retained placental fragments.** Inspect the placenta for any signs that a cotyledon or piece of membrane is missing. If missing pieces are suspected the uterine cavity requires uterine exploration. Sonography may be considered to look for retained fragments. Methylergonovine maleate (Methergine) IM or p.o. (see Drug Guide 8) is ordered or prostaglandins may be used.

3. **Lacerations.** A visual examination of the cervix is made and deep cervical lacerations are sutured to stop the bleeding.

4. **Hematomas.** Small hematomas are managed with ice packs and ongoing observation. They usually reabsorb naturally. Larger hematomas or those increasing in size are incised and drained to achieve hemostasis. Vaginal packing is inserted to achieve hemostasis if needed. Since incision and drainage may predispose to infection, antibiotics are ordered. Replace blood and clotting factors as needed.

Critical Nursing Assessments

1. Assess BP, pulse, and respirations every 15 minutes × 4, then every 30 × 2 after normal birth. If vaginal bleeding is noted, assess BP, pulse, and respirations q15min.
   Be alert for: Hypotension and tachycardia can be signs of hypovolemia, along with tachypnea, pallor, cyanosis, and cold and clammy skin.

2. Assess fundal status for height and firmness (see Procedure 9: Fundal Assessment). Uterus should be firm and at or below the umbilicus. A well-contracted fundus rules out uterine atony.

3. Assess amount of blood loss/vaginal bleeding, any blood clots expressed. **Assessment technique:** Visual assessment, do pad counts within a given time period or weigh the perineal pads (one mL of blood weighs 1 gram).

4. Examine perineum and buttocks for discoloration, bulging, tender areas. If woman is still recovering from regional anesthesia frequent visualization of perineum/buttocks is essential. Palpate obvious masses for tenderness and fluctuation.

5. Examine vagina or rectum for protruding masses. **Assessment technique:** Position woman on her side, raise her upper buttock, and instruct her to bear down.
   Be alert for: Bulging purplish mass may become apparent at the introitus or soft mass may be palpable upon rectal exam.

6. Assess for bladder distention (hinders effective uterine contractions and involution process).
7. Assess intake and output q8hrs.
   Be alert for: Urine output needs to stay at > 30 mL/hr to perfuse kidneys well.
8. Assess laboratory results.
   Be alert for: Decreasing hematocrit (500 mL blood loss may be seen as a 4-point decrease in hematocrit) and an increase in prothrombin time or partial thromboplastin time, and a decrease in fibrinogen.
9. Assess woman's coping responses, level of understanding of her condition, and emotional status.

Sample Nursing Diagnoses

- Fluid volume deficit related to blood loss secondary to uterine atony, retained placental fragments, lacerations, or hematoma formation
- Infection: High risk related to trauma and hemorrhage (See Nursing Care Plan 7: Hemorrhage in Third Trimester and at Birth.)

Critical Nursing Interventions

1. Gently massage boggy uterus while supporting lower uterine segment (see Figure 8–1) to stimulate contraction and express clots.
   Be alert for: Forceful massage can tire the uterus, resulting in uterine atony, and can cause pain, so be gentle.
2. Monitor type and amount of bleeding and associated consistency of the uterus.
   Be alert for: Dark red blood and relaxed uterus indicate uterine atony or retained placental fragments. Bright red vaginal bleeding and contracted uterus indicate laceration hemorrhage.
3. Monitor vital signs. Note any signs of hypovolemic shock (tachycardia, tachypnea, decreased blood pressure, pallor, oliguria, restlessness, and lethargy).
4. Maintain IV and start second IV with 14-, 16-, or 18-gauge needle to administer blood products if necessary. Send blood for type and cross match if not already done in the birthing area.

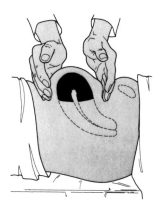

Figure 8–1   *Uterine massage.*

5. Administer oxytocics per order. Carefully note uterine tone and blood pressure response to medication.

6. Monitor intake and output hourly. Insert Foley catheter to ensure accurate output determination.

7. Provide oxygen via mask or nasal cannula at 7–10 L/min for signs of respiratory distress.

8. Position woman either flat with legs elevated or Trendelenburg per agency protocol to increase blood flow to vital organs.

9. Administer pain medications for discomfort as ordered.

10. Review the following critical aspects of the care you have provided:

    • Have I effectively monitored her fundal and lochia status? Did I quickly identify and intervene when there was continued relaxation of the uterus and expression of clots? Did I carry out the uterine massage as gently as possible?

    • Are woman's vital signs stable? Is woman showing any signs of hypovolemia?

    • Is woman complaining of discomfort anywhere along the genital tract? Have I provided adequate comfort measures for her, such as cold/warm packs, perineal care, sitz baths, or pain medication?

    • Have I assisted in decreasing the woman and her family's anxieties by keeping them informed about her status?

Evaluation

See Nursing Care Plan 7: Hemorrhage in Third Trimester and At Birth.

SUBINVOLUTION

Overview

Subinvolution is the failure of the uterus to follow the normal pattern of involution and is one of the most common causes of late postpartum hemorrhage. Primary causes of subinvolution are retained placental fragments or membranes, endometritis, or pelvic infection. Myomas and uterine fibroids are also contributing causes. Usually the signs and symptoms of subinvolution are not apparent until about four to six weeks postpartum. The client, who may not know that her uterus is not involuting properly, may have prolonged blood loss and develop anemia before seeking assistance from a health-care professional.

The fundus remains higher in the abdomen/pelvis than expected. Lochia often fails to progress from rubra to serosa to alba. The lochia may remain rubra or return to rubra several days postpartum. The amount of lochia may be more profuse than expected. Leukorrhea and backache may occur if infection is present. The woman may also relate a history of irregular or excessive bleeding after the birth.

Medical Management

1. **Uterine examination.** Bimanual uterine exam shows an enlarged, softer than normal uterus.
2. **Drug therapy.** Oral Methergine 0.2 mg or Ergotrate 0.2 mg q3–4 hrs for 24–48 hours is given to stimulate uterine contractility (see Drug Guide 8: Methylergonovine Maleate [Methergine]). Oral antibiotics are ordered if metritis (infection) is present or invasive procedures are done.
3. **Uterine curettage.** If treatment is not effective or if retained placental fragments and polyps are the cause, a dilatation and curettage (D & C) may be done. Polyps can form from fibrotic retained tissues.

Critical Nursing Assessments

1. Assess characteristics of lochial pattern since birth.
   Be alert for: Lochia pattern: Lochia doesn't progress from rubra to serosa or returns to rubra days after the birth.
2. Assess whether mother has felt feverish or has had a temperature.
   Be alert for: Elevation in temperature can occur if infection is cause of subinvolution.
3. Assess woman's level of understanding regarding her condition, the signs of subinvolution, and when she should call her health-care provider.

Sample Nursing Diagnoses

- Pain related to stimulation of uterine contraction secondary to administration of oxytocic medications
- Infection: High risk related to bacterial invasion of uterus secondary to dilatation and curettage
- Knowledge deficit regarding delayed postpartum bleeding secondary to failure of normal involution process
- Fluid volume deficit related to continued blood loss

Critical Nursing Interventions

1. During discharge teaching, review normal involution process and progression of lochia from rubra to serosa to alba, and stress that the woman should report any continued bleeding that does not go away with rest and medication and that covers the surface of one perineal pad two to six weeks after birth.
2. Discuss the importance of increasing the length and number of rest periods; see if she can have a support person with her during the 24-hour oxytocic medication period.
3. Review with the woman the treatment regimen, the importance of taking her medications as directed, and any adverse effects that should be reported to her health-care provider.
4. Inform the lactating woman that she can continue to breastfeed. Low-dose Methergine poses no threat to baby and breast–feeding can assist in involution.

5. If woman has history of elevated blood pressure, teach her the early signs of adverse effects of oxytocic medication on her blood pressure. These include nausea, vomiting, headache, and complaints of abdominal cramping or signs of circulatory stasis, including itching, tingling, numbness, and cold fingers and toes.

Sample Nurse's Charting

7:30 PM T 99.2° F, P 92, R 16, BP 124/76. Fundus soft 1 FB above symphysis pubis and midline. Tender to palpation. Lochia rubra with small clots. Complains of fatigue, lochia flow return to rubra, and soaking surface of one peripad/day 15 days after birth. Is breastfeeding and expresses concern over continued rubra lochia and progressive fatigue. S. Paulski, RNC

Evaluation

- Woman knows the signs of delayed uterine involution and when to report them to her health-care provider.
- Woman understands the treatment regimen and takes her medications as ordered.
- Woman has support since she has increased fatigue and anxiety related to the failure of uterus to return to normal.

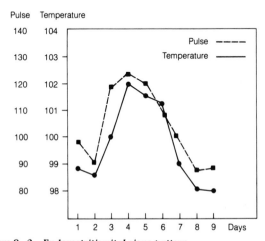

Figure 8–2   Endometritis vital signs pattern.

TYPES OF REPRODUCTIVE TRACT INFECTIONS

Type/Cause	Signs/Symptoms	Treatment
Localized Infection of External Genitalia Episiotomy or sutured laceration; infected traumatized perineum, vulva, vagina, or abdominal incision	Fever, localized pain, edema, redness, seropurulent discharge Late: skin discoloration, shock	Oral antibiotics, removal of stitches to promote drainage, use of gauze to keep lesion open, sitz baths, perineal heat lamp, analgesics
Endometritis (Metritis) Infection of total endrometrium or placental site	Sawtooth fever pattern (low grade to 103° F [39.4° C] see Figure 8–2), chills, rapid pulse. Headache, backache, malaise, loss of appetite, cramps. Large, boggy, tender uterus. Foul-smelling discharge. Dark brown and/or profuse lochia	IV antibiotics (cephalosporin), oxytocics to stimulate contraction and lochial drainage, semi-Fowler's position and/or ambulation to promote drainage, blood and lochial culture, D & C for retained placental tissue, hydration (oral/IV)
Parametritis (Pelvic Cellulitis) Infection of tissues around uterus via the lymphatics (often following endometritis)	Prolonged high fever (102–104° F, [39.4–40° C]), chills, abdominal tenderness on one or both sides. Pain when uterus is moved during pelvic exam. Vaginal, rectal, abdominal abscesses	Broad spectrum antibiotics (IV/PO). Hydration (up to 2000 mL/day), blood transfusion for decreasing hemoglobin, bed rest, analgesics

Critical Nursing Assessments

1. Assess BP, pulse, and respirations every two to four hours. Tachycardia is associated with endometritis.
2. Assess temperature every four hours unless elevated, then q2hr. **Tip:** Remember that a low-grade fever is common during the first 24 hours after birth. Be alert for elevated temp. (greater than 100.4° F [38° C]) patterns.

3. Assess fundal height, tone, and sensation (see Procedure 9: Fundal Assessment). Note any discomfort or pain that is greater than anticipated, and note protracted afterpains.

4. Assess perineum every eight hours. Inspect perineum using good light source. **Assessment technique:** Have woman lie on her side with her top leg slightly forward and ahead of the bottom leg (see Figure 8–3). After donning disposable gloves, lift the buttock to expose the perineum and the anus. If no episiotomy is present the perineum is described as "intact." Assess episiotomy or sutured laceration for redness, edema, ecchymosis, discharge, approximation of edges (skin edges together) and tenderness (REEDA Scale).

5. Assess lochia for type, amount, and odor (see Procedure 5: Evaluation of Lochia After Birth).

6. Assess laboratory results for above normal postpartum levels, especially the white blood cell count. **Tip:** Normal postpartum leukocyte levels are already increased (15,000–30,000/mm^3) so be alert for > 30,000/mm^3.

7. Assess hydration status.

Sample Nursing Diagnoses

- Infection: High risk related to broken skin or traumatized tissues
- Altered parenting related to mother's malaise and other symptoms of infection (see Nursing Care Plan 15: Puerperal Infection)

Critical Nursing Interventions

1. Monitor temperature every four hours and identify trends. **Be alert for:** Low-grade fever (< 101° F [38.3° C]) with rapid onset indicates localized infection. Irregular fever (sawtooth pattern), varying from 101–103° F (38.3–39.4° C) indicates endometritis. Persistent high fever (102–104° F [38.8–40° C]) and chills indicate parametritis.

2. Monitor lochial changes for signs of failure of normal involution.

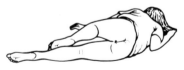

Figure 8–3   Episiotomy is inspected. Woman is on her side, and her upper leg is forward.

3. Instruct mother on and perform proper perineal and hygienic measures to promote healing and prevent contamination of the perineum, such as washing hands frequently and after each peripad change, perineal care (see Chapter 7), and use of sitz baths and the perineal heat lamp. Encourage a diet high in protein and vitamin C.

4. Obtain cultures of lochia, wound, and urine (to rule out asymptomatic urinary tract infection). **Tip:** With episiotomy infections, lochia may have a foul odor and appear yellow.

5. Administer antibiotics, oxytocics (see Drug Guide 10: Oxytocin [Pitocin], and Drug Guide 8: Methylergonovine Maleate [Methergine]), and analgesic spray as prescribed.

6. Assist mothers with endometritis to ambulate and lie in semi-Fowler's position to facilitate lochial drainage.

7. Maintain mother-infant interaction. Assist mother to balance her need for rest and her need for time with her baby.

8. If parametritis occurs, provide bed rest and maintain IV fluids. Monitor intake and output and urine specific gravity.

Evaluation

See Nursing Care Plan 15: Puerperal Infection.

MASTITIS

Overview

Mastitis refers to an inflammation of the breast commonly caused by *Staphylococcus aureus* from the infant's nose and throat. Contributing factors include clogged milk ducts, bruised tissue, unclean hands, and cracked or fissured nipples. Mastitis usually occurs in the 3rd or 4th week postpartum. A breast abscess may be a complication.

Medical Management

1. **Drug therapy.** Antibiotics are ordered for a full ten-day course even if symptoms subside within a few days. Antipyretics such as acetaminophen are used.

2. **Breast–feeding.** Breast–feeding is stopped only in the presence of large amounts of nipple drainage. In the presence of a yeast infection, the mother and baby are both treated with nystatin for 14 days.

3. **Laboratory tests.** Infectious mastitis is usually indicated by elevated leukocyte and bacterial counts.
4. **Breast abscess management.** If a breast abscess forms, the breast milk and any drainage is cultured. The abscessed area is incised, drained, and packed with sterile gauze.

Critical Nursing Assessments

1. Examine breast for localized redness, tenderness, and swelling. On palpation, it may be very hard and hot and the lump may feel like a hard "moth ball."
2. Inspect nipple for fissures or cracks (entry points for infection).
   Be alert for: If nipples are inflamed and painful consider a yeast or fungus infection. Breast abscesses appear as hardened, painful local areas of inflammation below the skin surface.
3. Assess mother's general physical status. Systemic symptoms include flulike symptoms: headache, malaise, muscle ache, rapid pulse, and temperature about 38.5° C (101.3° F).
4. Assess mother's dietary and sleep patterns, and level of stress. Decreases in diet and sleep and/or excessive stress and activity can decrease mother's resistance to infection.
5. Assess feeding history for precipitating factors such as ineffective emptying of breasts, engorgement, breast compression from tight clothing or bra, or sudden change in feeding pattern such as baby sleeping through the night or use of supplemental feedings.
6. Inspect baby's mouth for white patches surrounded by redness on the buccal membrane, which indicate *Candida albicans*, or thrush.

Sample Nursing Diagnoses

- Pain related to development of mastitis
- Knowledge deficit related to appropriate breast–feeding practices
- Infection: high risk related to cracked and traumatized breast tissue or nipples
- Ineffective breast–feeding related to interrupted breast–feeding schedule

Critical Nursing Interventions

Preventive measures

1. Discuss predisposing factors.
2. Use good handwashing technique.
3. Instruct mother about breast care: handwashing before handling breasts or nipples, cleansing of breast with water only (to maintain protective oils), wearing supportive bra at all times (to avoid milk stasis in lower lobes), changing bra and breast pads frequently.
4. Reinforce mother's knowledge about breast–feeding techniques, such as position, frequency, removal of baby from breast.
5. Provide special attention to mothers who have blocked milk ducts, as this places them at increased risk for mastitis.

If the woman has mastitis

1. Administer medications as ordered. Oral pain medications are given 20 minutes before feeding to ease discomfort.
2. Teach mother to increase feeding frequency, increase fluid intake (six to eight 8-oz glasses a day), have friends or relatives assist with care in order to increase rest periods, breast-feed first on unaffected breast until letdown occurs (promotes complete emptying of both breasts), express milk at least every three hours, and massage caked areas toward nipple during feeding (see Figure 8–4).
3. Mother's temperature should be monitored every four hours until infection resolves.
4. Instruct mother that if there is no improvement within 12–14 hours or if fever persists, she should notify her health-care provider. If mother is on antibiotics and the baby develops diarrhea, she should let her physician know.

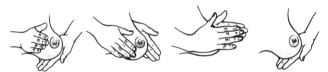

Figure 8–4 Breast massage. Caked areas of breast are massaged toward the nipple.

5. Provide support if mother needs to temporarily discontinue breast–feeding and instruct her on expression of milk (see Procedure 14: Methods of Breast Pumping and Milk Storage).

Evaluation

- The mother is able to identify predisposing factors, signs and symptoms of impending mastitis, and preventive measures.
- Mother knows proper management if mastitis should occur. Mother is supported in her decision to breast–feed and knows how to resume if it is necessary to stop.

URINARY TRACT INFECTION

Overview

Most postpartal urinary tract infections (UTIs) are caused by gram-negative organisms such as *Escherichia coli*, which invade the urethra and bladder and cause cystitis. Bladder bacteria then may ascend to the kidney as a result of vesicoureteral reflux during voiding, causing pyelonephritis. Clinical signs may not appear for several days and then present with dysuria, urinary urgency and frequency, suprapubic or lower abdominal pain, lower back discomfort, and possibly hematuria. In addition to the signs and symptoms of cystitis, pyelonephritis presents as cloudy urine and systemic signs of high fever, chills, nausea and vomiting (N & V), malaise, fatigue, severe flank pain, and costovertebral angle tenderness (CVAT). Cystitis management must continue after symptoms disappear, since this infection tends to recur.

Medical Management

1. **Urinalysis.** Urinalysis is obtained and analyzed for protein, blood, and organisms. Urine that contains an increase in WBCs, (> 100,000/mL organisms or too numerous to count) and protein and/or blood indicates UTI. Urine culture and sensitivities are obtained so organism-specific antibiotics can be identified. Urine cultures are obtained one week after therapy is completed and at four to six week intervals for at least a year to monitor for recurring infections.

2. **Fluid and drug management.** Fluid intake is increased to three to four L/day to dilute the urine and initiate flushing out of the infected urine. Therapeutic doses of vitamin C or cranberry juice are used to acidify the urine. Urine acidification decreases bacterial growth and increases the action of urinary tract antiseptics. Short-acting sulfonamides such as sulfisoxazole (Gantrisin) 1 gram qid are ordered for ten days except in term pregnancy, when Septra or Bactrim may be given. Urinary tract antiseptics (Aso Gantrisin) or systemic antibiotics (Ampicillin 500 mg q6hr for ten days) can also be used.

3. **Pyelonephritis management.** If woman develops pyelonephritis, she may be hospitalized for aggressive treatment and monitoring to prevent permanent kidney damage. Intravenous medications are given and an indwelling bladder catheter may be put in place. Relief of symptoms is usually obtained in 24 to 48 hours.

Critical Nursing Assessments

1. Assess bladder function for frequency, urgency, and amount of urine output. Inspect urine for color (hematuria), odor, appearance (concentrated or dilute).
2. Assess for painful or burning urination.
3. Assess for complaints of suprapubic or lower abdominal discomfort or lower back pain, severe flank pain.
4. Palpate for costovertebral tenderness.
5. Assess vital signs q4hrs and observe for signs of systemic involvement.
6. Assess intake and output q8hrs.

Sample Nursing Diagnoses

- Altered patterns of urinary elimination related to urinary tract infection
- Injury: High risk related to urinary tract infection
- Knowledge deficit related to urinary tract infection, its treatment, and possible sequelae

Critical Nursing Interventions

1. Take vital signs and monitor for fever.
2. Perform clean-catch, midstream urinalysis.

3. Encourage woman to void q2–3hrs and empty bladder completely. Provide ice pack for perineum within one hour after birth to decrease edema formation and facilitate voiding.

4. If taking cranberry juice, woman should drink at least 240 mL a day to be effective.

5. Provide comfort measures such as back massage and analgesics for back and flank pain; antispasmodics for dysuria and cramping, antiemetics for N & V, and oral hygiene to promote comfort. If woman has a fever provide tepid water baths and antipyretics.

6. If woman is taking sulfonamide drugs, instruct her that breast–feeding should be discontinued and teach her how to pump her breasts (see Procedure 14: Methods of Breast Pumping and Milk Storage).
   Be alert for: Sulfonamides are secreted in breastmilk and combine with proteins to create neonatal jaundice; therefore, pumped milk should be discarded while mother is on these medications.

7. Monitor baby for diarrhea and yeast infections (candidiasis) while mother is taking ampicillin.

8. Instruct mother that her urine may change color with prescribed medication.
   Be alert for: Aso Gantrisin can turn urine red or red orange, Furadantin creates brown urine, may cause N & V and diarrhea, and should be taken with food or milk to decrease gastric irritation.

9. Reinforce instruction on prophylactic hygienic practice, ie, wiping from front to back, voiding when she feels the urge to void, wearing cotton underclothing, and voiding after intercourse. Encourage woman to drink two glasses of water immediately after intercourse in order to increase urine output and flush out contaminants that may have entered the urethra.

Evaluation

- Mother understands any special instructions for taking medications and need for follow-up urine culture.
- Mother knows hygienic, nutritional, and fluid requirements to avoid urinary tract infections and any symptoms to report to health-care provider.

THROMBOEMBOLIC DISEASE

Overview

Thromboembolic disease refers primarily to superficial thrombophlebitis (thrombus formed due to inflammation), which primarily forms in saphenous veins, appears on third or fourth postpartal day, and shows clinical improvement within 48 hours of therapy. Thrombophlebitis often presents as a slight temperature elevation over the area of vein inflammation, mild calf pain, visible and palpable veins, and possibly a positive Homan's sign. Deep vein thrombosis is seen in woman with history of thrombosis and increases the likelihood of pulmonary emboli development. Deep vein thrombosis may be seen as a sudden onset of severe leg pain (pain may worsen if leg is in a dependent position), edema and paleness of affected leg, systemic signs of elevated temperature, pulse and chills, and possible positive Homan's signs. Deep vein thrombosis may take up to four to six weeks to resolve after the acute symptoms stop.

Medical Management

1. **Superficial thrombophlebitis.** Bedrest with leg elevation is ordered. Moist heat therapy is applied to facilitate drainage and decrease venous stasis. Elastic support hose are to be worn after acute inflammation subsides.

2. **Deep vein thrombosis.** In addition to treatment for superficial thrombophlebitis, anticoagulant therapy is ordered. Heparin via continuous IV of 1 unit/mL of estimated blood volume or subcutaneous 5000 to 7500 units q4–6hrs is ordered dependent on activated partial thromboplastin time (APTT). The desired APTT lab value is 1½–2½ X control in seconds. No aspirin or ibuprofin analgesic medications can be taken while on anticoagulant therapy.

   Special alert: One-percent protamine sulfate is used as the antidote for anticoagulant overdose.

Critical Nursing Assessments

1. Assess vital signs, especially oral temperature q4hrs. Be alert for and report temperature > 100.4° F.

2. Assess calves, thighs, and groin area (especially left side) bilaterally for increase in size, color, warmth, peripheral pulses, and positive Homans' sign. **Assessment technique for Homans' sign:** Dorsiflex foot with knee in extended position (see Figure 8–5). If pain occurs in foot or leg with foot dorsiflexion, it is a positive Homans' sign.

3. Assess CBC, platelet count, prothrombin time, and partial prothrombin time results.

Sample Nursing Diagnoses

- Altered peripheral tissue perfusion related to venous stasis
- Altered tissue perfusion related to pulmonary embolism secondary to dislodgement of deep vein thrombosis (see Nursing Care Plan 18: Thromboembolic Disease).

Critical Nursing Interventions

1. Monitor vital signs.
   Be alert for: elevated temperature, which may be associated with inflammation.

2. Inspect and palpate calf, thigh, and groin area daily for heat, color, tenderness, and peripheral pulses.
   Be alert for: increasing redness, swelling, or pain.

3. Monitor any signs of deep vein thrombosis.
   Be alert for: sudden onset of severe leg or thigh pain, elevated temperature, or chills. Report these signs to physician immediately.

4. Assist mother to stay on bed rest with her leg fully elevated on pillows. Do not use knee gatch on bed and avoid any pressure on popliteal space (to prevent pelvic pooling and impedance of blood flow). While mother is on bed rest,

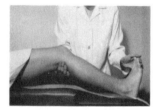

Figure 8–5   Homans' sign: With the woman's knee flexed to decrease the risk of embolization, the nurse dorsiflexes the foot. Pain in the foot or leg is a positive Homans' sign.

have her use footboard, do passive exercises, and change position frequently.

5. Apply warm packs to affected leg (vasodilatation facilitates blood flow and decreases pain). Be sure to wrap packs to prevent burns and remove for ten minutes each hour.

6. Administer antibiotics per order.

7. Administer heparin as ordered after obtaining APTT results. Monitor APTT and Hct to evaluate bleeding and adequacy of heparinization. Have 1% protamine sulfate on hand for heparin overdose.

8. Initiate progressive ambulation after acute inflammation subsides.

9. Apply support hose (compresses superficial veins and increases deep venous flow).

10. Monitor and report signs of pulmonary emboli.
    Be alert for: signs such as vague chest pain, anxiety, resp. rate > 16 breaths/minute, pallor, tachypnea, and possible changes in lung sounds (rales and friction rub).

11. Instruct mother on measures to prevent venous stasis:

    - Avoid crossing legs at the knee while sitting.
    - Elevate the feet while sitting when possible.
    - Ambulate periodically throughout the day.
    - Drink at least six 8-oz. glasses of water/day.

12. Instruct mother regarding anticoagulant therapy:

    - Take medication at the same time each day.
    - Keep appointments so that clotting times can be monitored and medication can be adjusted.
    - Maintain current eating habits (include green vegetables) and life-style.
    - Avoid any injuries that may cause bleeding, such as contact sports, stiff toothbrushes, or shaving legs with a straight razor.
    - Be aware of signs of heparin overdose such as bleeding gums, ecchymosis, nose bleed, hematuria, and melena.
    - Note any blood in the stools; it should be reported to the physician.
    - Wear a Medic-Alert bracelet indicating use of anticoagulants.

13. Review the following critical aspects of the care you have provided:

- Have I administered the correct dose of heparin at the designated times after first reviewing the APTT results?
- Have I been alert for any signs of heparin overdose?
- What can I do to assist the woman to maintain bed rest?
- Is mother able to eat a diet that assists her coagulation status?
- Have I assessed the woman's understanding of her thrombolic status and answered her questions? Have I given her opportunities to practice preventive measures?

Evaluation

See Nursing Care Plan 18: Thromboembolic Disease.

ONGOING MANAGEMENT OF SELECTED PERINATAL COMPLICATIONS

Pregnancy-Induced Hypertension (PIH)

The postpartum goal is to prevent eclamptic seizures and neurologic sequelae.

Effect of postpartum on PIH	Critical Nursing Interventions
Postpartum diuresis decreases serum magnesium sulfate levels, thereby increasing the possibility of seizures.	Monitor vital signs (VS) closely for 48 hours after birth (vital signs should remain stable then begin to slowly decrease). Monitor urine output (>30 mL/hr) and deep tendon reflexes (DTRs).
	Administer IV magnesium sulfate for 24 hours after birth.
	Check urine for protein and specific gravity qhr.
	Administer diuretic as ordered. Do not give oxytocics due to their hypertensive properties

Effect of postpartum on PIH	**Critical Nursing Interventions**
	Minimize environmental stimuli until status improves.
	Have seizure precautions in place.
Magnesium sulfate causes uterine relaxation, which increases the possibility of uterine atony; PIH decreases blood volume and lowers platelet counts, which can lead to postpartum hemorrhage.	Monitor for signs of postpartum hemorrhage. Carefully massaging the uterus is important.
	Encourage frequent voiding to keep bladder empty and avoid uterine atony.
	Emotional support is essential during critical illnesses.

Diabetes

The goal is to maintain normal blood glucose levels, prevention of postpartum complications (PIH, hemorrhage, infection) and enhance parent-infant interaction.

Effect of Postpartum on Diabetes	**Critical Nursing Interventions**
Loss of placental insulin inhibitory hormone (human chorionic somatomammotrophin [hCS], progesterone) drops insulin requirement sharply. Some women do not require insulin for the first day or so.	Draw blood glucose immediately after birth. Monitor urine for glucose and ketones q2hr × 24 hours. Administer insulin on sliding scale based on blood or urine glucose test per physician order.
Increased use of glucose during postpartum.	Monitor for hypoglycemia (see Chapter 2). Maintain IV glucose for 24 hours after birth then restart diabetic diet.
Increased postpartum complications, such as PIH.	Monitor VS for at least 48 hours. Be alert for PIH symptoms (see Chapter 2).
Hemorrhage due to uterine atony and increased amniotic fluid.	Monitor uterine involution.
Any infection complicates diabetic regulation and increases risk of acidosis.	Maintain excellent handwashing for self. Stress personal hygiene to avoid infections.

Effect of Postpartum on Diabetes

Altered parent-infant interaction due to baby requiring special observation.

Critical Nursing Interventions

Promote flexible visiting policy.

Keep parents informed of baby's progress and status.

If mother is breast–feeding have her increase her caloric intake by 400–500 Kcal/day (20% protein); adjust insulin dosage as needed per physician order. Provide for pumping or breast–feeding opportunities q2–4 hours around the clock.

DRUG GUIDE

Betamethasone (Celestone Solupan®)

Overview of Maternal-Fetal Action

"Betamethasone is a glucocorticoid which acts to accelerate fetal lung maturation and prevent hyaline membrane disease by inhibiting cell mitosis, increasing cell differentiation, promoting selected enzymatic actions, and participating in the storage and secretion of surfactant" (Bishop 1981). The best results are obtained when the fetus is between 30 and 32 weeks' gestation. It may be used as early as 26 weeks and as late as 34 weeks (Briggs et al 1986).

To obtain optimal results, birth should be delayed for at least 24 hours after the end of treatment. If birth does not occur, the effect of the drug disappears in about one week. A female fetus seems more likely than a male to obtain the most prophylactic effect (Briggs et al 1986).

Route, Dosage, Frequency

Prenatal maternal intramuscular administration of 12 mg of betamethasone is given once a day for 2 days. Repeated treatment will be needed on a weekly basis until 34 weeks of gestation (unless birth occurs).

Contraindications

Inability to delay birth for 24 to 48 hours

Adequate L:S ratio

Presence of a condition that necessitates immediate delivery (eg, maternal bleeding)

Presence of maternal infection, diabetes mellitus, hypertension

Concomitant use of tocolytic agents, which may increase risk of maternal pulmonary edema (Bishop 1981)

Gestational age greater than 34 completed weeks.

Maternal Side Effects

Bishop (1981) reports that suspected maternal risks include (a) initiation of lactation; (b) increased risk of infection; (c) augmentation of placental insufficiency in hypertensive women; (d) gastrointestinal bleeding; (e) inability to use estriol levels to assess fetal status; (f) pulmonary edema when used concurrently with tocolytics (such as ritodrine)

May cause Na^+ retention, K^+ loss, weight gain, edema, indigestion

Increased risk of infection if PROM present (Briggs et al 1986).

Effects of Fetus/Neonate

Lowered cortisol levels between 1 and 8 days following childbirth (Giacoia & Yaffe 1982)

Possible suppression of aldosterone levels up to 2 weeks following birth (Giacoia & Yaffe 1982)

Hypoglycemia

Increased risk of neonatal sepsis (Briggs et al 1986)

Animal studies have shown serious fetal side effects such as reduced head circumference, reduced weight of the fetal adrenal and thymus glands, and decreased placental weight (Briggs et al 1986). Human studies have not shown these effects, however.

Nursing Considerations

Assess for presence of contraindications.

Provide education regarding possible side effects.

Administer deep into gluteal muscle, avoid injection into deltoid (high incidence of local atrophy).

Periodically evaluate BP, pulse, weight, and edema.

Assess lab data for electrolytes.

Bromocriptine (Parlodel)

Overview of Obstetric Action

Bromocriptine is a dopamine agonist that acts to suppress lactation by stimulating the production of prolactin-inhibiting factor at the hypothalamic level. This results in decreased secretion of prolactin by the pituitary gland. The drug may also directly inhibit the pituitary by preventing the release of prolactin from the hormone-producing cells (Foster 1982). When administered postpartally it helps suppress milk production and decrease breast leakage and pain. It may also be used for suppression after lactation has already begun.

Route, Dosage, and Frequency

The usual dose is 2.5 mg orally two times per day. The total daily dose generally does not exceed 7.5 mg. The medication is usually taken for 2–3 weeks. Research regarding the efficacy of parenteral administration suggests that a single intramuscular dose of a microencapsulated form of bromocriptine may be effective in suppressing lactation when administered following birth. This would be useful following obstetric surgery or for women experiencing severe vomiting (Peters et al 1986).

Maternal Contraindications

Maternal hypotension, desire to breast-feed, pregnancy.

Maternal Side Effects

Hypotension is the primary side effect. To prevent problems associated with hypotension, administration should be delayed until the new mother's vital signs are stable. Other side effects include nausea, headache, dizziness, and occasionally faintness and vomiting.

Nursing Considerations

Administration should be delayed until maternal blood pressure is stable. Blood pressure should be carefully monitored if bromocriptine is administered concurrently with any antihypertensives. Taking bromocriptine with meals may help decrease the possibility of nausea. Early resumption of ovulation has occurred in women taking bromocriptine; the woman should be informed of this and receive information about contraceptives (Foster 1982). The woman should be advised that engorgement may occur when medication is stopped.

Clomid (Clomiphene Citrate)

Overview of Action

Clomid stimulates follicular growth by increasing secretion of FSH and LH. Ovulation is expected to occur five to ten days after last dose. Used when anovulation is caused by hypothalamic suppression, luteal phase dysfunction, oligo-ovulation and in vitro fertilization.

Route, Dosage, Frequency

Administered orally. Fifty mg/day to 250 mg/day from day 5 to day 9 (total of five days) of the menstrual cycle. Usually start with 50 mg/day and increase dose 50 mg each time (Kennedy & Adashi 1987). May need to give estrogen simultaneously if decrease in cervical mucus occurs.

Contraindications

Presence of ovarian enlargement, ovarian cysts, hyperstimulation syndrome, liver disease, visual problems, pregnancy.

Side Effects

Antiestrogenic effects may cause decrease in cervical mucus production.

Other side effects include: vasomotor flushes; abdominal distention and ovarian enlargement secondary to follicular growth and development and multiple corpus luteum formation; bloating, pain, soreness, breast discomfort; nausea and vomiting; visual symptoms (spots, flashes); headaches; dryness or loss of hair; multiple pregnancies.

Nursing Considerations

Determine if couple has been advised to have sexual intercourse every other day for one week beginning five days after the last day of medications.

Instruct couple on use of BBT chart to assess if ovulation has occurred. Also inform couple that plasma progesterone, cervical mucus, and vaginal cytology may be done.

Remind couples that if the woman doesn't have a period she must be checked for the possibility of pregnancy before another trial of Clomid is started.

Danazol (Danocrine)

Overview of Action

Danazol is a testosterone derivative with a mild androgenic effect. The drug has an antigonadotropic effect that results in the suppression of both follicle-stimulating hormone (FSH) and luteinizing hormone (LH). As a consequence, ovulation is suppressed and amenorrhea develops. Danazol also reduces levels of sex steroids by inhibiting the enzymes responsible for their production, and binds steroid hormone receptors on endometrial tissue implants (Hill & Herbert 1988). This results in atrophy of endometrial tissue implants and endometrium within the uterus. Dose-related menstrual changes have been associated with this drug. At lower dosages (50–100 mg), menstrual bleeding may be regular or irregular. With dosages of 200–400 mg, 40% to 90% of women experience amenorrhea. Progress of endometriosis is stopped and the woman's pain is relieved. The drug may also be used to treat fibrocystic breast disease.

Route, Dosage, Frequency

Endometriosis: 400 mg, orally, two times per day for three to six months. Therapy is begun if pregnancy test is negative or during woman's menstrual period. Treatment may be extended for nine months or restarted if symptoms recur.

Breast disease: 400 mg/day orally. Long-term effects of treatment not known.

Contraindications

Pregnancy

Breast-feeding women

Impaired kidney, heart, or liver function

Undiagnosed abnormal vaginal bleeding

Side Effects

Vaginal bleeding	Acne
Vasomotor instability	Oily skin and hair
Hirsutism	Weight gain
Reduced libido	Decreased breast size
Voice changes, hoarseness	Irritability, depression

Edema

Muscle cramps

Headaches

Nausea

Clitoral enlargement

Sleep disorders, fatigue

Gastroenteritis

Signs of atrophic vaginitis

Alopecia

Amenorrhea

Changed lab values including: reduced high-density lipoprotein (HDL); increased low-density lipoprotein (LDL); increased liver enzyme levels (serum glutamic-oxaloacetic transaminase [SGOT], serum glutamic-pyruvic transaminase [SGPT], creatinine phosphokinase [CPK], lactic dehydrogenase [LDH])

Nursing Considerations

1. Inform woman about potential side effects; stress that menses and ovulation usually resume within two to three months after discontinuing therapy.

2. Continue routine breast examinations and report any enlarged or hardened breast nodules.

3. Obtain baseline and other liver function tests as ordered.

4. Voice changes should be reported immediately and the medication stopped to avoid permanent damage.

5. Observe woman for signs of virilization.

6. Since ovulation may not be suppressed, a back-up, nonhormonal form of birth control should be used if the woman wishes to avoid conception (Govoni & Hayes 1988).

Erythromycin (Ilotycin) Ophthalmic Ointment

Overview of Neonatal Action

Erythromycin (Ilotycin) is used as prophylactic treatment of ophthalmia neonatorum, which is caused by the bacteria *Neisseria gonorrhoeae*. Preventive treatment of gonorrhea in the newborn is required by law. Erythromycin is also effective against ophthalmic chlamydial infections. It is either bacteriostatic or bactericidal depending on the organisms involved and the concentration of drug.

Route, Dosage, Frequency

Ophthalmic ointment (0.5%) is instilled as a narrow ribbon or strand, ¼-inch long, along the lower conjunctival surface of each eye, starting at the inner canthus. It is instilled only once in each eye. Administration may be done in the birthing area or later in the nursery so that eye contact is facilitated and the bonding process immediately after birth is not interrupted. After administration, gently close eye and manipulate to ensure spread of ointment (Milan & McFeely 1990; Pawlak & Herfert 1990).

Neonatal Side Effects

Sensitivity reaction; may interfere with ability to focus and may cause edema and inflammation. Side effects usually disappear in 24–48 hours.

Nursing Considerations

Wash hands immediately prior to instillation to prevent introduction of bacteria.

Do not irrigate the eyes after instillation. Use new tube or single-use container for ophthalmic ointment administration shortly after birth.

Observe for hypersensitivity.

Teach parents about need for eye prophylaxis. Educate them regarding side effects and signs that need to be reported to the physician/CNM.

Magnesium Sulfate (MgSO₄)

Overview of Obstetric Action

$MgSO_4$ acts as a CNS depressant by decreasing the quantity of acetylcholine released by motor nerve impulses and thereby blocking neuromuscular transmission. This action reduces the possibility of convulsion, which is why $MgSO_4$ is used in the treatment of preeclampsia. Because magnesium sulfate secondarily relaxes smooth muscle, it may decrease the blood pressure, although it is not considered an antihypertensive, and may also decrease the frequency and intensity of uterine contractions.

Route, Dosage, Frequency

MgSO$_4$ is generally given intravenously to control dosage more accurately and prevent overdosage. An occasional physician still prescribes intramuscular administration. However it is painful and irritating to the tissues and does not permit the close control that IV administration does.

IV: The intravenous route allows for immediate onset of action and avoids the discomfort associated with IM administration. It must be given by infusion pump for accurate dosage.

Loading Dose: 4 g MgSO$_4$ as a 20% solution is administered over a 3–5 minute period (Scott & Worley 1990; Cunningham et al 1989). (One authority recommends a loading dose of 6 g MgSO$_4$ in 100 mL D$_5$W infused over a 15–20 minute period [Sibai 1990].)

Maintenance Dose: Based on serum magnesium levels and deep tendon reflexes, 2 g/hr is administered.

Maternal Contraindications

Extreme care is necessary in administration to women with impaired renal function because the drug is eliminated by the kidneys and toxic magnesium levels may develop quickly.

Maternal Side Effects

Most maternal side effects are related to magnesium toxicity. Sweating, a feeling of warmth, flushing, nausea, slurred speech, depression or absence of reflexes, muscular weakness, hypothermia, oliguria, confusion, circulatory collapse, and respiratory paralysis are all possible side effects. Rapid administration of large doses may cause cardiac arrest.

Effects on Fetus/Neonate

The drug readily crosses the placenta. Some authorities suggest that transient decrease in FHR variability may occur, while others report that no change occurred. Similarly some report low Apgar scores, hypotonia, and respiratory depression in the newborn, while others report no ill effects. Sibai (1987) suggests that the majority of ill effects observed in the newborn may actually be related to fetal growth retardation, prematurity, or perinatal asphyxia.

Nursing Considerations

1. Monitor the blood pressure closely during administration.

2. Monitor respirations closely. If the rate is less than 14–16/min, magnesium toxicity may be developing, and further assessments are indicated. Many protocols require stopping the medication if the respiratory rate falls below 12/min.

3. Assess knee jerk (patellar tendon reflex) for evidence of diminished or absent reflexes. Loss of reflexes is often the first sign of developing toxicity (Sibai 1990).

4. Determine urinary output. Output less than 100 mL during the preceding 4-hour period may result in the accumulation of toxic levels of magnesium.

5. If the respirations or urinary output fall below specified levels or if the reflexes are diminished or absent, no further magnesium should be administered until these factors return to normal.

6. The antagonist of magnesium sulfate is calcium. Consequently an ampule of calcium gluconate should be available at the bedside. The usual dose is 1 g given IV over a period of about 3 minutes.

7. Monitor fetal heart tones continuously with IV administration.

8. Continue $MgSO_4$ infusion for approximately 24 hours after delivery as prophylaxis against postpartum seizures.

Note: Protocols for magnesium sulfate administration may vary somewhat according to agency policy. Consequently individuals are referred to their own agency protocols for specific guidelines.

Meperidine Hydrochloride (Demerol)

Overview of Obstetric Action

Meperidine hydrochloride is a narcotic analgesic that interferes with pain impulses at the subcortical level of the brain. In addition, it enhances analgesia by altering the physiologic response to pain, suppressing anxiety and apprehension, and creating a euphoric feeling. Meperidine hydrochloride is used during labor to provide analgesia. Peak analgesia occurs in 40 to 60 minutes with intramuscular and in 5 to 7 minutes with intravenous administration. Duration is 2 to 4 hours. Administration after labor has reached the active phase does not appear to delay labor or decrease uterine contraction frequency or duration. Meperidine HCl crosses the placental barrier and appears in cord blood within 2 minutes and after maternal intravenous injection can be detected in amniotic fluid 30 minutes after IM injection (Briggs et al 1990).

Route, Dosage, Frequency

IM: 50 to 100 mg every 3 to 4 hours

IV: 25 to 50 mg by slow intravenous push every 3 to 4 hours

Maternal Contraindications

Hypersensitivity to meperidine, asthma

CNS depression

Respiratory depression

Fetal distress

Preterm labor if birth is imminent

Hypotension

Respirations <12 per minute

Concurrent use with anticonvulsants may increase depressant effects

Maternal Side Effects

Respiratory depression

Nausea and vomiting, dry mouth

Drowsiness, dizziness, flushing

Transient hypotension

Increased intracranial pressure (Skidmore-Roth 1991)

May precipitate or aggravate seizures in women prone to convulsive activity (Giacoia & Yaffee 1982)

Effect on Fetus/Neonate

Neonatal respiratory depression may occur if birth occurs 60 minutes or longer after administration of the drug to the mother; incidence of respiratory depression peaks at 2 to 3 hours after administration (Briggs et al 1990).

Neonatal hypotonia, lethargy, interference of thermoregulatory response

Neurologic and behavioral alterations for up to 72 hours after birth; presence of meperidine in neonatal urine up to 3 days following birth (Briggs et al 1990).

May have depressed attention and social responsiveness for first 6 weeks of life (Briggs et al 1990)

Nursing Considerations

Assess the woman's history, labor and fetal status, maternal blood pressure and respirations to identify contraindications to administration.

Intramuscular doses should be injected deeply to avoid irritation to subcutaneous tissue.

Intravenous doses should be diluted and administered slowly, just as the contraction diminishes, to minimize the effect of rapid absorption on the fetus.

Stop intravenous solution while injecting the analgesic.

Use IV port nearest the patient for injection of the analgesic. Slowly restart the IV to prevent injecting a bolus of the analgesic.

If the IV line is being used for other drug administration or other drugs are mixed in the IV solution, flush the line to prevent incompatibility.

Provide for the woman's safety by instructing her to remain on bed rest and by keeping side rails up and placing call bell within reach.

Evaluate effect of drug.

Observe for maternal side effects.

Assess for respiratory depression, notify physician/CNM if respirations are <12/min (Skidmore-Roth 1991).

Observe newborn for respiratory depression, be prepared to initiate resuscitative measures and administer antagonist naloxone if needed.

Methylergonovine Maleate (Methergine)

Overview of Obstetric Action

Methylergonovine maleate is an ergot alkaloid that stimulates smooth muscle tissue. Because the smooth muscle of the uterus is especially sensitive to this drug, it is used postpartally to stimulate the uterus to contract. This contraction clamps off uterine blood vessels and prevents hemorrhage. In addition, the drug has a vasoconstrictive effect on all blood vessels, especially the larger arteries. This may result in hypertension, particularly in a woman whose blood pressure is already elevated.

Route, Dosage, and Frequency

Methergine has a rapid onset of action and may be given intramuscularly, orally, or intravenously.

Usual IM dose: 0.2 mg following expulsion of the placenta. The dose may be repeated every 2–4 hours if necessary.

Usual oral dose: 0.2 mg every 4 hours (six doses).

Usual IV dose: Because the adverse effects of Methergine are far more severe with IV administration, this route is seldom used. If Methergine is given intravenously, the rate should *not* exceed 0.2 mg/min, and the client's blood pressure should be monitored prior to administration and frequently afterward until it is stable.

Maternal Contraindications

Pregnancy, hepatic or renal disease, cardiac disease and hypertension, contraindicate this drug's use (Karch & Boyd 1989).

Maternal Side Effects

Hypertension (particularly when administered IV), nausea, vomiting, headache, bradycardia, dizziness, tinnitus, abdominal cramps, palpitations, dyspnea, chest pain, and allergic reactions may be noted.

Effects on Fetus/Neonate

Because Methergine has a long duration of action and can thus produce tetanic contractions, it should never be used during pregnancy as it may result in fetal trauma or death.

Nursing Considerations

1. Monitor fundal height and consistency and the amount and character of the lochia.

2. Assess the blood pressure before administration.

3. Observe for adverse effects or symptoms of ergot toxicity.

Naloxone Hydrochloride (Narcan)

Overview of Neonatal Action

Naloxone hydrochloride (Narcan) is used to reverse respiratory depression due to acute narcotic toxicity. It displaces morphinelike drugs from receptor sites on the neurons; therefore, the narcotics can no longer exert their depressive effects. Naloxone reverses narcotic-induced respiratory depression, analgesia, sedation; hypotension, and pupillary constriction.

Route, Dosage, Frequency

Intravenous dose is 0.01 mg/kg, usually through umbilical vein, although naloxone can be given intramuscularly. Neonatal dose is supplied as 0.02 mg/mL solution (0.5–1.0 mL for preterms and 2 mL for full-terms). Reversal of drug depression occurs within 1 to 2 minutes. The duration of action is variable (minutes to hours) and depends on amount of drug present and rate of excretion. Dose may be repeated in 5 minutes. If no improvement after two or three doses, naloxone administration should be discontinued. If initial reversal occurs, repeat dose as needed. Some institutions use 0.1 mg/kg of 0.4 mg/mL Narcan preparation.

Neonatal Contraindications

Must be used with caution in infants of narcotic-addicted mothers as it may precipitate acute withdrawal syndrome. Respiratory depression resulting from nonmorphine drugs such as sedatives, hypnotics, anesthetics, or other nonnarcotic CNS depressants.

Neonatal Side Effects

Excessive doses may result in irritability and increased crying, and possibly prolongation of PTT

Tachycardia

Nursing Considerations

Monitor respirations closely—rate and depth.

Assess for return of respiratory depression when naloxone effects wear off and effects of longer-acting narcotic reappear.

Have resuscitative equipment, O_2, and ventilatory equipment available.

Monitor bleeding studies.

Note that naloxone is incompatible with alkaline solutions.

Oxytocin (Pitocin)

Overview of Obstetric Action

Oxytocin (Pitocin) exerts a selective stimulatory effect on the smooth muscle of the uterus and blood vessels. Oxytocin affects the myometrial cells of the uterus by increasing the excitability of the muscle cell, increasing the strength of the muscle contraction, and supporting propagation of the contraction (movement of the contraction from one myometrial cell to the next). Its effect on the uterine contraction depends on the dosage used and on the excitability of the myometrial cells. During the first half of gestation, little excitability of the myometrium occurs and the uterus is fairly resistant to the effects of oxytocin. However, from midgestation on, the uterus responds increasingly to exogenous intravenous oxytocin. When at term, cautious use of diluted oxytocin, administered intravenously, results in a slow rise of uterine activity.

The circulatory half-life of oxytocin is 3–4 minutes. It takes approximately 40 minutes for a particular dose of oxytocin to reach a steady-state plasma concentration (Nugent 1989).

The effects of oxytocin on the cardiovascular system can be pronounced. There may be an initial decrease in the blood pressure, but with prolonged administration, a 30% increase in the baseline blood pressure may be noted. Cardiac output and stroke volume are increased. With doses of 20 mU/min or above, the antidiuretic effect of oxytocin results in a decrease of free water exchange in the kidney and a marked decrease in urine output (Marshall 1985).

Oxytocin is used to induce labor at term and to augment uterine contractions in the first and second stages of labor. Oxytocin may also be used immediately after birth to stimulate uterine contraction and thereby control uterine atony.

Oxytocin is not thought to cross the placenta because of its molecular weight and the presence of oxytocinase in the placenta (Giacoia & Yaffe 1982).

Route, Dosage, Frequency

For induction of labor: Add 10 units Pitocin (1 mL) to 1000 mL of intravenous solution. (The resulting concentration is 10 mU oxytocin per 1 mL of intravenous fluid.) Using an infusion pump, administer IV, starting at 0.5 mU/min and increasing the rate stepwise at no less than every 30–60 minutes until good contractions (every 2–3 minutes, each lasting 40–60 seconds) are achieved.

Maternal Contraindications

Severe preeclampsia-eclampsia (PIH)

Predisposition to uterine rupture (in nullipara over 35 years of age, multigravida 4 or more, overdistention of the uterus, previous major surgery of the cervix or uterus)

Cephalopelvic disproportion

Malpresentation or malposition of the fetus, cord prolapse

Preterm infant

Rigid, unripe cervix; total placenta previa

Presence of fetal distress

Maternal Side Effects

Hyperstimulation of the uterus results in hypercontractility, which in turn may cause the following:

Abruptio placentae

Impaired uterine blood flow → fetal hypoxia

Rapid labor → cervical lacerations

Rapid labor and birth → lacerations of cervix, vagina, perineum, uterine atony, fetal trauma

Uterine rupture

Water intoxication (nausea, vomiting, hypotension, tachycardia, cardiac arrhythmia) if oxytocin is given in electrolyte-free solution or at a rate exceeding 20 mU/min. Hypotension with rapid IV bolus administration postpartum.

Effect on Fetus/Neonate

Fetal effects are primarily associated with the presence of hypercontractility of the maternal uterus. Hypercontractility causes a decrease in the oxygen supply to the fetus, which is reflected by irregularities and/or decrease in FHR. Hyperbilirubinemia.

Trauma from rapid birth.

Nursing Considerations

Explain induction or augmentation procedure to client.

Apply fetal monitor and obtain 15- to 20-minute tracing and NST to assess FHR before starting IV oxytocin.

For induction or augmentation of labor, start with primary IV and piggy-back secondary IV with oxytocin.

Ensure continuous fetal and uterine contraction monitoring.

The maximum rate is 40 mU/min (ACOG 1988). Decrease oxytocin by similar increments once labor has progressed to 5–6 cm dilatation (ACOG 1988).

0.5 mU/min = 3 mL/hr	8 mU/min = 48 mL/hr
1.0 mU/min = 6 mL/hr	10 mU/min = 60 mL/hr
1.5 mU/min = 9 mL/hr	12 mU/min = 72 mL/hr
2 mU/min = 12 mL/hr	15 mU/min = 90 mL/hr
4 mU/min = 24 mL/hr	18 mU/min = 108 mL/hr
6 mU/min = 36 mL/hr	20 mU/min = 120 mL/hr

Protocols may vary from one agency to another.

For augmentation of labor: Prepare and administer IV Pitocin as for labor induction. Increase rate until labor contractions are of good quality. The flow rate is gradually increased at no less than every 30 minutes to a maximum of 10 mU/min (Cunningham et al 1989). In some settings, or in a situation when only limited fluids may be administered, a more concentrated solution may be used. When 10 U Pitocin is added to 500 mL IV solution the resulting concentration is 1 mU/min = 3 mL/hr. If 10 U Pitocin is added to 250 mL IV solution the concentration is 1 mU/min = 1.5 mL/hr.

For administration after expulsion of placenta: One dose of 10 units Pitocin (1 mL) is given intramuscularly or by slow intravenous push or added to IV fluids for continuous infusion.

Assess FHR, maternal blood pressure, pulse, and uterine contraction frequency, duration, and resting tone before each increase in oxytocin infusion rate.

Record all assessments and IV rate on monitor strip and on client's chart. Record oxytocin infusion rate in mU/min and mL/hour. For example: 0.5 mU/min (3 mL/hr)

Record all client activities (such as change of position, vomiting), procedures done (amniotomy, sterile vaginal examination), and administration of analgesics on monitor strip to allow for interpretation and evaluation of tracing.

Assess cervical dilatation as needed.

Apply nursing comfort measures.

Discontinue IV oxytocin infusion and infuse primary solution when (a) fetal distress is noted (bradycardia, late or variable decelerations; (b) uterine contractions are more frequent than every 2 minutes; (c) duration of contractions exceeds more than 60 seconds; or (d) insufficient relaxation of the uterus between contractions or a steady increase in resting tone are noted (ACOG 1988); in addition to discontinuing IV oxytocin infusion, turn client to side, and if fetal distress is present, administer oxygen by tight face mask at 6–10 L/min; notify physician.

Maintain intake and output record.

Postpartum Epidural Morphine

Overview of Obstetric Action

Epidural morphine is used to provide relief of pain associated with cesarean birth, extensive episiotomies (mediolaterals), or third- and fourth-degree lacerations. Epidural morphine pain relief results directly from its effect on the opiate receptors in the spinal cord (it depresses pain impulse transmission). Morphine binds opiate receptors, thereby altering both the perception of and emotional response to pain. Women experience little or no discomfort or pain during recovery and for up to 24 hours afterward. There is no motor or sympathetic block or associated hypotension. Onset of analgesia is slower, but duration is longer.

Route, Dosage, Frequency

Five to seven and one-half mg of morphine is injected through a catheter into the epidural space, providing pain relief for about 24 hours.

Maternal Contraindications

Allergy to morphine, narcotic addiction, or chronic debilitating respiratory disease (Inturrisi et al 1988).

Maternal Side Effects

Late onset respiratory depression (rare but may occur 8–12 hours after administration), nausea and vomiting (occurring between four and seven hours after injection), itching (begins within three hours and lasts up to ten hours), urinary retention, and, rarely, somnolence. Side effects can be managed with naloxone.

Neonatal Effects

No adverse effects since medication is injected after birth of baby.

Nursing Considerations

Assess client's sensitivity to narcotics on admission.

Monitor and evaluate analgesic effect. Ask client about comfort level and notify anesthesiologist of inadequate pain relief.

Check catheter for obvious knots, breaks, and leakage at insertion site and catheter hub.

Assess for pruritus (scratching and rubbing, especially around face and neck).

Administer comfort measures for narcotic-induced pruritus, such as: lotion, back rubs, cool/warm packs, or diversional activities. If the itching can be tolerated, naloxone should be avoided, especially since it counteracts the pain relief.

If allergic reaction (urticaria, edema, or respiratory difficulties) occurs, administer naloxone or diphenhydramine per physician order.

Provide comfort measures for nausea/vomiting, such as frequent oral hygiene or gradual increase of activity; administer naloxone, trimethobenzamide (Tigan) or metoclopramide HCl per physician order (Henrikson and Wild 1988).

Assess postural blood pressure and heart rate before ambulation.

Assist client with her first ambulation and then as needed.

Assess respiratory function every hour for 24 hours, then q2–8 hrs as needed. Also assess level of consciousness and mucous membrane color. May need to monitor client via apnea monitor for 24 hours.

Monitor urinary output and assess bladder for distention. Assist client to void.

Rh$_o$ (D) Immune Globulin (Human) (RhoGAM, Gamulin Rh, HypoRho-D, MICRhoGAM, Mini-Gamulin RH)

Overview of Obstetrical Action

Rh$_o$ (D) immune globulin is a concentrated solution of immunoglobulin (IgG) that contains anti-Rh$_o$ (D) from human fractionated plasma. It functions by suppressing the immune response of nonsensitized Rh$_o$ (D)-negative women who are exposed to Rh$_o$ (D or D^u) positive blood. It prevents maternal isoimmunization by lysis of fetal Rh-positive red blood cells (RBCs) that may be circulating in the maternal blood stream after birth. RhoGAM prevents hemolytic disease of the newborn. In addition, it is given to Rh-negative women exposed to Rh-positive blood after abortion, miscarriage, and amniocentesis.

Route, Dosage, Frequency

IM injection in deltoid. Single-dose vials. One standard dose (300 μg) vial given for antepartum prophylaxis at approximately 28 weeks to Rh-negative woman unless father of the baby is known to be Rh-negative, for Rh-negative unimmunized woman undergoing amniocentesis, and for postpartum prophylaxis within 72 hours of birth if lab tests indicate no sensitization has occurred. Multiple dose is required when fetomaternal hemorrhage is > 30 mL. Microdose preparation (50 μg) is given to unsensitized Rh-negative woman who aborts before 13 weeks.

Maternal Contraindications

Previous sensitization, hypersensitization, Rh$_o$ (O)-positive/D^u-positive client (Mosby's Nursing Drug Reference 1991).

Maternal Side Effects

Irritation at injection site, fever, lethargy, and myalgia. Potential allergic reaction, rare systemic reactions.

Nursing Considerations

Note the blood type and Rh status of all pregnant women.

Send Rh blood workup on mother and baby and cord blood for type and cross match on baby.

If large fetomaternal transfusion is suspected, it may be necessary to send blood for Betke-Kleihauer or D^u test, which detect 20 mL or more of Rh-positive fetal blood in the maternal circulation.

Confirm that the following criteria for administration are present: Mother must be Rh negative with no Rh antibodies present (negative indirect Coomb's test) in order to receive Rh immune globulin.

Client teaching: Instruct Rh-negative woman that the drug needs to be given after subsequent births if the baby is Rh positive. She should carry information on Rh status and dates of RhoGAM injections with her at all times.

Check preparation with another nurse. Assure correct vial is used for the client (each vial is cross matched to the specific woman and must be carefully checked).

Administer IM only in deltoid; inject entire contents of vial, and aspirate prior to injecting.

Assess for tenderness at injection site and any other side effects.

Do not administer discolored/precipitated solutions.

Keep solutions stored in refrigerator.

Record lot number, route, dose, client education, and any other data per agency policy.

Ritodrine (Yutopar)

Overview of Obstetric Action

Ritodrine is a sympathomimetic β_2-adrenergic agonist which is FDA approved for use in treatment of preterm labor. It exerts its effect on beta$_2$ receptors, which are found in uterine smooth muscle, bronchioles, and diaphragm. Stimulation of beta$_2$ receptors results in uterine relaxation, bronchodilation, vasodilation, and muscle glycogenolysis. As muscles in the vessel walls relax, hypotension is induced. The body compensates by increasing maternal heart rate and pulse pressure.

Ritodrine causes a potassium shift, which may cause hypokalemia but not total body potassium depletion. There may also be an increase in blood glucose and plasma insulin levels and stimulation of glycogen release from muscles and the liver (NAACOG 1984).

Route, Dosage, Frequency

Add 150 mg of ritodrine to 500 mL IV fluid and administer as a piggyback to a primary IV. The resulting dilution is 0.3 mg/mL. Note: Some authorities recommend a saline solution and others believe a dextrose solution reduces the incidence of pulmonary edema (Niebyl et al 1986). The initial dose is 0.1 mg/min (20 mL/hr on an adult infusion pump). The dose is increased 0.05 mg/min (10 mL/hr on an adult infusion pump) every 10 minutes until contractions cease. Maximum dosage is 0.35 mg/min (70 mL/hr on an adult infusion pump). When contractions cease, the infusion rate may be decreased by 0.5 mg/min (10 mL/hr on an adult infusion pump). The infusion may be maintained at a low rate for a period of hours to assure that contractions do not begin again. Before the intravenous infusion is discontinued, PO administration is begun (Pauerstein, 1987).

Gonik and Creasy (1986) recommend administration of oral ritodrine 30 minutes before ending IV ritodrine. The initial PO dose is 10–20 mg every 2 hours, and the time between doses may be increased to 3–4 hours based on uterine response and maternal pulse. The maternal pulse is maintained in the 90–100 BPM range.

This dosage can be administered safely to a maximum of 120 mg over 24 hours. The length of therapy varies.

Current research is directed toward the use of a single injection of ritodrine for other obstetric problems. Rapid relaxation of the uterus may be needed in the presence of tetanic contractions and cord prolapse (Ingemarsson et al 1985b). It has also been suggested for use with fetal bradycardia to improve the heart rate (Ingemarsson et al 1985a) and to inhibit labor in order to manage fetal distress (Caritis et al 1985).

Maternal Contraindications

Preterm labor accompanied by cervical dilatation greater than 4 cm, chorioamniotitis, severe preeclampsia-eclampsia, severe bleeding, fetal death, significant IUGR contraindicate use of ritodrine, as do any of the following:

Hypovolemia, uncontrolled hypertension

Pulmonary hypertension

Cardiac disease, arrhythmias

Diabetes mellitus (use with caution)

Concurrent therapy with glucocorticoids (use with caution)

Gestation less than 20 weeks

Hyperthyroidism (Givens 1988)

Chronic hepatic or renal disease

Maternal Side Effects

Tachycardia, occasionally premature ventricular contractions (PVCs), increased stroke volume, slight increase in systolic and decrease in diastolic pressure, palpitations, tremors, nervousness, nausea and vomiting, headache, erythema, hypotension, shortness of breath (Bealle et al 1985)

Decreased peripheral vascular resistance, which lowers diastolic pressure → widening of pulse pressure

Hyperglycemia (usually peaks within 3 hours after initiation of therapy) (Pauerstein 1987)

Metabolic acidosis

Hypokalemia (causes internal redistribution)

Pulmonary edema in women treated concurrently with glucocorticoids, and who have fluid overload (Skidmore-Roth 1989).

Increased concentration of lactate and free fatty acids
ST segment depression, T wave flattening, prolongation of QT interval (Hendricks et al 1986)

Increase in plasma volume as indicated by decreases in hemoglobin, hematocrit, and serum albumin levels (Philipsen 1981)

Possible neutropenia with long-term IV therapy (Wang & Davidson 1986)

Effects on Fetus/Neonate

Fetal tachycardia, cardiac dysrhythmias

Increased serum glucose concentration

Fetal acidosis

Fetal hypoxia

Neonatal hypoglycemia, hypocalcemia, ↑ WBC

Neonatal paralytic ileus, irritability, tremors

Neonatal hypotension at birth

May decrease incidence of neonatal respiratory distress syndrome (Lipshitz 1981)

Nursing Considerations

Position woman in left side-lying position to increase placental perfusion and decrease incidence of hypotension.

Complete a history and assessment to identify possible presence of infection and maternal-fetal contraindications to treatment.

Explain procedure, which will include electronic fetal monitor, IV, frequent assessments, possible use of cardiac monitor, blood samples, intake and output, and daily weight, and potential for development of side effects, especially increase in pulse and fetal heart rate.

Monitor uterine activity and fetal heart rate by electronic fetal monitor.

Assess maternal BP and pulse every 10 minutes while dosage is being increased and while woman is being stabilized (Givens 1988). As long as dosage is being increased, some agency protocols recommend taking maternal BP and pulse prior to dose increase. Notify physician if maternal pulse > 120 bpm. (Note: Expect increase of 20–40 bpm. Maternal pulse may exceed 120 bpm for a brief period of time (Pauerstein 1987).

Assess respiratory rate and auscultate breath sounds with maternal vital signs. Note signs of pulmonary edema (rales and rhonchi). When oral therapy is begun, maternal BP, pulse, and respirations may be taken with each PO dose.

Monitor FHR with maternal assessments (Note: Expect increase of approximately 10 bpm. The rate should not exceed 180 bpm. Notify physician of rate > 180 bpm).

Apply antiembolism stockings to prevent pooling of blood in extremities.

Encourage passive range of motion in legs every 1–2 hours.

Assess hydration status by evaluating intake/output, skin turgor, mucous membranes, and urine concentration.

Maintain intake and output records. Intake is usually limited to between 1500 and 2500 mL/day (Pauerstein 1987) and 90–100 mL/hr (Shortridge 1983).

Intake and output are assessed hourly during initial IV therapy and every 4 hours during maintenance therapy (Givens 1988).

Weigh daily at same time after woman has emptied bladder, using same scale and same clothing.

Observe woman closely for problems associated with hypo-kalemia (muscle weakness, cardiac arrhythmia) and pulmonary edema (dyspnea, wheezing, coughing, rales or rhonchi, or tachypnea). Discontinue therapy if pulmonary edema or cardiac problems develop.

Assess lab data regarding electrolytes, glucose, and WBC (Givens 1988).

Have beta blocking agent available as antidote for betasym-pathomimetic therapy. Propranolol (Inderal) 0.25 mg IV is usually used (Shortridge 1983). It should be given by a physician and injected over at least 1 minute to reduce the potential for lowering the blood pressure and precipitating cardiac standstill. Cardiac monitoring should be continuous.

Provide psychosocial support. The threat of preterm labor produces anxiety. Provide information and counseling for the woman and partner, and encourage questions. Assist them in making life-style changes such as more frequent rest periods, cessation of employment, and possible changes in sexual activity. If woman is discharged on oral therapy, teach her to take medications on time to ensure optimum effect, to observe for signs of preterm labor, and to assess her pulse with each dose. The woman needs to report pulse above 120, palpitations, tremors, agitation, nervousness, chest pain, and any difficulty breathing.

If birth occurs when woman is on ritodrine therapy, assess new-born for presence of side effects (NAACOG 1984).

It is recommended to discontinue ritodrine in the presence of any of the following: Maternal heart rate above 140 bpm or fetal heart rate above 200 bpm, more than 6 maternal or fetal premature ventricular contractions/min, maternal systolic pressure above 180 mm Hg or diastolic below 40 mm Hg, chest pain, shortness of breath (Bealle et al 1985).

Rubella Virus Vaccine (Meruvax 2)

Overview of Obstetrical Action

Rubella vaccine is a live attenuated virus that stimulates active immunity against the rubella virus. Rubella acquired during pregnancy may result in congenital rubella syndrome (CRS), with associated fetal anomalies. The greatest risk period for the fetus is from one week prior to four weeks after conception. Women who have not had rubella or who are serologically negative (ie, titer of 1:10 or less) are candidates for the vaccination to prevent fetal anomalies in future pregnancies. It should be given in the immediate postpartum period and/or if avoidance of pregnancy for at least three months can be assured. Nursing mothers can be vaccinated since live, attenuated rubella virus is not communicable nor is it excreted in breast milk. If mother receives both rubella vaccine and RhoGAM, antibody formation to rubella may be suppressed by the RhoGAM injection. Mother may be retested for maternal rubella immune status in three months (Varney 1987).

Route, Dosage, Frequency

Single-dose vial; inject subcutaneously in outer aspect of the upper arm (deltoid).

Maternal Contraindications

Women with allergies to ducks or duck eggs (may have a hypersensitivity reaction and require adrenalin), women with allergy to neomycin (vaccine contains neomycin), women on immunosuppression drugs (corticosteroids, irradiation, alkylating agents, or antimetabolites), or women who have received a blood transfusion, plasma transfusion, or serum immune globulin within the previous three months. If pregnancy status is unknown, do not give vaccine, as it may be teratogenic.

Maternal Side Effects

Burning or stinging at the injection site. Two to four weeks later, a transient rash over the body, arthralgia, malaise, sore throat, or headache may occur.

Nursing Considerations

Instruct women to **avoid pregnancy for three months** following vaccination.

Provide information on contraceptives and their use.

Check if woman has signed an informed consent form (per agency protocol) and received written information about the vaccine, its side effects, and risks.

Ascertain whether mother is to receive RhoGAM as well as rubella and instruct mother that a rubella titer should be re-drawn in about three months.

Sodium Bicarbonate

Overview of Neonatal Action

Sodium bicarbonate is an alkalizing agent. It buffers hydrogen ions caused by accumulation of lactic acid from anaerobic metabolism occurring during hypoxemia. Sodium bicarbonate thereby raises the blood pH, reversing the metabolic acidosis. Sodium bicarbonate should *only* be used to correct severe metabolic acidosis in asphyxiated newborns once adequate ventilation has been established.

Note: Sodium bicarbonate dissociates in solution into sodium ion and carbonic acid, which can split into water and carbon dioxide. The carbon dioxide must be eliminated via the respiratory tract.

Route, Dosage, Frequency

For resuscitation and severe asphyxiation: intravenous push via umbilical vein catheter for quick infusion. Dosage is 2 mEq/Kg: 4 mL of 0.5 mEq/mL (4.2%) or 2 mL of mEq/mL (8.4%). 8.4% solution diluted at least 1:1 with sterile water to decrease the osmolarity; infuse at rate no faster than 1 mEq/kg/min. Can repeat every 15 minutes if needed for total of 4 doses. For marked metabolic acidosis: a pH of less than 7.05 and a base deficit of 15 mEq/L or more should be corrected using a 0.5 mEq/mL solution of sodium bicarbonate at a rate of 1 mEq/kg/min or slower. Calculate total dosage by the following formula:

$$mEq = 0.3 \times weight\ (kg) \times base\ deficit\ in\ mEq/L$$

Neonatal Contraindications

Inadequate respiratory ventilation that causes a rise in PCO_2 and a decrease in pH

Presence of edema; metabolic or respiratory alkalosis; and hypocalcemia, anuria, or oliguria

Neonatal Side Effects

Hypernatremia, hyperosmolarity, fluid overload

Intracranial hemorrhage (rapid infusion of bicarbonate increases serum osmolarity, causing a shift of interstitial fluid into the blood and capillary rupture)

Nursing Considerations

Assess for any contraindications.

Monitor intake and output rates.

Assess adequacy of ventilation by monitoring respiratory status, rate, and depth; ventilate as necessary.

Dilute bicarbonate prior to administration into umbilical vein catheter (for resuscitation) or peripheral IV to prevent sloughing of tissue.

Evaluate effectiveness of drug by monitoring arterial blood gases for PCO_2, bicarbonate concentration, and pH determination.

Incompatible with acidic solutions.

Administration with calcium creates precipitates.

Vitamin K₁ Phytonadione (AquaMEPHYTON)

Overview of Neonatal Action

Phytonadione is used in prophylaxis and treatment of hemorrhagic disease of the newborn. It promotes liver formation of the clotting factors II, VII, IX, and X. At birth the neonate does not have the bacteria in the colon that is necessary for synthesizing fat-soluble vitamin K_1, therefore the newborn may have decreased levels of prothrombin during the first 5–8 days of life reflected by a prolongation of prothrombin time.

Route, Dosage, Frequency

Intramuscular injection is given in the vastus lateralis thigh muscle. A one-time only prophylactic dose of 0.5–1.0 mg is given in the birthing area or upon admission to the newborn nursery. If the mother received anticoagulants during pregnancy, an additional dose may be ordered by the physician and is given at 6–8 hours post first injection.

Neonatal Side Effects

Pain and edema may occur at injection site. Possible allergic reactions such as rash and urticaria.

Nursing Considerations

Observe for bleeding (usually occurs on second or third day). Bleeding may be seen as generalized ecchymoses or bleeding from umbilical cord, circumcision site, nose, or gastrointestinal tract. Results of serial PT and PTT should be assessed.

Observe for jaundice and kernicterus especially in preterm infants.

Observe for signs of local inflammation.

Protect drug from light.

REFERENCES

American College of Obstetricians and Gynecologists: *Induction and Augmentation of Labor.* Technical Bulletin No. 110. Washington, DC, 1988.

Bealle MH et al: A comparison of ritodrine, terbutaline, and magnesium sulfate for the suppression of preterm labor. *Am J Obstet Gynecol* 1985; 153:854.

Bishop EH: Acceleration of fetal pulmonary maturity. *Obstet Gynecol* 1981; 58(Suppl):48.

Briggs GC et al: *Drugs in Pregnancy and Lactation.* 2nd ed. Baltimore: Williams and Wilkins, 1986.

Briggs GG, Freeman RK, Yaffe SJ: *Drugs in Pregnancy and Lactation,* 3rd ed. Baltimore: Williams & Wilkins, 1990.

Caritas SN et al: Evaluation of the pharmacodynamics and pharmacokinetics of ritodrine when administered as a loading dose. *Am J Obstet Gynecol* 1985; 152:1026.

Cunningham FG, MacDonald PC, Gant NF: *Williams Obstetrics,* 18th ed. Norwalk, CT: Appleton & Lange, 1989.

Foster S: Bromocriptine: Suppressing lactation. *MCN* March/April 1982; 7:99.

Giacoia GP, Yaffee S: Perinatal pharmacology, in Sciarri JJ (ed) *Gynecology and Obstetrics.* Vol 3. Philadelphia: Harper & Row, 1982.

Giacoia GP, Yaffe S: Perinatal pharmacology. In: *Gynecology and Obstetrics,* Vol. 3. Sciarri JJ (editor). Philadelphia: Harper & Row, 1982, Ch 100.

Givens SR: Update on tocolytic therapy in the management of preterm labor. *J Perinatal Neonatal Nurs* 1988; 2:1.

Gonik B, Creasy RK: Preterm labor: Its diagnosis and management. *Am J Obstet Gynecol* 1986; 154:3.

Govoni LE, Hayes JE: *Drugs and Nursing Implications,* 6th ed. Norwalk, CT: Appleton-Century-Crofts, 1988.

Hendricks SK et al: Electrocardiographic changes associated with ritodrine-induced maternal tachycardia and hypokalemia. *Am J Obstet Gynecol* 1986; 154:921.

Henrikson ML, Wild LR: A nursing process approach to epidural analgesia. *JOGNN* 1988; 17(5):316.

Hill GA, Herbert CM: Endometriosis—Drug therapy or surgery? *Female Patient* October 1988; 13:69.

Ingemarsson I et al: Single injection of terbutaline in term labor. I. Effect on fetal pH with prolonged bradycardia. *Am J Obstet Gynecol* 1985a; 153:859.

Inturrisi M, Camenga CF, Rosen M: Epidural morphine for relief of postpartum, postsurgical pain. *JOGNN* July/August 1988; 17:238.

Karch A, Boyd E: *Handbook of Drugs.* Philadelphia: Lippincott, 1989.

Kennedy JL, Adashi EY: Ovulation induction. *Obstet Gynecol Clin North Am* December 1987; 14(4):831.

Lipshitz J: Beta-adrenergic agonists. *Semin Perinatol* July 1981; 5:252.

Marshall C: The art of induction/augmentation of labor. *JOGNN* January/February 1985; 14:22.

Milan EM, McFeely EJ: *Memory Bank for Neonatal Drugs.* Baltimore: Williams & Wilkins, 1990.

Mosby's Nursing Drug Reference. St. Louis: Mosby, 1991.

NAACOG: Preterm labor and tocolytics. *OGN Nurs Practice Resource* September 1984; 10.

Niebyl J (moderator): Symposium: Tocolytics: When and how to use them. *Contemp OB/GYN* June 1986: 27:146.

Nugent CE: Induction of labor. In: *Gynecology and Obstetrics,* Vol. 2. Dilts PV, Sciarri JJ (editors). Philadelphia: Lippincott, 1989, Ch 71.

Pauerstein CJ: *Clinical Obstetrics.* New York: Wiley, 1987.

Pawlak RP, Tabor Herbert LA: *Drug Administration in the NICU: A Handbook for Nurses,* 2nd ed. Petaluma, CA: Neonatal Network, 1990.

Peters F et al: Inhibition of lactation by long-acting bromocriptine. *Obstet Gynecol* 1986; 67:82.

Philipsen T, et al: Pulmonary edema following ritodrine-saline infusion in preterm labor. *Obstet Gynecol* 1981; 58:304.

Scott JR, Worley RJ: Hypertensive disorders of pregnancy. In: *Danforth's Obstetrics and Gynecology,* 6th ed. Scott JR et al (editors). Philadelphia: Lippincott, 1990.

Shortbridge LA: Using ritodrine hydrochloride to inhibit preterm labor. *Am J Mat Child Nurs* January/February 1983; 8:58.

Sibai BM: Preeclampsia-eclampsia: Valid treatment approaches. *Contemp OB/GYN* August 1990; 35:84.

Sibai BM: Pre-eclampsia-eclampsia: Valid treatment approaches. *Contemp OB/GYN* August 1990; 35:84.

Sibai BM: Seeking the best use for magnesium sulfate in pre-eclampsia-eclampsia. *Contemp. OB/GYN* January 1987; 29:155.

Skidmore-Roth L: Mosby's 1991 Nursing Drug Reference. St. Louis: Mosby Year Book, 1991.

Wang R, Davidson BJ: Ritodrine-induced neutropenia. *Am J Obstet Gynecol* 1986; 154:924.

Varney H: *Nurse Midwifery,* 2nd ed. Boston, Blackwell Scientific Publications, 1987.

Amniocentesis: Nursing Responsibilities

Nursing action	Rationale
Objective: Prepare woman.	
Explain procedure.	
Reassure woman.	Information will decrease anxiety.
Have woman sign consent form.	Signing indicates woman's awareness of risks and consent to procedure.
Have woman empty bladder.	Emptying bladder decreases risk of bladder perforation.
Objective: Prepare equipment.	
Collect supplies:	
22-gauge spinal needle with stylet	
10-mL syringe	
20-mL syringe	
Three 10-mL test tubes with tops (amber-colored or covered with tape)	Amniotic fluid must be shielded from light to prevent breakdown of bilirubin.
Objective: Monitor vital signs.	
Obtain baseline data on maternal BP, pulse, respiration, and FHR.	Status of woman and fetus is assessed.
Monitor every 15 minutes.	

Objective: Locate fetus and placenta.

Provide assistance as physician palpates for fetal position. Assist with real-time ultrasound.

Real-time ultrasound is used to identify fetal parts and placenta and locate pockets of amniotic fluid. Amniocentesis is usually performed laterally in the area of fetal small parts where pockets of amniotic fluid are usually seen.

Objective: Cleanse abdomen.

Prep abdomen with Betadine or other cleansing agent.

Objective: Collect specimen of amniotic fluid.

Obtain test tubes from physician; provide correct identification; send to lab with appropriate lab slips.

Incidence of infection is decreased.

Objective: Reassess vital signs.

Determine woman's BP, pulse, respirations, and FHR; palpate fundus to assess fetal and uterine activity; monitor woman with external fetal monitor for 20–30 minutes after amniocentesis.

Have woman rest on left side.

Fetus may have been inadvertently punctured. Uterine contractions may ensue following procedure; treatment course should be determined to counteract any supine hypotension and to increase venous return and cardiac output.

Objective: Complete client record.

Record type of procedure done, date, time, name of physician performing test, maternal-fetal response, and disposition of specimen.

Client records will be complete and current.

(continued)

Amniocentesis: Nursing Responsibilities (*continued*)

Nursing Action	Rationale
Objective: Educate woman.	Client will know how to recognize side effects or conditions that warrant further treatment.
Reassure woman; instruct her to report any of the following side effects:	
1. Unusual fetal hyperactivity or lack of movement	
2. Vaginal discharge—clear drainage or bleeding	
3. Uterine contractions or abdominal pain	
4. Fever or chills	

Assessment for Amniotic Fluid

Nursing Action	Rationale
Objective: Assemble equipment.	
Gather Nitrazine test tape and a pair of disposable gloves.	Nitrazine test tape reacts to alkaline fluids and confirms presence of amniotic fluid.
May need microscope and glass slide if determining ferning of obtained fluid.	Microscope is used to detect ferning pattern.
Objective: Prepare woman.	
Explain the procedure, indications for the procedure, and information that may be obtained. Determine whether she has noted the escape of any clear fluid from the vagina.	Explanation of the procedure decreases anxiety and increases relaxation.
Objective: Test fluid.	
Prior to doing a vaginal exam that uses lubricant, put on gloves. With one gloved hand, spread the labia, and with the other hand place a small section (approx. 2 inches long) against the vaginal opening. You may also place the test tape against any clothing or pads that have been soaked with possible amniotic fluid.	Contamination of the Nitrazine test tape with lubricant can make the test unreliable.
	Enough fluid needs to be placed on the test tape to make it wet. Amniotic fluid is alkaline, and an alkaline fluid turns the Nitrazine test tape a dark blue. If the test tape remains a beige color, the test is negative for amniotic fluid.

(*continued*)

Assessment for Amniotic Fluid (*continued*)

Nursing Action	Rationale
Compare the color on the test tape to the guide on the back of the Nitrazine test tape container to determine the test results.	
Amniotic fluid may also be obtained by speculum exam. Some labor and birth nurses are using this technique. If fluid is present in sufficient amount to draw some into a syringe, a small amount of fluid can be placed on a glass slide, allowed to dry, and then looked at under a microscope. A ferning pattern confirms the presence of amniotic fluid.	Obtaining a specimen by speculum exam reduces the contamination of the fluid with other substances such as blood.
Objective: Record information on client's record.	
Record on labor record, eg, SROM, Nitrazine positive	Nurse documents status of membranes, intact or ruptured.

Deep Tendon Reflexes and Clonus Assessment

Nursing Action	Rationale
Objective: Assemble and prepare equipment.	
Obtain a percussion hammer. If one is not available, the side of the hand is also useful in assessing DTRs.	A percussion hammer permits accurate delivery of a brisk tap.
Objective: Prepare woman.	
Explain the procedure, indications for the procedure, and information that will be obtained. At a minimum the patellar reflex should be checked. Most nurses check a second reflex such as the biceps, triceps, or brachioradialis.	Explanation decreases anxiety and increases cooperation. Deep tendon reflexes (DTRs) are assessed to gain information about CNS status and to assess the effects of $MgSO_4$ if the woman is receiving it.
Objective: Elicit reflexes.	
Biceps reflex. The woman's arm is flexed at the elbow with the nurse's thumb placed on the biceps tendon. The nurse's thumb is struck in a slightly downward motion and response is assessed. Normal response is flexion of the arm.	Correct positioning and technique is essential to elicit the reflex. The correct position causes the muscle to be slightly stretched. Then when the tendon is stretched with the tap, the muscle should contract.
Patellar reflex. The woman is positioned with her legs hanging over the edge of the bed (feet should not be touching the floor). She may also lie supine with her	

(*continued*)

Deep Tendon Reflexes and Clonus Assessment (*continued*)

Nursing Action	Rationale
knees slightly flexed and supported by the nurse. The nurse briskly strikes the patellar tendon, which is located just below the patella. Normal response is extension or a thrusting forward of the foot. *Objective:* Grade reflexes. Reflexes are graded on a scale of 1+ to 4+. See Table 3–1.	Normally reflexes are 1+ or 2+. With CNS irritation hyperreflexia may be present; with high magnesium levels reflexes may be diminished or absent.

Table 3–1 Deep Tendon Reflex Rating Scale

Rating	Assessment
4+	Hyperactive; very brisk, jerky, or clonic response; abnormal
3+	Brisker than average; may not be abnormal
2+	Average response; normal
1+	Diminished response; low normal
0	No response; abnormal

Objective: Assess for clonus.

With the knee flexed and the leg supported, vigorously dorsiflex the foot, maintain the dorsiflexion momentarily and then release. (Figure 8–5).

Normal response: The foot returns to its normal position of plantar flexion. Clonus is present if the foot "jerks" or taps against the examiner's hand. If so, the number of taps or beats of clonus is recorded.

Objective: Report and record findings.

For example: DTRs 2+, no clonus or DTRs 4+, 2 beats clonus.

Clonus indicates more pronounced hyperreflexia and is indicative of CNS irritability.

Provides a permanent record.

Endotracheal Suctioning

Nursing Action	Rationale
Objective: Minimize potential for pulmonary infection through cross-contamination.	
Assess respiratory status to determine necessity for suctioning.	Infant should be suctioned only as often as necessary to maintain patent airway and adequate oxygenation.
Gather all necessary equipment: catheters, suction machine, disposable sterile suction tubing, saline (no preservatives), sterile syringe/needle, and gloves (not powdered). Ensure that gloves, catheters, and liquefying solutions are sterile.	In healthy individual, lower respiratory tract is free of pathogenic organisms.
Maintain sterile technique throughout entire suctioning procedure.	
Discard catheter, glove, and saline after each procedure.	Once equipment is moistened and contaminated with body flora and mucus, it becomes a culture bed for noxious organism growth.
Set wall suction for not more than 80 mm Hg.	Mucosal hemorrhages and tissue invagination occur more frequently when higher pressure is used.

Objective: Alleviate partial or total airway obstruction in support of cell oxygenation.

Monitor transcutaneous readings during suctioning procedure and supplement with increased oxygen as needed.

Suctioning physically removes oxygen from airways. In addition, it mechanically occludes airways and therefore diminishes potential for oxygenation. It usually stimulates coughing and increases work of breathing, thereby increasing tissue demand for oxygen.

Position and immobilize infant.

It is quite difficult to suction alert infant successfully without restraint. An assistant should be employed to ensure effective, atraumatic suctioning in infants.

Using sterile technique, don sterile glove; hook up appropriate suction catheter; lubricate tip.

"Whistle-tip" catheter should be used for respiratory tract suctioning, because it tends to be less traumatizing to tissues.

Catheter size should be no more than $1/2$ the size of lumen to be suctioned in order to minimize hypoxemia due to airway obstruction.

Place sterile normal saline in a sterile specimen cup or unit dose plastic container.

Prelubrication of catheter is essential to minimize tissue trauma with subsequent obstructive edema.

If infant is intubated:

1. Disconnect source of oxygenation from newborn just prior to entry of suction catheter.

Suction applied while entering airway increases removal of oxygen from airways.

(*continued*)

Endotracheal Suctioning (*continued*)

Nursing Action	Rationale
2. Assistant should stabilize endotracheal tube while suctioning.	During suctioning, tube can be easily dislodged and increases potential for tissue invagination once catheter tip passes end of tube. Passing the suction catheter more than 1 cm beyond the endotracheal tube risks damaging the carina and creating pneumothoraces (Figure 4–1).
3. Insert catheter without applied suction into tube the distance from the proximal airway to no more than 1 cm below the end of the endotracheal tube. (This can be determined by noting cm markings on tube or by using calculations for oral-carinal distance.)	

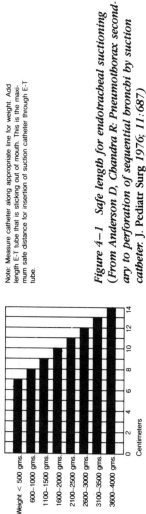

Note: Measure catheter along appropriate line for weight. Add length E-T tube that is sticking out of mouth. This is the maximum safe distance for insertion of suction catheter through E-T tube.

Figure 4–1 Safe length for endotracheal suctioning (From Anderson D, Chandra R: Pneumothorax secondary to perforation of sequential bronchi by suction catheter. J. Pediatr Surg 1976; 11:687)

Weight < 500 gms.
600–1000 gms.
1100–1500 gms.
1600–2000 gms.
2100–2500 gms.
2600–3000 gms.
3100–3500 gms.
3600–4000 gms.

Centimeters
0   2   4   6   8   10   12   14

4. Apply suction by placing thumb of assistive hand over vent port or Y-connector (Figure 4–2).

Placing thumb over venting device closes negative pressure system, which allows atmospheric pressure to push secretions and debris into catheter, facilitating their removal.

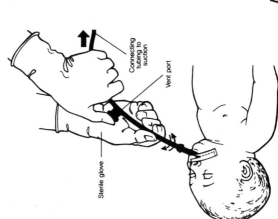

Connecting tubing to suction

Vent port

Sterile glove

Figure 4–2 Suctioning with endotracheal tube

(*continued*)

Endotracheal Suctioning (*continued*)

Nursing Action	Rationale
5. Slowly withdraw catheter in a pill-rolling rotation.	Rotating catheter in a slow, steady fashion maximizes catheter access to secretions while minimizing potential for tissue invagination.
6. Clear catheter with sterile saline.	
7. After each suction attempt, ventilate for a few breaths to reinflate atelectatic areas.	Hypoxia insult with a drop in PaO_2 occurs during suction efforts. Suction, the application of negative pressure to the airway, decreases by 50% the pulmonary compliance and tidal volume.
	Suction creates pulmonary atelectasis.
8. If tenacious secretions are encountered, instill normal saline with syringe (needleless) into tube prior to suctioning.	Instillation of normal saline liquefies and loosens secretions.
If infant is not intubated:	
After having failed to get infant to cough voluntarily in effective manner, follow procedure for suctioning intubated infant with these exceptions:	Suctioning to clear airways should be employed only when infant is unable to clear own airways effectively by use of cough reflex. It should be considered a last resort.
1. Enter airway via nasopharynx, advancing catheter into trachea on inspiration.	Inspiration opens glottis and tends to entrain catheter along with inspired air. Achieving coordination with inspiration is often quite easy with pediatric clients, because they are frequently crying involuntarily during
2. Attempt to liquefy tenacious secretions by humidification via mist tent, face mask, or hand-held nebulizer.	

Action	Rationale
	procedure. Instillation of liquefying agents directly into trachea in unintubated infant is not possible. Indirect means must be used.
Objective: Minimize iatrogenic hypoxemia secondary to suctioning.	
Suction only when absolutely necessary.	Always assess need for suctioning. There should never be standing orders such as "Suction every hour."
Limit each catheter insertion to no more than 10 sec. Reoxygenate newborn (monitoring transcutaneous readings) between each insertion and at conclusion of procedure.	Limiting suction time and frequent reoxygenation counterbalance the mechanical obstruction of airway and removal of available oxygen.
Remove catheter with suction applied as soon as infant begins to cough.	Holding catheter in airway while infant coughs can deprive infant of needed inspiratory volume at end of cough because of airway obstruction by catheter.
During procedure, assess infant for signs of bradycardia.	Suctioning can cause vagal response in form of bradycardia, which, if unchecked, can lead to asystole.
Objective: Record information on infant's record. Record infant's response during and after the procedure. Also record amount and type of secretions obtained.	Provides record of infant's response to procedure.

Evaluation of Lochia After Birth

Nursing Action	Rationale
Objective: Prepare woman.	
Explain the procedure, the reason for carrying out the procedure, and information that will be obtained.	Explanation of procedure decreases anxiety and increases relaxation
Objective: Obtain and evaluate maternal vital signs.	
Assess maternal temperature, blood pressure, and pulse.	Provides information regarding physiologic status
Objective: Accurately evaluate the amount of lochia after birth.	
Put on disposable gloves prior to the assessment.	Universal precautions and body substance isolation require use of gloves when exposed to body secretions such as lochia.
Lower perineal pad so amount of lochia can be visualized.	Allows nurse to view amount of lochia collected during the assessment
Palpate uterine fundus by placing one hand on the fundus and the other hand just over the symphysis pubis and	The fundus is located in the midline at the umbilicus or 1 to 2 fingerbreadths below the umbilicus.

press downward. With the other hand, palpate the uterine fundus.	Downward pressure exerted just above the symphysis will prevent excessive downward movement of the uterus during assessment.
Determine firmness of fundus.	The uterus needs to remain firmly contracted to prevent excessive blood loss.
If fundus is boggy, massage by rubbing in circular motion.	Manual pressure stimulates uterine contractions.
Evaluate the color and amount of lochia, and observe for the presence of clots. The following guidelines may be used to evaluate and describe the amount of lochia:	Provides information regarding expected status. After birth, a moderate amount of lochia rubra, without clots, is expected.
Small: smaller than a 4-in. stain on the pad; 10 to 25 mL	
Moderate: smaller than a 6-in. stain; 25 to 50 mL	
Large: larger than 6-in. stain; 50 to 80 mL (Luegenbiehl et al 1990)	
If blood loss exceeds above guidelines, the perineal pads and the chux may be weighed to more accurately estimate blood loss.	An estimate may be obtained by using the equivalent of 1 g of weight equals 1 mL. Weighing the pads and chux can provide important information, as amounts of blood loss may be underestimated due to the expectation that some blood loss is to be expected.

Exchange Transfusion: Nursing Responsibilities*

Nursing Action	Rationale
Objective: Prepare infant.	
1. Identify baby.	To prepare correct infant.
2. Keep newborn NPO for four hr preceding exchange transfusion or aspirate stomach.	To decrease chance of regurgitation and aspiration by neonate.
3. May administer salt-poor albumin (1 g/kg body weight) one hr before exchange transfusion.	To increase binding of bilirubin. Do not give to severely anemic or edemic neonate or to neonate with congestive heart failure, because of hazard of hypervolemia.
4. Assess vital signs.	To provide a baseline.
5. Position neonate in supine position, soft restraints; provide warmth under radiant warmer and have warm blankets available.	To provide maximum visualization, thermoregulation and prevent chilling.
6. Clean abdomen by scrubbing.	To reduce number of bacteria present.
7. Attach monitor leads to infant.	To assess pulse and respiration.
Objective: Prepare equipment.	
1. Have resuscitation equipment available (oxygen, bag and mask, intubation equipment, 10% glucose IV solution and sodium bicarbonate).	To provide life support measures if necessary.

2. Obtain blood and check it with physician for type, Rh, and age.	To ensure using correct blood.
3. Attach blood tubing.	To allow infusion.
4. Apply blood warmer.	To reduce chill.
5. Open exchange transfusion and umbilical vein trays. Pour prep solution into basins.	To maintain sterility.
6. Prepare gown and gloves for physician.	
Objective: Monitor infant status before and during procedure.	
Assess pulse, respirations, color, and activity state.	To recognize possible problems such as apnea, bradycardia, cardiac arrhythmia, or arrest and provide data on neonate's response to treatment.
Objective: Record blood exchange and medications used.	
1. Using blood exchange sheet, record time, amount of blood in, amount of blood out, medications and baby's response, and any other pertinent information.	Donor blood is given at rate of 170 mL/kg of body weight. It replaces 85% of infant's own blood.
2. Inform physician when 100 mL of blood has been used.	Calcium gluconate is given IV after each 100 mL of blood if indicated to decrease cardiac irritability.

*Exchange transfusion is a therapeutic procedure for hyperbilirubinemia of any etiology.

(*continued*)

Exchange Transfusion: Nursing Responsibilities (*continued*)

Nursing Action	Rationale
Objective: Assess neonate response after transfusion.	To provide information on status of neonate and identification of complications such as hypocalcemia, hyperkalemia, hypernatremia, hypoglycemia and acidosis, sepsis, shock, thrombus formation, and transfusion mismatch reaction.
After the exchange, carefully monitor the following for 24–48 hr:	
1. Vital signs	
2. Neurologic signs (lethargy, increased irritability, jitteriness, convulsion)	
3. Amount and color of urine (hematuria)	
4. Presence of edema	
5. Signs of necrotizing enterocolitis	
6. Infection or hemorrhage at infusion site	
7. Signs of increasing jaundice	
8. Neurologic signs of kernicterus	
9. Calcium, glucose, and bilirubin levels	
10. Other complications such as hypokalemia, septicemia, shock, and thrombosis	

Objective: Prepare blood samples.

Label tubes and send to laboratory with appropriate laboratory slips.

To follow routines of your institution.

Retype and cross-match 2 units of blood two hours postexchange.

To provide for possible future exchange.

Objective: Record information on infant's record.

Record infant's response during and after the exchange procedure.

Recording of infant's responses assists in identifying possible complications.

Fetal Heart Rate Auscultation

Nursing Action	Rationale
Objective: Assemble equipment.	
Obtain a fetoscope or Doppler.	Fetoscope is a special type of stethoscope that amplifies sound.
	Doppler uses ultrasound.
Objective: Prepare woman.	
Explain the procedure, indications for the procedure, and the information that will be obtained.	Explanation of the procedure decreases anxiety and increases relaxation.
Objective: Auscultate FHR.	
Perform Leopold's maneuver to identify the fetal presentation and position.	Assists in locating the fetal back where FHR is most likely to be heard.
Uncover the woman's abdomen.	It is more difficult to auscultate through cloth.
If using a fetoscope, place the metal band on your head; the diaphragm should extend out from your forehead.	The metal band conducts sound.
If using a Doppler, place ultrasonic gel on the diaphragm. Note: some Dopplers have a plastic cap over the diaphragm that will need to be removed to expose the diaphragm.	The gel is used to maintain contact with the maternal abdomen and to enhance conduction of ultrasound.

Place the bell of the fetoscope or the Doppler diaphragm on the maternal abdomen, about half-way between the umbilicus and symphysis pubis and in the midline. If the FHR is not heard, move the fetoscope out about an inch, in an ever-widening circle until the FHR is heard. When using the Doppler, you may need to tilt the diaphragm slightly in order to hear the FHR. If tilting the diaphragm does not locate the FHR, move the fetoscope in the same manner as described above.	The FHR is most likely to be heard over the fetal back. In LOA or ROA, the fetal back will be located in this portion of the maternal abdomen.
Objective: Differentiate maternal pulse from fetal heart rate.	
Place your index finger over the woman's radial pulse to differentiate maternal heart rate from fetal heart rate.	Ensures that the FHR, not the woman's pulse, is being heard.
Count the FHR. Note that the FHR has a double rhythm and just one sound is counted. Palpate for uterine contractions while you are auscultating FHR.	The FHR has the same "Lub dup" sound of adult heart sounds. The response of the FHR to uterine contractions is important in evaluating FHR changes.
Count FHR during a uterine contraction and continue for an additional 30 seconds to identify FHR response.	Counting during and just after the contraction evaluates fetal response to the contraction.
Determine FHR baseline by counting FHR for 30 to 60 seconds between uterine contractions to identify average baseline rate. Note if the rate is regular or irregular. If the rate changes (abruptly or gradually) recount for a brief period (5 or 10 seconds) to correctly identify an increasing or slowing rate.	The FHR baseline is the rate between contractions.

Increases or decreases in the FHR need to be described as accurately as possible. |

(*continued*)

Fetal Heart Rate Auscultation (*continued*)

Nursing Action	Rationale
Tell the parents what the FHR is; offer to help them listen if they would like to.	
Objective: Provide systematic evaluation.	
Auscultate between, during and for 30 seconds following a uterine contraction. For low-risk women, NAACOG 1990 recommends an auscultation frequency of every 1 hour in latent phase, every 30 minutes in active phase, and every 15 minutes in the second stage. For high-risk women, the recommended frequency is every 30 minutes in latent phase, every 15 minutes in active phase, and every 5 minutes in the second stage.	Evaluation provides the opportunity to assess the fetal status and response to the labor process.
Objective: Record information on client record.	
Document FHR data (rate and rhythm), characteristics of uterine activity, and any actions taken as a result of the FHR.	Complete documentation is mandatory.

Sample nurse's entry:

		Nurse's entry documents FHR rate, rhythm, and response to UC.
1/1/92	FHR 140 by auscultation, regular rhythm. Maternal pulse 78. UC q 3 min × 60 sec, strong. No increase or decrease in FHR noted during or following UC. J. Smith RN	
0700		

Sample nurse's entry for baseline and slowing of FHR after uterine contraction.

		Nurse's entry documents FHR rate, response to UC, nursing intervention, and fetal response.
1/1/92	FHR 136 by auscultation with slowing noted during the acme of UC and for 10 seconds following the UC. Client turned to left side. Maternal pulse 80. FHR 140, regular rhythm with no decrease during or following the next two UC. UC q 3 × 60 sec, strong. J. Smith RN	
0800		

Fetal Monitoring: Electronic

Nursing Action	Rationale
Objective: Prepare woman.	
Explain the procedure, the indications for the EFM, and the information that will be obtained. Explain the monitor so that parents will know what they are seeing and hearing.	Explanation of the procedure decreases anxiety and increases relaxation.
Place the external fetal monitor. Turn on the monitor.	
Place two elastic belts around the woman's abdomen. Place the "toco" over the uterine fundus in the midline and secure it with a belt so that it fits snugly. Note the UC tracing. The resting tone tracing (without uterine contraction) should be recording on the 10 or 15 mm Hg pressure line.	The uterine fundus is the area of greatest contractility. If the tracing is on the 0 line, there may be a constant grinding noise.
Apply ultrasonic gel to the diaphragm of the ultrasound transducer. Place the diaphragm on the maternal abdomen between the umbilicus and symphysis pubis, in the midline. Listen for the FHR (which will have a "whip-like" sound). When FHR is located, attach the elastic belt snugly.	Ultrasonic gel is used to maintain contact with the maternal abdomen. The ultrasonic beam is directed toward the fetal heart. Firm contact is necessary to maintain a continuous tracing.

Objective: Identify the tracing.

Place the following information on the beginning of the fetal monitor paper: date, time, client name, gravida, para, membrane status, physician name. (Note: Each birthing area may have specific guidelines regarding additional information that is to be included.)

Assures accurate identification.

Objective: Evaluate EFM tracing.

For high-risk women, NAACOG (1988) recommends evaluating the EFM tracing every 15 minutes in the first stage, and every 5 minutes in the second stage. For low-risk women specific time intervals have not been recommended by NAACOG. However, evaluation every 15—30 minutes in the first stage, and every 5—15 minutes in the second stage (as long as FHR has reassuring characteristics) is frequently done. The time interval for evaluation needs to be shortened if any nonreassuring characteristics occur.

Evaluation provides the opportunity to assess the fetal status and response to the labor process. Presence of reassuring characteristics is associated with good fetal outcome. Rapid identification of nonreassuring characteristics allows interventions to be initiated and then to determine the fetal response to the interventions.

Objective: Record information on client record.

Sample nurse's entry:

1/1/92 FHR BL 135—140. STV and LTV present. Two acceler-
0700   ations of 20 bpm × 20 sec with fetal movement in
        10 minutes. UC q 3 min × 50—60 sec of moderate
        intensity by palpation. No decelerations noted.

Nurse's entry documents reassuring FHR characteristics and response to UCs.

(*continued*)

Fetal Monitoring: Electronic (*continued*)

Nursing Action

Sample nurse's entry if slowing is noted.

0730   FHR BL 135–144. STV and LTV present. Late deceleration noted with decrease of FHR to 130 bpm for 20 sec. UC q 3 min × 50–60 sec of moderate intensity by palpation. Client turned to left side. No further deceleration with three subsequent UC. Two accelerations of 20 bpm × 20 sec noted with fetal movement. Client instructed to remain on left side.

Rationale

Nurse's entry documents FHR rate, presence of variability, response of FHR to UC, the intervention used and subsequent positive fetal response to the intervention.

Fundal Assessment

Nursing Action	Rationale
Objective: Prepare woman.	
Explain procedure; have the woman void; position woman flat in bed with head comfortably positioned on a pillow; if the procedure is uncomfortable, woman may flex legs.	Having the woman void assures that a full bladder is not causing any uterine atony. Having woman flat prevents falsely high assessment of fundal height. Flexing the legs relaxes the abdominal muscles. The uterus may be tender if frequent massage has been necessary.
Objective: Determine uterine firmness.	
Gently place one hand on the lower segment of the uterus; using the side of the other hand, palpate the abdomen until the top of the fundus is located. Determine whether the fundus is firm. If it is not firm, massage until firm.	Provides support for uterus. Provides a larger surface for palpation and is less uncomfortable for the woman. A firm fundus indicates that the muscles are contracted and bleeding will not occur.
Objective: Determine the height of the fundus.	
Measure the height of the top of the fundus in finger-breadths. (See Figure 9–1.)	Fundal height gives information about the progress of involution.

(*continued*)

Fundal Assessment (*continued*)

Nursing Action	Rationale

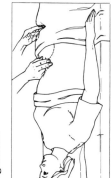

Figure 9–1 Measurement of descent of fundus: The fundus is located two fingerbreadths below the umbilicus.

Objective: Ascertain position.

Determine whether fundus is deviated from the midline. If not in midline, locate position. Evaluate bladder for distention. Ascertain voiding pattern; use measuring device to measure urine output for next few hours (until normal elimination status is established).

Fundus may be deviated when bladder is full.

Objective: Correlate uterine status with lochia.

Observe lochia for amount, presence of clots, color, and odor.

As normal involution occurs, the lochia decreases in amount and changes from rubra to serosa. Increased amounts of lochia may be associated with uterine relaxation; failure to progress to next type of lochia may indicate uterine relaxation or infection.

Objective: Record findings.

Fundal height is recorded in fingerbreadths; example:
2 FB ↓ U; 1 FB ↑ U.

If massage had been necessary it could be recorded as:
Uterus: Boggy → firm c̄ light massage.

A complete note illustrating normal findings might be:
Fundus firm, 1 FB ↓ U, lochia rubra, scant amount.

Allows for consistency of reporting among care givers.

Gavage Feeding

Nursing Action

Objective: Ensure smooth accomplishment of the procedure.

Gather necessary equipment including:

1. No. 5 or No. 8 Fr. feeding tube
2. 10–30 mL syringe
3. ¼-in. paper tape
4. Stethoscope
5. Appropriate formula
6. Small cup of sterile water

Explain procedure to parents.

Rationale

Considerations in choosing size of catheter include size of the infant, area of insertion (oral or nasal), and rate of flow desired. The very small infant (less than 1600 g) requires a 5 Fr. feeding tube; an infant greater than 1600 g may tolerate a larger tube. Orogastric insertion is preferred over nasogastric insertion as most infants are obligatory nose breathers. If nasogastric insertion is used, a No. 5 catheter should be used to minimize airway obstruction. The size of the catheter will influence the rate of flow. The syringe is used to aspirate stomach contents prior to feeding, to inject air into the stomach for testing tube placement, and for holding measured amount of formula during feeding. Tape is used to mark tube for insertion depth as well as for securing tube during feeding. Stethoscope is needed to auscultate rush of air into stomach when testing tube placement.

Objective: Insert tube accurately into stomach.

Position infant on back or side with head of bed elevated.

Take tube from package and measure the distance from the tip of the ear to the nose to the xiphoid process, and mark the point with a small piece of paper tape (Figure 10–1).

This position allows easy passage of the tube.

This measuring technique ensures enough tubing to enter stomach.

If inserting tube nasally, lubricate tip in cup of sterile water. Shake excess drops to prevent aspiration.

Water should be used, as opposed to an oil-based lubricant, in case the tube is inadvertently passed into a lung.

Stabilize infant's head with one hand, and pass the tube via the mouth (or nose) into the stomach, to the point previ-

Any signs of respiratory distress signal likelihood that tube has entered trachea. Orogastric insertion is less likely to

Sterile water may be used to lubricate feeding tube when inserted nasally. With oral insertion, there are enough secretions in the mouth to lubricate the tube adequately. The cup of sterile water may also be used to test for placement by placing the end of the tube into the water to check for air bubbles from the lungs. However, this test may not be accurate as air may also be present in the stomach.

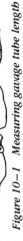

Figure 10–1 Measuring gavage tube length

(continued)

Gavage Feeding (*continued*)

Nursing Action

ously marked. If the infant begins coughing or choking or becomes cyanotic or aphonic, remove the tube immediately.

If no respiratory distress is apparent, lightly tape tube in position, draw up 0.5–1.0 mL of air in syringe, and connect it to tubing. Place stethoscope over the epigastrium and briskly inject the air (Figure 10–2).

Rationale

result in passage into the trachea than nasogastric insertion.

Nurse should hear a sudden rush of air as it enters stomach.

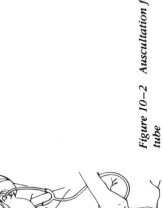

Figure 10–2   Auscultation for placement of gavage tube

Aspirate stomach contents with syringe, and note amount, color, and consistency. Return residual to stomach unless otherwise ordered to discard it.

Residual formula should be evaluated as part of the assessment of infant's tolerance of gavage feedings. It is not discarded, unless particularly large in volume or mucoid in nature, because of the potential for causing an electrolyte imbalance.

If only a clear fluid or mucus is found upon aspiration and if any question exists as to whether the tube is in the stomach, the aspirate can be tested for pH.

Stomach aspirate tests in the 1–3 range for pH.

Objective: Introduce formula into stomach without complication.

Hold infant for feeding or position on right side if infant cannot be held.

Positioning on side decreases the risk of aspiration in case of emesis during feeding.

Separate syringe from tube, remove plunger from barrel, reconnect barrel to tube, and pour formula into syringe.

Feeding should be allowed to flow in by gravity. It should not be pushed in under pressure with a syringe.

Elevate syringe 6–8 in. over infant's head. Allow formula to flow at slow, even rate.

Raising column of fluid increases force of gravity. Nurse may need to initiate flow of formula by inserting plunger of syringe into barrel just until formula is seen to enter feeding tube. Rate should be regulated to prevent sudden stomach distention, with possibility of vomiting and aspiration.

Continue adding formula to syringe until desired volume has been absorbed. Then rinse tubing with 2–3 mL sterile water.

Rinsing tube ensures that infant receives all of formula. It is especially important to rinse tube if it is going to be left in place, because this decreases risk of clogging and bacterial growth in tube.

(*continued*)

Gavage Feeding (*continued*)

Nursing Action

Remove tube by loosening tape, folding the tube over on itself, and quickly withdrawing it in one smooth motion. If tube is to be left in, position it so that infant is unable to remove it.

Objective: Maximize feeding pleasure of infant.

Whenever possible hold infant during gavage feeding. If it is too awkward to hold infant during feeding, be sure to take time for holding afterward.

Offer a pacifier to infant during feeding.

Rationale

Folding tube over on itself minimizes potential for aspiration of fluid, which would otherwise flow from tubing as it passes epiglottis. A tube left in place should be replaced at least every 24 hours.

Feeding time is important to infant's tactile sensory input.

Infants fed for long periods by gavage can lose their sucking reflex. Sucking during feeding comforts and relaxes infant, making formula flow more easily. One study showed that infants allowed to suck during feedings were able to nipple sooner and were discharged earlier than a control group of infants who did not suck during tube feedings.

Glucose Chemstrip Test Using Accu-Check II Machine

Nursing Action

Objective: Assemble equipment
Gather the following equipment:

1. Lancet (do not use needles)
2. Alcohol swabs
3. 2 × 2 sterile gauze squares
4. Small Band-Aid ™
5. Glucose strips and bottle
6. Gloves

Wash hands before and after touching infant and equipment; then apply gloves.

Objective: Prepare infant's heel for procedure

Select clear, previously unpunctured site. Clean site by rubbing vigorously with 70% isopropyl alcohol swab, followed by dry gauze square. Grasp lower leg and heel so as to impede venous return slightly.

Rationale

All necessary equipment must be ready to ensure that blood sample is collected at time and in manner necessary. Do not use needles because of danger of nicking periosteum. Warm heel for five to ten sec prior to heel stick with a warm wet wrap or specially designed chemical heat pad to facilitate flow of blood.

To implement universal precautions and prevent nosocomial infections.

Selection of previously unpunctured site minimizes risk of infection and excessive scar formation. Friction produces local heat, which aids vasodilation. Impeding venous return facilitates extraction of blood sample from puncture site.

(continued)

Glucose Chemstrip Test Using Accu-Check II Machine (*continued*)

Nursing Action

Objective: Minimize trauma at puncture site.

Blot dry site completely before lancing.

With quick piercing motion, puncture lateral heel with microlancet, being careful not to puncture too deeply (Figure 11–1). Toes are acceptable sites if necessary.

Rationale

Alcohol is irritating to injured tissue and may also produce hemolysis.

The lateral heel is the site of choice because it precludes damaging the posterior tibial nerve and artery, plantar artery, and important longitudinally oriented fat pad of the heel, which in later years could impede walking. This is especially important for infant undergoing multiple heel stick procedures. Optimal penetration is 4 mm.

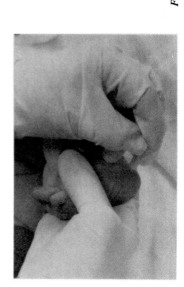

Figure 11–1 Glucose Chemstrip test (heel stick)

Objective: Ensure accurate blood sampling.

After puncture is made, allow first drop of blood to touch both test pads on Chemstrip, making sure to cover both yellow and white squares completely (Figure 11–2).

The first drop of blood is used for accuracy.

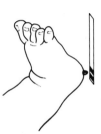

Right   Wrong

Figure 11–2 Glucose strip drop of blood

If Dextrostix reagent strip was used, first drop of blood would be discarded.

The first drop is usually discarded because it tends to be minutely diluted with tissue fluid from puncture.

Objective: Read reagent strip via Accu-Check II machine.

If using Accu-Check II machine,

(*continued*)

Glucose Chemstrip Test Using Accu-check II Machine (*continued*)

Nursing Action

Immediately press the TIME button. The meter will count to 60 but emit 3 high beeps on 57, 58, 59 then one low beep on 60. This is a warning to prepare for wiping the blood from the test strip. Wipe blood from test strips with clean dry cotton ball using moderate pressure when display reads 60. Do not leave any blood on test pad.

Machine will continue to count to 120 seconds. While meter is counting, turn test strip on side, with the test pads facing the On/Off button, and insert the reacted test strip into the test strip adaptor. *The strip must be inserted before the display reads* 120.

When the display reads 120, a high beep will be emitted, followed by the blood sugar value on the display screen in mg/dL. Read the blood sugar value on the display screen.

HHH = blood sugar > 500 mg/dL. Wait an additional minute and take the reacted test strip out of the meter and compare it to the color chart on the side of the Chemstrip bG vial to estimate results up to 800 mg/dL.

Rationale

For accurate results, directions must be followed closely, and reagent strips must be fresh. False low readings may be caused by the following:

1. Timing
2. Blood left on test strip

LLL = blood sugar is lower than the reading range of the instrument (less than 10 mg/dL). Values below 20 mg/dL have not been confirmed clinically.

Objective: Prevent excessive bleeding.

Apply folded gauze square to puncture site and secure firmly with bandage.

A pressure dressing should be applied to puncture site to stop bleeding.

Check puncture site frequently for first hour after sample.

Active infants sometimes kick or rub their dressings off and can bleed profusely from puncture site, especially if bandage becomes moist or is rubbed excessively against crib sheet.

Objective: Record findings on infant's record.

Record test results. Report immediately any results under 45 mg/dL or over 175 mg/dL.

Recording of infant's results assists in identifying possible complications.

Heelstick for Newborns

Nursing Action	Rationale
Objective: Assemble and prepare equipment. Have following equipment available: 2 × 2 or cotton balls Band–Aid Micro lancet Gloves Alcohol and Betadine Heparinized capillary tubes (2) Heel warmer Lab slips and labels	
Objective: Prepare infant's heel for procedure.	
Wash hands.	Handwashing is the single most important step in the prevention of infection.
Apply heel warmer or moist, warm washcloth	Increases capillary dilation and decreases venous stasis. Venous stasis results in higher hemoglobin and hematocrit values. Should be kept on heel 10–15 minutes.
Remove heel warmer	
Glove	Decreases spread of infection. Maintains universal precautions.
Cleanse foot with Betadine and allow to dry, than cleanse with alcohol.	Cleanses skin of bacteria.

Objective: Obtain blood for capillary hematocrit.

Use sterile microlancet stick. For proper puncture sites on lateral aspect of heel, see Procedure 11: Glucose Chemstrip Test.

Wipe away first drop of blood with a 2 × 2 or cotton ball.

Obtain specimen as quickly as possible using a squeeze/release technique.

Hold the heparinized capillary at a 45° angle to puncture site. Avoid air bubbles. Fill each tube two-thirds full and plug one end with clay. Put pressure on site with 2 × 2 until bleeding stops.

Apply Band–Aid if needed.

Cuddle infant after procedure.

Send specimen to lab with slip, or run test on unit per agency policy.

Objective: Report and record findings.

Record time, site of puncture, and infant's response.

Hematocrit is done to detect ratio of red blood cells (RBCs) to plasma in the blood. Use microlancet only one time. Be careful to avoid accidental puncture of medial plantar artery or injury to nerves.

First drop of blood is hemolysed.

Decreases trauma to surrounding tissues. Blood coagulates quickly.

Air bubbles or clots may cause inaccurate results.

Protects from infection and further trauma.

Provides sense of comfort and safety.

Provides a permanent and continuous record of hematocrits drawn for lab quality assurance; decreases repeated punctures at one site and scar formation.

Installation of Ophthalmic Ilotycin Ointment

Nursing Action	Rationale
Objective: Provide newborn prophylactic eye care	
Wash hands prior to instillation.	Prevents introduction of bacteria.
Clean infant's eyes of any drainage.	Removal of exudate allows instillation of ointment.
Retract lower eyelid outward with forefinger to allow instillation of ¼-inch long strand of ointment along lower conjunctival surface, starting at inner canthus.	Maximizes absorption of ointment.
Repeat process on other eye.	
Instill only a single dose per eye.	Prophylaxis requires only a single dose.
Do not irrigate eyes.	Irrigation will remove ointment.
Assess for sensitivity reaction such as: edema, inflammation, drainage.	May interfere with ability to focus and the bonding process.
Inform parents about rationale for eye prophylaxis, that instillation can be done in the birthing area or admission nursery, it may interfere with newborn's ability to focus on parents' face, and that there may be temporary side effects.	Preventive treatment of gonorrhea and chlamydia infection, which can cause blindness. Required by law. Side effects usually disappear in 24 to 48 hours.
Objective: Record completion of procedure	
Document the instillation of the prophylaxis eye medication	Provides a permanent record to meet the legal requirements.

Methods of Breast Pumping and Milk Storage

Breast-Pumping—Manual Expression

Advantages

1. Collection container only equipment needed.
2. Technique easily learned.

Disadvantages

1. Time-consuming
2. Less effective than pumping

Procedure

1. Assemble sterilized container and wash hands and breasts.
2. Perform gentle breast massage to stimulate the letdown reflex.
3. Position thumb and index finger about ½ inch behind nipple where milk sinuses are located.
4. Push fingers straight back toward chest and then squeeze them together with a slight rolling motion, lifting nipple outward. Avoid sliding fingers away from original position.
5. Rotate fingers around nipple to empty other milk sinuses. (Helpful hint: Practice technique on one breast while baby is nursing on other breast so infant will stimulate letdown reflex.)
6. Express milk into sterilized container.
7. Store as directed (see milk storage section).
8. Switch breasts as soon as flow in each breast decreases.

(*continued*)

Methods of Breast Pumping and Milk Storage (*continued*)

Breast Pumping—Using Breast Pumps

Advantages

1. Milk has a higher fat content when pumped with a breast pump than when expressed manually because more complete emptying of breasts allows access to hindmilk.

2. Increased volume obtained

3. Less potential for milk contamination

Disadvantages

1. More expensive—cost varies depending on equipment chosen.

2. Increased possibility of nipple trauma due to incorrect use or high pressures.

Procedures

Hand (Cylinder) Pump

1. Collect equipment. All equipment including hand pump, tubing, and collection bottles should be cleaned and/or sterilized between uses.

2. Wash hands and breasts.

3. Apply gentle massage or heat to breasts to stimulate flow of milk.

4. Alternate breasts as soon as flow decreases.

5. Place flange on breast and secure with one hand. If flange is not angled, mother should lean forward.

6. Suction is created by sliding outer cylinder away from breast, starting with short frequent pulls with other hand to initiate milk flow.

7. Empty breast milk into plastic storage container.

8. Repeat on opposite breast.

9. Store milk as directed.

Battery-Operated Pumps

1. Follow steps 1 through 4 as for hand pump method.
2. Place flange on breast.
3. Turn on and regulate suction by depressing button or bar with one hand to achieve gentle, continuous suction.
4. Milk flows gently into storage container.
5. Repeat on other breast.
6. Store milk as directed.
7. Clean equipment.

Electric Pump

1. Follow steps 1 through 4 as for hand pump method.
2. After assembling pump, place flange over breast. If using double pump with Y connector, overall production is increased and pumping time is decreased by half.
3. Turn machine on with pressure setting on low and gradually increase pressure setting as tolerance permits.
4. Pump creates a rhythmic suck-release pattern closely approximating sucking action of baby.

(continued)

Methods of Breast Pumping and Milk Storage (*continued*)

Procedure

5. Milk is expressed directly into storage container.

6. Seal and store milk as directed.

7. Clean equipment.

Milk Storage

1. Although milk may be stored in small plastic or glass bottles or disposable plastic bottle liners, the most recommended collection container is the rigid polypropylene plastic container, which maintains the stability of all constituents in human milk and is easier and safer to use (Lawrence 1989).

2. Label milk with name, date, and time.

3. Once collected and sealed, milk may be stored in refrigerator for no more than 48 hours, freezer compartment of refrigerator for 2 weeks, or deep freezer for 6 months.

4. Warm refrigerated milk in warm water for 10 to 15 minutes just prior to use. Do not microwave or heat on stove.

5. Discard all unused milk. Breast milk cannot be refrozen.

6. Freshly pumped milk can be added to already frozen milk by chilling it in refrigerator for 30 to 60 minutes prior to adding it to prevent the top layer of frozen breast milk from defrosting.

7. Thaw frozen milk in refrigerator up to 24 hours prior to use or in water just before feeding, gradually increasing temperature from cool to warm. Do not microwave or heat on stove.

8. Frozen breast milk may take on a yellow color which does not indicate spoilage.

9. If pumping and transporting milk, place milk in insulated pouch or cooler with ice to prevent spoilage.

Methods of Bottle Sterilization

Terminal sterilization

Advantages

1. Safest, most efficient method
2. More easily learned

Disadvantages

1. Prolonged cooling period (1 hr)
2. Not suitable for disposable bottles

Procedure

1. Assemble equipment and wash hands.

2. Thoroughly wash bottles, caps, and nipples in warm soapy water; squeeze some water through holes to rid them of accumulated milk; rinse well.

3. Wash the lid of the formula can (if using a liquid) and prepare formula according to directions.

4. Fill the bottles with the desired amount of formula and loosely apply the nipples and caps; one or two bottles of water may be prepared at the same time.

5. Place the prepared bottles in a large kettle or bottle sterilizer and add the appropriate amount of water (as specified on the sterilizer or 2–3 in. if a kettle is used).

6. Cover the sterilizer, bring the water to a gentle boil, and boil for 25 min. at 212°F.

7. Remove from heat but let the bottles remain in the sterilizer with the lid on until the sides of the pan are cool to the touch.

8. Remove the bottles, tighten the lids, and refrigerate until needed.

Aseptic method of sterilization

Advantages

1. May be modified for use with disposable bottles

Disadvantages

1. Difficult to learn, contamination more likely

Procedure

1. Same as steps 1 and 2 of terminal method.

2. Place all equipment needed (bottles, nipples, caps, can opener, tongs, measuring pitcher, and spoon) in a large kettle or sterilizer; cover with water, and boil for 5 min.

3. In another pan boil the amount of water necessary to make the formula (boil for 5 min).

4. Drain the water from the sterilizer pan and let the equipment cool 1 hour.

5. Remove the measuring pitcher, being certain to touch only the handle.

6. Use the sterilized can opener to open a can of formula after first washing the lid with soapy water and rinsing well; pour the formula into the prepared measuring pitcher, and add the correct amount of boiled water; mix with the prepared spoon.

7. Use tongs to remove the bottles from the sterilizer and fill them with the desired amount of formula; (one or two bottles of water may also be prepared by boiling enough additional water).

(*continued*)

Methods of Bottle Sterilization (*continued*)

Procedure

8. Use the tongs to set the nipples on the bottles; then apply the caps, touching only the edges.

9. Refrigerate until needed.

To modify for disposable bottles:
Complete all steps as directed except *do not boil the bottles* with the other equipment and allow the water to cool for 15–20 min before preparing the formula (the plastic bag may melt if the formula is too hot).

Dishwasher Sterilization

Advantages

1. Easy

Disadvantages

1. May not have access to dishwasher

2. Hot water tank needs to be set at 120°F or medium heat setting.

Procedure

1. Place bottles, caps into dishwasher rack.

2. Wash on hot water cycle then machine dry.

3. Spoon dry formula powder into bottles, cap with nipples, invert, and store at room temperature. Add tap water at time of feeding.

4. If liquid formula is used, add unboiled tap water to the liquid formula after dishwasher sterilization of bottles; refrigerate filled, capped bottles until needed.

5. Clean nipples separately with hot, soapy water; rinse thoroughly; then boil for 5 minutes. Cool for one hour. Nipples become softened if sterilized in dishwasher.

6. Sterilize disposable bottles in the top rack of dishwasher; clean nipples as in step 5 above.

Pelvic Exam: Nursing Responsibilities

Nursing Action	Rationale
Objective: Assemble and prepare equipment.	
Prepare and arrange following equipment so that they are easily accessible:	
1. Various-sized vaginal specula, warmed with water or on a heating pad prior to insertion.	Examination is facilitated. Warmed speculum assists in lubrication and facilitates initial insertion when culture and smears are to be taken. Do not use lubricant on speculum prior to insertion. This may alter findings or cultures.
2. Gloves.	
3. Water soluble lubricant.	
4. Materials for Pap smear and cultures.	
5. Good light source.	
Objective: Prepare woman.	
Explain procedure.	Explanation of procedure decreases anxiety.
Instruct woman to empty her bladder and to remove clothing below waist. She may be encouraged to keep her shoes on and will be given a disposable drape or sheet to place on her lap. Encourage her to sit on the end of the examining table with the drape across her lap prior to examination. Provide a warm environment either through over-	Comfort is promoted during internal examination. She may feel more comfortable with shoes on rather than supporting her weight with bare heels against cold stirrups.

head heat lights or through central heat. If a woman has never had a pelvic examination before, show her the equipment and explain the procedure prior to examination.

Position woman in lithotomy position with thighs flexed and adducted. Place her feet in stirrups. Buttocks should extend slightly beyond end of examining table.

Drape woman with a sheet, leaving flap so perineum can be exposed.

Objective: Provide support to woman as physician or nurse practitioner carries out examination.

Explain each part of examination as it is performed: inspection of external genitals, vagina, and cervix: bimanual examination of internal organs. Instruct woman to relax and breathe slowly.

Objective: Relaxation is promoted.

Advise woman when speculum is to be inserted and ask her to bear down.

When speculum is inserted, woman may feel intravaginal pressure. Bearing down helps open vaginal orifice and relax perineal muscles.

Lubricate examiner's finger well prior to bimanual examination.

Lubrication decreases friction and eases insertion.

Objective: Provide for woman's comfort at end of examination.

(continued)

Pelvic Exam: Nursing Responsibilities (*continued*)

Nursing Action	Rationale
Move to the end of the examining table and face woman's perineum. Cover the woman with the drape. Apply gentle pressure to the woman's knees and encourage her to move toward the head of the table. Offer your hand to the woman, remove her heels from the stirrups, and assist the woman to a sitting position. Be sure that she is not dizzy and that she is sitting or standing safely before you leave the room.	Supine position may create postural hypotension.
Provide tissues to wipe lubricant from perineum.	Upon assuming sitting position, vaginal secretions along with lubricant may be discharged.
Provide privacy for woman to dress.	Comfort and sense of privacy is promoted.

RhIgG Administration

Nursing Action	Rationale
Objective: Confirm that RhIgG immune globulin is indicated.	Sensitization occurs when an Rh negative woman is exposed to Rh positive blood. She develops antibodies to the Rh positive blood. These antibodies can attack the fetal red blood cells causing profound anemia. If both the direct and indirect Coombs' tests are negative, sensitization has not occurred and RhIgG immune globulin (RhIgG) is indicated.
Confirm that mother is Rh negative by checking her prenatal or intrapartal record. Then confirm that sensitization has not occurred—maternal indirect Coombs' negative.	
Confirm that infant is Rh positive. (A sample of the infant's cord blood is generally sent to the lab immediately after birth for typing and cross-matching.) If infant is Rh positive, confirm that sensitization has not occurred—direct Coombs' negative.	
Objective: Confirm that the woman does not have a history of allergy to immune globulin preparations.	
Review entries on medication allergies in client chart and ask woman specifically whether she has had any allergic reactions to medications, globulins, or blood products.	RhIgG immune globulin is made from the plasma portion of blood. Allergic reactions are possible.

(continued)

RhIgG Administration (*continued*)

Nursing Action	Rationale
Objective: Explain purpose and procedure. Have consent signed.	The woman should clearly understand the purpose of the procedure, its rationale, and the procedure itself, including any risks. Generally the primary side effects are erythema and tenderness at the injection site and allergic responses.
Many agencies require informed consent before administering RhIgG immune globulin.	
Objective: Obtain correct medication.	
RhIgG is available from the blood bank or pharmacy according to agency policy. Lot numbers for the drug and the cross match should be the same.	Because blood products are involved in the preparation careful verification is essential.
Objective: Confirm client identity and administer medication in deltoid muscle.	

Medication is administered intramuscularly within 72 hours of childbirth. The normal dose of 300 mg provides passive immunity following exposure of up to 15 mL of transfused RBCs. If a larger bleed is suspected (as in cases of severe abruptio placentae) additional doses may be administered at one time using multiple sites, or at regular intervals, as long as all doses are given within 72 hours of childbirth.

The medication causes passive immunity to occur and "tricks" the body into believing that it is not necessary to develop antibodies. Immunization is indicated any time there is a potential for maternal exposure to Rh positive blood. It is given prophylactically at 28 weeks' gestation, within 72 hours after the birth of an Rh positive Coombs' negative child, and following any spontaneous or therapeutic abortion, ectopic pregnancy, or amniocentesis.

Objective: Complete education for self-care.

Provide opportunities for the woman to ask questions and express concerns.

Many women, especially primigravidas, are not aware of the risks for an Rh positive fetus of a sensitized Rh negative mother. They must understand the importance of receiving medication for each pregnancy to ensure continued protection.

Objective: Complete client record.

Chart according to agency procedure. Most agencies chart lot number, route, dose, client education.

Provides a permanent record.

Sterile Vaginal Exam

Nursing Action	Rationale
Objective: Assemble and prepare equipment.	
Have following equipment easily accessible:	Examination is facilitated and can be done quickly.
● Sterile disposable gloves	
● Lubricant	
● Nitrazine test tape prior to first examination	
Objective: Prepare woman.	
Explain procedure, indications for carrying out procedure, and information being obtained.	Explanation of procedure decreases anxiety and increases relaxation.
Position woman with thighs flexed and abducted; instruct her to put heels of feet together.	Prevents contamination of area during examination and allows for visualization of external signs of labor progress.
Drape so that only the perineum is exposed.	Provides as much privacy as possible.
Encourage woman to relax her muscles and legs during procedure.	
Objective: Use aseptic technique during examination.	
If leakage of fluid has been noted or if woman reports leakage of fluid, use Nitrazine test tape before doing vaginal exam.	Nitrazine test tape registers a change in pH if amniotic fluid is present (unless a lubricant has already been used).

Put on both gloves; using thumb and forefinger of left hand, spread labia widely; insert well-lubricated second and index fingers of right hand into vagina until they touch the cervix.

Avoid contaminating hand by contact with anus; positioning of hand with wrist straight and elbow tilted downward allows fingertips to point toward umbilicus and find cervix.

Objective: Determine status of fetal membranes.

Palpate for movable bulging sac through the cervix; observe for expression of amniotic fluid during exam.

If intact, bag of waters feels like a bulge.

Objective: Determine status of labor progress during and after contractions.

Carry out vaginal examination during and between contractions

Examination varies. Assessment of dilatation is more accurate during contractions.

Objective: Identify degree of cervical dilatation.

Palpate for opening or what appears as a depression in the cervix.

Estimation of the diameter of the depression identifies degree of dilatation.

Estimate diameter of cervical opening in centimeters (0–10 cm).

One finger represents approximately 1.5–2 cm cervical dilatation.

Objective: Identify degree of cervical effacement.

Palpate the shortening of the surrounding circular ridge of tissue; estimate degree of shortening in percentages

Effacement results from the lengthening of muscle fibers around the internal os as they are taken up into the lower uterine segment. The endocervix becomes part of the lower uterine segment (Varney 1987).

(*continued*)

Sterile Vaginal Exam (*continued*)

Nursing Action	Rationale
Objective: Determine presentation and position of presenting part.	
As cervix opens, palpate for presenting part and identify its relationship to the maternal pelvis.	Presenting part is easier to palpate through a dilated cervix, and differentiation of landmarks is easier.
Objective: Determine station.	
Locate lowest portion of presenting part (excluding caput) (−5 to +5).	Identification of station provides information as to degree of descent.
Objective: Inform woman about progress in labor.	
Discuss findings of the vaginal examination and correlate them to woman's progress in labor.	Assists in identifying progress and reinforces need for frequency of procedure. Information is reassuring and supportive for woman and family.
Objective: Record information on client's record.	
Record on labor record, eg, 4 cm 50% or 8 cm. complete.	Nurse's entry documents progress of labor.

Suctioning of the Newborn

Nursing Action

Objective: Assess infant.

Objective: Remove secretions from oral/nasal pharynx.

If using DeLee mucus trap, attach it to mechanical suction or have safeguard against aspiration attached.

Using a #10 French catheter attached to suction, check negative pressure suction.

Place catheter into newborn's mouth first. Place finger over control and gently rotate catheter as secretions are withdrawn with suction.

Repeat suction of oropharynx if necessary to clear secretions.

Avoid deep suctioning, especially soon after birth.

If using bulb syringe, deflate the bulb prior to inserting it into the mouth and/or the nose.

Rationale

If the infant shows signs of respiratory distress the nurse must ensure patency of the airway.

Ensure infant's secretions are not suctioned into mouth of resuscitator.

#10 French is correct size for oral suction of average-size newborn. Negative pressure not to exceed 80–100 cm H_2O.

No suctioning episode should be longer than six seconds to prevent respiratory depression. Gentle rotation prevents trauma to mucous membranes.

Repeated suctioning must provide recovery time of at least 10–15 seconds to prevent respiratory depression.

Deep suction can stimulate the vagus nerve, causing a decrease in heart rate.

This prevents blowing the contents further into the nose and/or throat.

(*continued*)

Suctioning of the Newborn (*continued*)

Nursing Action	Rationale
Immediately after birth, insert bulb into mouth first and then into the nares.	Suctioning after birth requires clearing the mouth first to prevent aspiration of contents. Then suction the nares of birth secretions.
For routine suctioning, insert bulb into the nares, then corners of the mouth.	Infants can show signs of respiratory distress if the nose is congested, since infants are obligatory nose breathers. Don't force bulb into the nares and/or mouth.
Gently release the compressed bulb.	Provides suction that will draw the secretions into bulb.
Empty the bulb of secretions by squeezing it hard onto a cloth or paper towel.	
Reassess the infant's respiratory status.	It may take several times before nares and/or mouth are cleared. Take care not to traumatize the infant. If color change or bradycardia occur, oxygen or resuscitative procedures may be needed.
Clean the inside and outside of the bulb after using it by rinsing with clear water.	Dry secretions become a medium for bacteria to grow.
Objective: Record information on client's record.	
Record procedure, method and how infant tolerated it.	
Document amount, color, consistency of aspirate, and if specimen was sent to lab for analysis.	

Temperature Stabilization of the Newborn

Nursing Action	Rationale
Objective: Prepare warming equipment	
Prewarm incubator or radiant warmer. Have warmed towels/lightweight blankets available	Change from warm, moist intrauterine environment to cool, dry, drafty environment stresses the immature thermoregulation mechanisms of newborn.
Maintain birthing room at 22°C (71°F) with relative humidity of 60% to 65%.	
Objective: Establish a stable temperature after birth	
Wipe newborn free of blood and excessive vernix, especially from the head, with prewarmed towels.	Prevents loss of body heat from large surface area through evaporation.
Place newborn under radiant warmer.	Creates a heat-gaining environment.
Wrap newborn in prewarmed blanket and transfer to mother.	Reduces convective heat loss. Facilitates immediate maternal-infant contact without compromising infant thermoregulation.
Place skin-to-skin with mother under warmed blanket.	Skin-to-skin contact with mother or father acts to maintain newborn's temperature.

(continued)

Temperature Stabilization of the Newborn (*continued*)

Nursing Action	Rationale
Objective: Maintain stable infant temperature	
Diaper newborn and place hat on head. Place newborn uncovered (except for diaper and hat) under radiant warmer.	Radiant heat warms outer surface skin so skin needs to be exposed.
Tape servocontrol probe on infant's anterior abdominal wall (metal side next to skin) and cover with aluminum heat deflector patch.	Aluminum cover prevents heating of probe directly and overheating of infant. Turn heater to servocontrol mode with abdominal skin temperature maintained at 36.5°C–37°C.
Monitor infant's axillary and skin probe temperature per institution protocol.	Rechecking temperature ensures that it is within desired range. Temperature indicator on the radiant warmer continually displays baby's probe temperature so nurse checks baby's axillary temperature to ensure that the machine accurately reports baby's temperature.
Once infant's temperature reaches 98.6°F (37°C), remove infant from radiant warmer. Dress infant in T-shirt, diaper, and stocking hat then wrap in two blankets (called double wrap). Place in open crib. Recheck axillary temperature in one hour.	It is important to monitor infant's ability to maintain own thermoregulation.
Objective: Rewarm infant gradually if temperature < 97°F (36.1°C)	

Assess temperature frequently	Early detection of hypothermia, which predisposes infant to cold stress.
Check axillary temperature per hospital routine usually every 2 to 4 hours.	
Place unclothed infant with diaper under radiant warmer with servocontrol probe on abdomen.	Rapid heating leads to hyperthermia.
Gradually rewarm infant back to normal temperature.	Hyperthermia caused by too-rapid warming is associated with apnea, increased insensible water loss, and increased metabolic rate.
Recheck temperature in 30 minutes, then hourly.	
Once infant's temperature reaches 98.6°F (37°C), remove from heater, dress, double-wrap with hat on, and place in open crib. Recheck temperature in 1 hour.	
Objective: Prevent drops in baby's temperature.	Prevents loss of heat by conduction, convection, radiation, and evaporation.
Keep infant clothing and bedding dry.	
Double-wrap with hat on.	
Use heat lamp during procedures.	
Reduce exposure to drafts.	
Warm objects coming in contact with infant, eg, stethoscopes.	
Encourage mother to snuggle with infant under blankets or breast-feed with light cover over infant.	

Nursing Care Plan

Care of Expectant Woman with Limited Resources

Client Assessment

Nursing History		**Social Assessment**
Elicit which of the following are present in her life:	Limited money for food	Educational level
Limited financial resources	Limited emotional support	Work setting
Lack of secure housing	Limited recreational opportunities	Primary language
Limited accessibility of transportation		

Nursing Diagnosis	Nursing Interventions	Rationale	Evaluation
Powerlessness related to limited resources	Provide opportunities for client to talk with health care providers to establish rapport and feeling of support.	A sense of rapport enhances the health care relationship and provides a basis for communication, support, and counseling.	The woman verbalizes increased sense of power and control over her life.
Client Goal: The client will experience in-	Provide opportunities for decision making to enhance self-esteem. Assist		

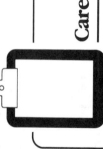

creased sense of control over her own life.	Provide information regarding community resources for available financial support; housing resources; food supplements such as WIC, food stamps; transportation resources such as city, bus, ride sharing; neighborhood community activities; church groups.	Knowledge of available resources will enhance the woman's ability to select those that will best meet her needs.
	Provide information regarding health care settings such as: community health clinic, prenatal classes through the clinic, and future well-baby/nurturing classes.	Prenatal care is available at low cost through community health clinics.
	Discuss resources for spiritual support such as church groups.	Depending on the support available, a church group may be a useful resource.
	Explore child-care potential in neighborhood such as baby-sitting cooperatives, day care.	
	Investigate community loan programs for maternity clothes, child-care equipment. Loan programs may be available in the Salvation Army or at thrift stores.	Some communities have a loan program for maternity needs.

The woman in establishing priorities in terms of her own needs, and assist her in locating resources to get needs met.

A sense of control over one's life may increase self-esteem.

Nursing Care Plan
Care of the Woman with
Acquired Immunodeficiency Syndrome (AIDS)

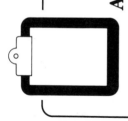

Client Assessment

Nursing History

1. Present pregnancy course
2. Estimated gestational age
3. Sensitivity to medications
4. History of infections

Physical Examination

1. Fetal size, fetal status (FHR), and fetal maturity
2. Observe for signs of fatigue and weakness, recurrent diarrhea, pallor, night sweats
3. Lymphadenopathy
4. Present weight and amount of weight gain or weight loss

Diagnostic Studies

1. Ultrasound
2. Fetal maturity studies (L/S ratio, PG, creatinine)
3. Hemoglobin and hematocrit
4. WBC
5. Testing for HIV-1 virus
6. T4 lymphocyte count (absolute T4)

5. Presence of nonproductive cough, fever, sore throat, chills, shortness of breath (*Pneumocystis carinii* pneumonia)
6. Dark purplish marks or lesions, especially on the lower extremities (Kaposi's sarcoma)
7. Oral, gingival lesions

7. ESR
8. Differential
9. Platelet count

Nursing Diagnosis	Nursing Interventions	Rationale	Evaluation
Altered nutrition: less than body requirements related to decreased appetite	Weigh woman. Obtain food history.	Establishes baseline weight. Identifying food likes and dislikes will assist in meal planning.	The woman maintains current weight or gains weight.
Client Goal: The woman will maintain current body weight or gain weight.	Plan high-protein, high-calorie diet.	Diet must take woman's needs and pregnancy needs into account.	
	Provide teaching regarding nutritional needs.	Nutritional education and support may assist the woman in planning her daily diet.	
Fear related to outcome of disease	Establish rapport. Provide opportunities to talk without interruption.	Establishment of rapport helps create a therapeutic relationship.	The woman has opportunities to talk with staff and contacts other sources of support.

(*continued*)

Care of the Woman with Acquired Immunodeficiency Syndrome (AIDS) (cont.)

Nursing Diagnosis	Nursing Interventions	Rationale	Evaluation
Client Goal: The woman will have opportunities to talk with nursing staff and other persons she identifies as supportive.	Provide support and counseling. Refer to community resources.		
Knowledge deficit related to appropriate precautions to prevent transmission of HIV infection	Provide information on transmission of HIV and measures to prevent infection.	Information regarding the ways in which the HIV virus is spread is an important basis for medical asepsis. As the woman understands more about the disease, she will be able to take precautions to protect against the spread of the HIV virus.	The woman is able to identify appropriate actions to prevent transmission of HIV and implements the actions as identified.
Client goal: Woman will be able to identify necessary precautions to prevent spread of HIV infection.	Discuss household safety issues (acceptable to use same dishes, safe to sleep in same bed, safe to use same bathroom, can hold and hug children. Sexual abstinence is safest; if not latex condoms should be used. Avoid sharing razors, toothbrushes. Use 10%		

	bleach solution to clean spills, disinfect bathroom. Use gloves to handle body fluids and so forth).		
	Discuss the implications of breast-feeding her infant.	Current information suggests that the virus may be spread in breast milk.	The woman does not develop a superimposed infectious disease.
Exchanging Infection: High risk related to suppressed immune status	Monitor for signs of infection (fever, cough, sore throat, night sweats, etc).	Any pathogen may be able to establish itself in an immuno-suppressed body. *Pneumocystis carinii* pneumonia is an infection frequently associated with AIDS.	
Client Goal: The woman will not develop infections during the hospital stay.	Maintain universal precautions.	Universal precautions with body secretions are advised for all clients who are hospitalized. In this case, the nurse and others will be protected from exposure to the woman's body secretions. In addition, the woman needs to be protected from other infectious agents.	

Nursing Care Plan
Cesarean Birth: Preparation and Immediate Recovery Period

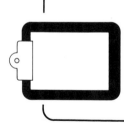

Client Assessment

Nursing History

Present pregnancy course
Estimated gestational age
Childbirth preparation
Sensitivity to medications and anesthetic agents
Past bleeding problems
Allergies
Last time woman ate and drank fluids

Physical Examination

1. Fetal size, fetal status (FHR), and fetal maturity
2. Maternal lung and cardiac status
3. Complete physical examination prior to administration of anesthetic

Diagnostic Studies

CBC
Hemoglobin and hematocrit
Type and cross-match for two units whole blood
Rh
Prothrombin time
Testing for syphilis
Urinalysis

Nursing Diagnosis	Nursing Interventions	Rationale	Evaluation
Nursing Diagnosis: Knowledge deficit related to the cesarean birth	Integrate cesarean birth information into childbirth preparation classes. Emphasize the similarities between vaginal and cesarean birth.	Couples may deny the possibility of an unplanned cesarean birth. Preparatory needs are basically the same for all couples anticipating childbirth.	Woman is able to discuss cesarean birth procedure and associated pre- and postoperative care.
Client Goal: The woman will discuss the cesarean birth procedure as measured by the following:	Minimize perceptions of "normal" versus "abnormal" birth.	A good knowledge base will allow for adaptive coping responses should birth occur.	
• Reason for cesarean	Provide factual information.	Information enables couples to make choices and participate in their birth experience.	
• Preoperative preparation			
• Postoperative care measures such as turn, cough, deep breathe, and need for frequent monitoring by nursing personnel	Encourage couple to discuss with obstetrician the approach and birth preferences in the event of a vaginal or cesarean birth.	Opportunity to discuss needs and desires minimizes unrealistic expectations, disappointment, and/or feelings of loss; promotes understanding of options, beliefs of birth attendant, and hospital policies; and allows couple to do anticipatory problem solving and develop effective coping behaviors.	
• Woman will demonstrate deep breathing, coughing, and splinting.			

(continued)

Cesarean Birth: Preparation and Immediate Recovery Period (*continued*)

Nursing Diagnosis	Nursing Interventions	Rationale	Evaluation
	Encourage expression of feelings.	Enables couple to work through fears, ambivalent or unresolved feelings, and potential grief associated with loss of vaginal birth.	
	Assess reaction to and interpretation of past cesarean birth or other surgical experiences.	Identifies need for information and opportunity to work through fears or unresolved feelings.	
	Encourage the development of mutual support by couples sharing their experiences and common concerns.	Decreases sense of being "different" or "alone" by realizing that their fears and concerns are not unique and feelings of anger or guilt are normal.	
	Describe preoperative procedure: • Abdominal prep • Insertion of in-dwelling bladder catheter • Insertion of IV	Explanation of pre- and post-operative measures decreases client anxiety and increases the woman's ability to participate in care.	

- Administration of pre-operative medications

Teach postoperative measures:

- How to deep breathe and cough
- Need for frequent position changes
- Frequency of monitoring vital signs

Create a safe, nonthreatening environment for couples to work through unresolved negative feelings.

Encourage couples to identify events that would make this birth experience more positive.

Cover most salient points of what to anticipate:

- What is going to happen to the woman's body and how it will feel

Negative feelings may contribute to distortion of information, impede learning, and affect expectations of upcoming birth experience.

Allow for anticipatory problem solving, and enhance ability to meet goals and expectations for birth event.

Knowing what to expect increases coping capability.

(continued)

Cesarean Birth: Preparation and Immediate Recovery Period (*continued*)

Nursing Diagnosis	Nursing Interventions	Rationale	Evaluation
	• What and why specific procedures will be done • How to handle discomfort associated with procedures • What the woman will see and hear during the cesarean		
	Provide couple with brief period of privacy.	They need an opportunity to pool their coping strengths to deal with the anxiety of the situation.	
	Inquire if couple has any questions about the decision.	Give opportunity for further clarification.	
	Prepare woman in stages, giving information and rationale for each procedure.	Crisis-altered cognitive grasp leads to information being misinterpreted or not being heard.	

Nursing Diagnosis: Impaired gas exchange related to decreased air exchange secondary to shallow breathing with incisional pain and ineffective cough	Avoid silence. Employ eye contact and therapeutic touch. As a part of preoperative teaching: ● Teach deep breathing and coughing. ● Teach abdominal splinting while deep breathing and coughing. ● Assess lung sounds.	Silence is often interpreted by the client as frightening and/or negative. Conveying a feeling of caring and reality orientation provides support. Promotes good air exchange. Provides support and decreases pain. Provides data on respiratory status.	Woman's respirations are between 14 and 20 per minute; lung sounds are clear; secretions are removed from respiratory track.
Client Goal: The woman will maintain effective respiratory function as measured by: ● Respirations between 14 and 20 per minute ● Secretions removed from respiratory tract	Explain that she will be turned every two hours and offer rationale. After surgery: assess respiratory rate	Provides aeration of lungs and assists in preventing pulmonary complications. Determines that respiratory rate is in normal range.	The woman is able to discuss the need for position changes and can demonstrate deep breathing and coughing. In the postpartal period she will be able to deep breathe and cough effectively, and her lungs remain clear.

(*continued*)

Cesarean Birth: Preparation and Immediate Recovery Period (*continued*)

Nursing Diagnosis	Nursing Interventions	Rationale	Evaluation
In the Postoperative Period			
Nursing Diagnosis: Pain related to incision, uterine involution, and contractions resulting from oxytocin administration	Administer analgesic medications. Provide quiet environment to enhance rest.	Provides relief of pain. Promotes comfort.	The woman has decreased pain as evidenced by reporting decreased pain on a 0 to 10 pain scale, is normotensive and eupneic, is able to move in bed and complete deep breathing and coughing with minimal discomfort.
Client Goal: The woman will have increased comfort as measured by: • Woman states pain has lessened. • Woman able to relax and rest.	Provide comfort measures such as the following: • Change position and support body parts. • Back rub. • Therapeutic touch. • Use music. • Modify environment.	Identified comfort measures. Use gate control theory.	
Nursing Diagnosis: Altered tissue perfusion related to excessive blood loss secondary to inadequate contraction of the uterus after birth	Evaluate firmness and position of fundus. Palpate fundus after pain medication is administered to promote patient comfort.	Provides opportunity to monitor involution. Palpation of fundus causes discomfort to the woman and is therefore frequently neglected and therefore becomes increasingly important.	

Client Goal: The woman will maintain normal tissue perfusion as measured by: • No excessive blood loss • Uterus remains contracted, in midline and below umbilicus • Skin warm, dry, and nonclammy • Normotensive	Fundus may be palpated from side of abdomen to avoid placing pressure on vertical incision. Administer oxytocin per physician order. Evaluate lochia.	Avoid tenderness at incisional site. Stimulates uterine contractions and thereby prevents bleeding. Lochia progresses from rubra to serosa to alba. Increase in flow indicates inefficient contraction of uterus and/or subinvolution.	The woman remains normotensive, uterus is well contracted in the midline and below the umbilicus, and blood loss is not excessive.
Nursing Diagnosis: Altered parenting	Provide information about the baby as soon as possible.	Interaction may be impaired because of recovery from anesthesia and discomfort in first few hours after birth.	
Client Goal: The parents will have opportunities to interact with their baby and will move into a positive attachment.	Provide opportunities for the parents to be with the baby as soon as possible. Provide opportunities to discuss feelings about the cesarean birth and the woman's self-image as a mother.	Feelings of failure associated with birthing experience can be generalized to ability to assume mothering role.	The woman is interacting with her newborn and engaging in care-taking behaviors.

Nursing Care Plan
Diabetes Mellitus

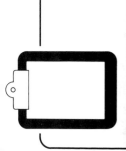

Client Assessment

Nursing History

1. Complete assessment: client and family
2. Identification of client's predisposition to diabetes
   a. Recurrent PIH
   b. Previous LGA infants (≥ 4000 g)
   c. Hydramnios
   d. Unexplained fetal death
   e. Obesity
   f. Family history of diabetes

Physical Examination

1. Length of gestation
2. Complaints of thirst and hunger
3. Recurrent monilial vaginitis or urinary tract infection (UTI)
4. Frequent urination beyond first trimester and prior to third trimester
5. Fundal height greater than expected for gestation
6. Obesity
7. Funduscopic examination to detect any vascular changes

Diagnostic Studies

1. Fasting plasma glucose (FPG)
2. 3-hour GTT
3. Urine test for glucose, ketones
4. Ultrasound to evaluate fetal growth and detect hydramnios
5. If woman has IDDM, glycosylated hemoglobin level (HbA_{1c}) determined
6. Serum fructosamine screening is now used in some centers
7. Maternal serum α-fetoprotein (AFP) screen

Third Trimester—Fetal Assessment

1. Serial NSTs
2. CST as necessary
3. Serial ultrasound
4. Biophysical profile to determine fetal maturity
5. Amniocentesis and L/S ratio as necessary

Nursing Diagnosis	Nursing Interventions	Rationale	Evaluation
Altered nutrition: High risk for more than body requirements related to imbalance between intake and available insulin.	Discuss importance of strict dietary control. Work with nutritionist and client to plan an individualized diet.	Dietary management is designed to ensure optimum fetal growth and normalize blood glucose levels. The greatest success occurs when a dietary plan is individualized to meet client needs and preferences.	Woman understands her prescribed diet, follows it carefully, and gains the optimum amount of weight for her prepregnant size.
Client Goal: The woman will understand and follow her prescribed diet as evidenced by weight gain within desired range, abil-	Recommended intake 30–35% kcal/kg body wt 12–20% protein 50–60% carbohydrate 20–30% fat	Recommended intake is designed to permit the following weight gain (Kitzmiller 1988): underweight 30+ lb desirable wt 24–30 lb	

(continued)

Diabetes Mellitus (*continued*)

Nursing Diagnosis	Nursing Interventions	Rationale	Evaluation
ity to discuss diet and plan menus, glycosylated hemoglobin (HbA$_{1c}$) levels in normal range.	Sodium intake may be restricted somewhat.	overweight 20–24 lb very overweight 15–20 lb	
Injury: High risk related to possible complications secondary to hypoglycemia or hyperglycemia	Determine insulin needs: 1. Check lab results of FPG and 2-hour postprandial. 2. Test blood four times daily using Dextrostix.	Sufficient insulin must be present to enable proper carbohydrate metabolism to take place; pregnancy requires a marked increase in circulating insulin to maintain normal blood glucose.	Woman avoids episodes of hyperglycemia or hypoglycemia, or, if they occur, they are detected early and treated successfully. Insulin requirements become stabilized.
Client Goal: Woman will avoid injury associated with hypoglycemia or hyperglycemia as evidenced by absence of signs or symptoms, blood glucose readings in normal range, and stabilization of insulin requirements.	Teach use of home blood glucose monitoring device; determine amount of insulin based on sliding scale. Administer regular or NPH insulin, or combination, as ordered.	Fasting glucose level tends to be lower than nonpregnant value. Effectiveness of insulin may be reduced by presence of hPL.	

(continued)

Teach early signs of hypoglycemia, including sweating, periodic tingling, disorientation, shakiness, pallor, clammy skin, irritability, hunger, headache, blurred vision, and, if untreated, coma or convulsions.

Insulin requirements fluctuate widely during pregnancy because of factors mentioned in text and because of lowered glucose tolerance, especially in second half of pregnancy, and fluctuate during intrapartal period because of depletion of glycogen stores during labor; fluctuations during puerperium are a result of involuntary process; in addition, conversion of blood glucose into lactose during lactation may cause marked changes in glucose tolerance and/or hypoglycemia.

Client needs to understand appropriate interventions because self-care at home in the event of hypoglycemia may save her life.

Rapid treatment of hypoglycemia is essential to prevent brain damage because the

Diabetes Mellitus (*continued*)

Nursing Diagnosis	Nursing Interventions	Rationale	Evaluation
		brain requires glucose to function (skeletal and heart muscles can derive energy from ketones and free fatty acids).	
	Treat within minutes of onset		
	a. Obtain immediate blood glucose level. If < 60 mg/dL, have client drink 8 oz milk (some agencies prefer to use ½ glass orange juice) and notify physician.	Provides baseline information on glucose levels. Liquids are absorbed from the GI tract faster than solids.	
	b. If woman is not alert enough to swallow give 1 mg glucagon subcutaneously or intramuscularly; notify physician.	Glucagon triggers the conversion of glycogen stored in the liver to glucose.	

c. If woman is in labor with intravenous lines in place, 10–20 mL of 50% dextrose may be given IV.

Standing order should be available; notify physician.

Teach woman early signs of hyperglycemia and treatment.

Woman can recognize signs and administer self-treatment.

Woman can also report any symptoms that may occur.

Observe for signs of hyperglycemia such as polyuria, polydipsia, dry mouth, increased appetite, fatigue, nausea, hot flushed skin, rapid deep breathing, abdominal cramps, acetone breath, headache, drowsiness, depressed reflexes, oliguria or anuria, stupor, coma.

Administer treatment; notify physician.

Administer insulin to restore body's normal metabolism of carbohydrate, protein, and fat.

(continued)

Diabetes Mellitus (*continued*)

Nursing Diagnosis	Nursing Interventions	Rationale	Evaluation
	a. Obtain frequent measurement of blood glucose; measure urine acetone.	Need to establish a baseline and to determine additional insulin dosage and prevent overtreatment; urine acetone indicates development of ketoacidosis.	
	b. Administer prescribed amount regular insulin subcutaneously or intravenously, or combination of routes.	Regular insulin is used because it acts immediately and is of short duration.	
	c. Replace fluids IV, orally, or both.	Fluids are depleted in the process of ketoacidosis; hypotension can result from decreased blood volume due to dehydration.	
	d. Measure intake and output.	Polyuria is an early sign of hyperglycemia; oliguria develops with hypotension and decreased bloodflow to kidneys.	

	e. Observe for symptoms of circulatory collapse; monitor BP and pulse.	Circulatory collapse can result from hypotension.	Woman implements self-care measures to avoid UTI. If UTI develops, treatment is effective and complications are avoided.
Injury: High risk related to signs of UTI secondary to glycosuria	Review preventive measures such as voiding frequently, voiding following intercourse, wiping from front to back, wearing cotton crotch underpants, drinking cranberry juice.	Preventive measures are designed to remove bacteria from the bladder, avoid contamination from the rectal area or outside sources, facilitate air flow in the perineal area, and acidify the urine.	
Client Goal: Woman will be able to identify signs of developing UTI and appropriate self-care measures to help prevent UTI. If signs of UTI do develop, therapy will be effective in preventing injury from complications.	Teach signs of developing UTI, including urgency, frequency, dysuria, and hematuria; low back pain with kidney involvement. Obtain clean-catch urine for culture and sensitivity.	Incidence of UTI is increased in diabetes, possibly because the existence of glycosuria provides rich medium for bacterial growth.	
	Administer prescribed antibiotics.	Antibiotic prescribed is specific to causative organism.	
	Encourage fluids to 2000–3000 mL/day. Measure intake and output.	Increased fluid intake promotes urinary removal of organisms.	

(continued)

Diabetes Mellitus (continued)

Nursing Diagnosis	Nursing Interventions	Rationale	Evaluation
Knowledge deficit related to the disease, its treatment, its implications for the woman, her unborn child, and the birth process	Provide teaching as indicated based on individualized assessment of couple's knowledge level:	Decreasing fear and increasing knowledge will make the client a more effective member of the antepartal-intrapartal health team.	Woman is able to discuss her condition and its implications, follows the recommendations of her care givers, and correctly carries out self-care activities related to her diabetes.
	1. Explain procedures.		
	2. Allow them to ask questions.		
Client Goal: Woman and her partner will understand the diabetes and its possible implications for her pregnancy as evidenced by their ability to administer insulin, to identify signs of hypo- or hyperglycemia, to discuss basic information about birth and anticipated therapy measures.	3. Develop a teaching plan to discuss and provide opportunities to practice administering insulin. Provide written information. Include partner so he can administer insulin if necessary.	Anticipatory guidance helps the couple prepare for the upcoming experience.	

4. Assess their level of knowledge of childbirth and use this to teach about what is happening.
5. Provide information about possible changes to expect during labor and birth due to DM. Explain about IV insulin, continuous monitoring of fetal status. Stress unchanged aspects of the experience.

Explain purpose of all scheduled tests and procedures:
1. Ultrasound as ordered to provide periodic assessment of fetal size.

Compliance is increased when client understands purpose of tests. Information about fetal growth and activity helps care givers evaluate placental functioning, anticipate the need

Woman cooperates with fetal testing schedule. Fetus responds well to tests and shows evidence of normal growth and placental functioning.

(continued)

Injury: High risk to fetus related to the effects of diabetes on uteroplacental functioning and fetal growth

Diabetes Mellitus (*continued*)

Nursing Diagnosis	Nursing Interventions	Rationale	Evaluation
Client Goal: Woman will be able to discuss rationale for fetal monitoring and testing, and will cooperate with fetal testing and assessment schedule.	2. Fetal activity diary 3. Serial NSTs 4. CST if indicated. 5. Measurement of L/S ratio and PG levels to determine fetal lung maturity. 6. Biophysical profile	for cesarean birth, determine fetal maturity, and decide on best time for birth.	
Altered family processes related to client's DM and the need for hospitalization. *Client Goal:* Family will deal successfully with the woman's illness, plan for changes necessary following discharge, and share their thoughts, feelings, and concerns with each other.	Encourage visits from family members and older siblings. Discuss with client and family changes that are necessary following discharge with regard to insulin, diet, exercise, and so forth. Assist family to make specific plans.	Illness in one family member impacts the entire family. Sometimes outside support is necessary to help the family deal with feelings and identify ways of dealing with the illness of a member.	Woman and family cope successfully with illness, make necessary plans for managing following discharge, and discuss their feelings in an open caring way.

Arrange for social services to visit or for homemaker assistance if necessary following discharge.
Give the family members information about the frustration that can occur when a family member is ill. Provide opportunities for them to discuss their feelings.
Offer suggestions for coping.

Nursing Care Plan
Fetal Distress

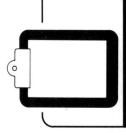

Nursing History

Assess client for presence of predisposing factors:

1. Preexisting maternal diseases
2. Maternal hypotension, bleeding
3. Placental abnormalities

Physical Examination

Asphyxia is suggested when one or more of the following are present:

1. FHR decelerations, decreased variability, tachycardia followed by bradycardia
2. Presence of meconium in amniotic fluid
3. Fetal scalp blood pH determination ≤7.20

Diagnostic Studies

Maternal hemoglobin and hematocrit

Urinalysis

Nursing Diagnosis	Nursing Interventions	Rationale	Evaluation
Nursing Diagnosis: Decreased cardiac output in fetus related to decreased uteroplacental perfusion secondary to maternal hypotension, circulating blood volume, and vasoconstriction associated with PIH	Observe and record the signs of fetal asphyxia:	Fetal asphyxia implies hypoxia (reduction in P_{O_2}), hypercapnia (elevation of P_{CO_2}), and acidosis (lowering of blood pH). Anaerobic glycolysis (breakdown of glycogen) takes place in the presence of hypoxia, and the end product of this process is lactic acid, resulting in metabolic acidosis.	FHR baseline remains in 120–140 range, short-term variability present, average long-term variability, no late or variable decelerations.
Client Goal: The FHR will remain in the range of 120–160 with short-term variability present, average long-term variability, accelerations with fetal movement, and no late or variable decelerations.	1. Presence of meconium in amniotic fluid	Fetal hypoxic episode leads to increased intestinal peristalsis and anal sphincter relaxation resulting in meconium release.	
	2. Decreased variability	Variability of FHR depends on intact sympathetic and para-	

(continued)

Fetal Distress (*continued*)

Nursing Diagnosis	Nursing Interventions	Rationale	Evaluation
		sympathetic nervous systems. When variability decreases, it indicates the fetus is no longer able to react or compensate for changes in the uterine environment.	
	3. Late decelerations in FHR	Vagal stimulation elicited through hypoxic brain tissues causes bradycardia.	
	4. Fetal hyperactivity	Fetus may initially become hyperactive in an attempt to increase circulation.	
	Initiate following interventions:		
	1. Administer O_2 to the woman with tight face mask at 6–10 L/min, per physician order.	Administration of O_2 may increase amount of oxygen available for transport to fetus. Tight face mask is used because laboring woman tends to breathe through her mouth.	

(*continued*)

2. Change maternal position (lateral, left side preferred).

Institute emergency measures for prolapse of cord:

1. Manually exert pressure on the presenting part; this must be done continuously; woman may be maintained in supine position, Trendelenburg position, knee-chest position, or on her side with a pillow to elevate her hips.

2. If occult prolapse is suspected, change maternal position to side-lying position.

3. Notify physician/nurse-midwife immediately.

Changed maternal position may relieve compression of the maternal vena cava and the cord, thereby facilitating O_2 exchange.

Fetal Distress (*continued*)

Nursing Diagnosis	Nursing Interventions	Rationale	Evaluation
Nursing Diagnosis: Fear related to knowledge of fetal distress *Client Goal:* The woman will have opportunity to ask questions and will verbalize whether she receives support.	Inform woman of fetal status. Explain treatment plan. Provide accurate information.	Anxiety is decreased when factual information is provided.	The woman verbalizes understanding of current problem and has no further questions.

Nursing Care Plan
Genetic Counseling for the Older Pregnant Woman

Nursing History:
Note age, gravida, parity, religious preference, LMP.

Physical Examination:
Pelvic examination to assess uterine changes associated with pregnancy.

Diagnostic Studies:
Urine hCG

Nursing Diagnosis Goals	Nursing Interventions	Rationale	Evaluation
Nursing Diagnosis: High risk knowledge deficit related to increase in genetic risks in the older pregnant woman.	Explain increased risks of Down syndrome after age of 35.	Cannot assume that all clients are aware of this risk.	Couple can describe increased risks of Down syndrome with pregnancy over the ages of 35 and 40. In addition, they are able to discuss problems and strengths related to indi-
	Share statistics that demonstrate incidence of problem in different age groups and how incidence increases at	Help client to develop a more realistic perspective of the increased risk with age.	

(continued)

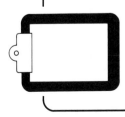

Genetic Counseling for the Older Pregnant Woman (*continued*)

Nursing Diagnosis	Nursing Interventions	Rationale	Evaluation
Goal: The couple will be able to identify genetic risks associated with pregnancy and the woman who is over the age of 35.	35 and dramatically increases over age 40.		viduals with Down syndrome and implications for their decision making.
	Discuss realities of having a Down syndrome baby and life-long prognosis for adults with Down syndrome.	Recent media attention to problem may not reflect a comprehensive perspective. Important for couples to understand life-long implications and variations in severity of problems.	
	Assess for concerns and questions. Clarify as appropriate.	Help to clarify any misunderstandings or questions the couple may still have.	
Nursing Diagnosis: Knowledge deficit related to amniocentesis.	Assess couple's knowledge and/or preconceived ideas related to amniocentesis.	Couple may have no knowledge about amniocentesis or may have misconceptions that increase their anxieties and fears about the procedure.	The couple will understand the process involved with amniocentesis as demonstrated through their questions and discussion.

Goal: The couple will have accurate information related to amniocentesis.	Clarify misconceptions about procedures with factual information.	Difficult for couple to listen if concerns and misconceptions are not addressed initially.
	Explain each step of procedure and effect on mother and fetus.	Most couples do not know what to expect and have fears about risks to mother and fetus.
	Assess for further questions or concerns.	New questions and concerns may arise as procedure is explained.

Nursing Care Plan

Hemorrhage in Third Trimester and at Birth

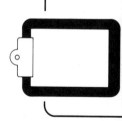

Client Assessment

Nursing History

Identify factors predisposing to hemorrhage:

1. Presence of preeclampsia-eclampsia (PIH)
2. Overdistention of the uterus
   a. Multiple pregnancy
   b. Hydramnios
3. Grandmultiparity
4. Advanced age
5. Uterine contractile problems
   a. Hypotonicity
   b. Hypertonicity

Physical Examination

Severe abdominal pain (central abruptio placentae)

External or concealed bleeding

Painless vaginal hemorrhage (placenta previa)

Shock symptoms (decreased blood pressure, increased pulse, pallor)

Uterine tetany or uterine atony

Portwine amniotic fluid with abruptio placentae

Degree of hemorrhage

Diagnostic Studies

Hemoglobin and hematocrit

Type and cross-match

Fibrinogen levels

Platelets

Prothrombin time

Activated partial thromboplastin time

Fibrin split products

6. Painless vaginal bleeding after seventh month
7. Presence of hypertension
8. Presence of diabetes
9. History of previous hemorrhage or bleeding problems, blood coagulation defects, abortions
10. Retained placental fragments
11. Cervical and/or vaginal lacerations

Changes in FHR
Increased resting tone of uterus between contractions

Determine religious preference to establish whether client will permit a blood transfusion.

Nursing Diagnosis	Nursing Interventions	Rationale	Evaluation
Nursing Diagnosis: Altered tissue perfusion (renal, cerebral, and peripheral) secondary to excessive blood loss	General interventions: Observe, record, and report blood loss. Evaluate woman experiencing decrease in blood volume using following parameters:	Monitoring the amount of blood loss aids in determining appropriate interventions.	Woman maintains normal tissue perfusion; BP remains between 110/70 and 138/88; pulse rate 60–90 beats/min; urine output > 30 mL/hr; urine clear, straw colored; specific gravity *(continued)*

Hemorrhage in Third Trimester and at Birth (continued)

Nursing Diagnosis	Nursing Interventions	Rationale	Evaluation
Client Goal: The woman will maintain adequate tissue perfusion as measured by the following: • BP between 110/70 and 138/88 • Pulse rate 60–90 • Urine output > 30 mL/hr • Skin warm and nonclammy	1. Monitor rate and quality of respirations frequently.	Initially respiratory rate increases as a result of sympathoadrenal stimulation, resulting in increased metabolic rate; pain and anxiety may cause hyperventilation.	1.010–1.025; skin warm, dry.
	2. Measure pulse rate.	Increased pulse rate is an effect of increased epinephrine.	
	3. Assess pulse quality by direct palpation. Determine pulse deficit by comparing apical-radial rates.	Reflects circulatory status. Thready pulse indicates vasoconstriction and reflects decreased cardiac output; peripheral pulses may be absent if vasoconstriction is intense. Bounding pulse may indicate overload.	
	4. Compare present BP with woman's baseline BP; note pulse pressure.	Hypotension indicates loss of large amount of circulatory fluid or lack of compensation in circulatory system.	

5. Monitor urine output (decrease to less than 30 mL/hr is sign of shock):
   a. Insert Foley catheter.
   b. Measure output hourly.
   c. Measure specific gravity to determine concentration of urine.

As cardiac output decreases, there is usually a fall in pulse pressure. Peripheral vasoconstriction may make accurate readings difficult.

Vasoconstrictor effect of norepinephrine decreases blood flow to kidneys, which decreases glomerular filtration rate and the output of urine. Inability to concentrate urine may indicate renal damage from vasoconstriction and decreased blood perfusion.

6. Inspect skin for presence of following:
   a. Pallor and cyanosis: *Pallor* in brown-skinned persons appears yellowish-brown; black-skinned individuals appear ashen gray; generally

Skin reflects amount of vasoconstriction. Pallor is determined by intensity of vasoconstriction.

Hemorrhage in Third Trimester and at Birth (*continued*)

Nursing Diagnosis	Nursing Interventions	Rationale	Evaluation
	pallor may be observed in mucous membranes, lips, and nail beds.		
	Cyanosis is assessed by inspecting lips, nail beds, conjunctiva, palms, and soles of feet at regular intervals; evaluate capillary refilling by pressing on nail bed and observing return of color; compare by testing your own nail bed.	Cyanosis occurs when the amount of unoxygenated hemoglobin in the blood is ≤ 5 g/dL blood.	
	b. Coldness c. Clamminess		
	Evaluate state of consciousness frequently.	Produced by slow blood flow.	
	Measure CVP: normal CVP is 5–10 cm H_2O.	Caused by sympathetic stimulation of sweat glands.	

(*continued*)

Intervention	Rationale
	Diminished cerebral blood flow causes restlessness and anxiety; as shock progresses, state of consciousness decreases.
Assess amount of blood loss: 1. Count pads. 2. Weigh pads and chux (1 g = 1 mL blood approximately). 3. Record amount in a specific amount of time (for example, 50 mL bright red blood on pad in 20 min).	Provides estimation of volume of blood returning to heart and ability of both chambers in right heart to propel blood. Low CVP indicates a decrease in the circulating volume of blood (hypovolemia). In obstetric clients, blood is replaced according to estimates of actual blood loss, rather than using parameters of increased and decreased BP.

Hemorrhage in Third Trimester and at Birth (continued)

Nursing Diagnosis	Nursing Interventions	Rationale	Evaluation
	Hypovolemia: Relieve decreased blood pressure by administration of whole blood.	Hypotension results from decreased blood volume.	
	While waiting for whole blood to be available, infuse isotonic fluids, plasma, plasma expanders, or serum albumin, per physician order.	Degree of hypovolemia may be assessed by CVP, hemoglobin, and hematocrit.	
	Marginal abruptio placentae: If abruptio placentae is diagnosed, nurse and physician will:		
	1. Evaluate blood loss. 2. Assess uterine contractile pattern, tenderness, and height.	Provides information on type of abruption and maternal and fetal status.	Bleeding often stops as shock develops but resumes as circulation is restored.

(*continued*)

3. Start continuous monitoring of uterine contractions by EFM.

4. Monitor maternal vital signs.

5. Assess fetal status per continuous EFM.

6. Assess cervical dilatation and effacement to determine labor progress if uterine contractions are present.

7. Rule out placenta previa.

8. Perform amniotomy and begin oxytocin infusion if labor does not start immediately or is ineffective.

9. Review and evaluate diagnostic lab blood tests (hemoglobin, hematocrit, PT, APPT, fibrin split products, fibrinogen).

Hemorrhage in Third Trimester and at Birth (*continued*)

Nursing Diagnosis	Nursing Interventions	Rationale	Evaluation
	Central abruptio placentae with severe blood loss:		
	1. Perform same assessments as for marginal abruptio placentae.		
	2. Monitor CVP.		
	3. Replace blood loss.		
	4. Effect immediate delivery.		
	5. Observe for signs and symptoms of disseminated intravascular coagulation (DIC).		
Nursing Diagnosis: Altered tissue perfusion: High risk related to blood loss secondary to uterine atony following birth	1. Assess contractility of uterus and amount of vaginal bleeding.	Muscle fibers that have been overstretched or overused do not contract well; contraction of muscle fibers over open placental site is essential; slight relaxation of uterus muscle	The woman's uterus remains firm, in the midline, and below the umbilicus.
	2. Postpartally, massage uterus every 15 min for one hour, every 30 min		

Client Goal: The woman's uterus will remain well contracted in the midline and below the umbilicus.	for one hour, every 60 min for two to four hours. Evaluate more frequently if uterus is boggy or not in the midline. Administer more oxytocin per protocol or physician/nurse-midwife order.	fibers leads to continuous oozing of blood.	
Nursing Diagnosis: Fear related to concern for own personal status and the baby's safety. Client Goal: The woman will have opportunities to verbalize concern.	Keep woman informed of present status. Provide accurate information. Provide opportunities for questions. Establish trusting relationship. Encourage woman to participate in decision making if at all possible.	As hemorrhage occurs, the safety of the mother and baby are threatened. Anxiety and fear may be lessened somewhat when the woman is informed, understands what is happening, and has some part in the decision-making process.	The woman verbalizes questions and receives support.
Nursing Diagnosis: Impaired fetal gas exchange: High risk related to decreased blood volume and hypotension	Assess and monitor fetal heart rate (range 120–160 beats/min).	Hemorrhage from woman disrupts blood flow pattern to fetus, possibly compromising fetal status.	Fetal heart rate baseline remains stable between 120–160 beats/min, short-term variability present, (continued)

Hemorrhage in Third Trimester and at Birth (*continued*)

Nursing Diagnosis	Nursing Interventions	Rationale	Evaluation
Client Goal: The FHR will remain within normal limits without signs of stress or distress.	Observe for meconium in amniotic fluid.	Hypoxia causes increased motility of fetal intestines and relaxation of abdominal muscles, with release of meconium into amniotic fluid.	long-term variability is average, no late or variable decelerations, fetal scalp blood pH is > 7.25.
	Assist in obtaining fetal blood sample (pH < 7.20 indicates severe jeopardy).		

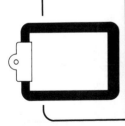

Client Assessment

Nursing Care Plan
Induction of Labor

Nursing History

Previous pregnancies
Present pregnancy course
Childbirth preparation
Estimated gestational age

Physical Examination

1. Examination of pregnant uterus (Leopold's maneuvers to determine fetal size and position)
2. Vaginal examination to evaluate cervical readiness
   a. Ripe cervix: Feels soft to the examining finger, is located in a medial to anterior position, is more than 50% effaced, and is 2–3 cm dilated

Diagnostic Studies

Fetal maturity tests (lecithin/sphingo-myelin ratio, creatinine concentrations, ultrasonography), NST, CST, FBPP

Maternal blood studies (complete blood cell count [CBC], hemoglobin, hematocrit, blood type, Rh factor)

Urinalysis

(continued)

Induction of Labor (*continued*)

Client Assessment
b. Unripe cervix: Feels firm to the examining finger, is long and thick, perhaps in a posterior position, with little or no dilatation
3. Presence of contractions
4. Membranes intact or ruptured
5. Fetal size (Leopold's maneuvers, ultrasound)
6. Fetal readiness
7. CPD evaluation
8. Maternal vital signs and FHR before beginning induction

Nursing Diagnosis	Nursing Interventions	Rationale	Evaluation
Nursing Diagnosis: Knowledge deficit related to induction procedure.	Assess the woman's feelings regarding induction. She may ask, "Will this work?" "How long will it take?" "Will it hurt more?"	Woman may be apprehensive about what will happen, or feel a sense of failure that she cannot "go into labor by herself."	The woman is able to discuss the induction procedure, feels comfortable asking questions as they arise, and has no further questions.

Client Goal: The woman will discuss the induction procedure, the benefits, and the potential risks.	Assess knowledge base regarding the induction process. Provide needed information (for example, when the cervix is ripe, contractions should begin in 30–60 minutes); length of labor depends on a number of factors.	After assessing knowledge base, appropriate information can be given to allay apprehension.
	Assess knowledge of breathing techniques; if woman does not have a method to use, teach breathing techniques before starting oxytocin infusion.	Use of breathing techniques during contractions will help relaxation; although a woman may be apprehensive about induction, teaching a new breathing method will be easier before contractions are present.
Nursing Diagnosis: Decreased cardiac output related to positional changes and the weight of the uterus on the vena cava	Position woman on her side; encourage her to avoid supine position. Monitor maternal blood pressure (BP) and pulse and FHR every 15–20 minutes.	Side-lying position maintains optimal blood flow to uterus and placenta.
		The woman's vital signs remain within normal limits.

(continued)

Induction of Labor (*continued*)

Nursing Diagnosis	Nursing Interventions	Rationale	Evaluation
Client Goal: The woman will maintain vital signs within normal range with no significant increase or decrease.	If she becomes hypotensive: 1. Keep the woman on her side, may change to other side. 2. Discontinue oxytocin infusion. 3. Increase rate of primary IV. 4. Monitor FHR. 5. Notify physician. 6. Assess for cause of hypotension.	Initial hypotension is secondary to peripheral vasodilatation induced by oxytocin, which causes diminished blood supply to placenta and resultant decrease in O_2 supply to fetus. Actions are directed toward improving blood flow and oxygenation of tissues.	
Nursing Diagnosis: Altered tissue perfusion (placenta) related to potential hypertonic contraction pattern	Apply monitor to obtain 15 minutes of tracing prior to starting induction.	Establishes baseline data.	The woman's contraction pattern is established with contractions every two to three minutes, lasting about 60–75 seconds with relaxation of the uterus between contractions.

(*continued*)

Client Goal: The woman will maintain normal contraction pattern as measured by: • Frequency of 2½–3 minutes • Duration of about 60 seconds • Relaxation of uterus between contractions	Administer oxytocin in electrolyte solution.	Oxytocin has slight antidiuretic effect, especially when administered in electrolyte-free solutions.
	Encourage voiding every 2 hours. Monitor and record fluid intake and output. Monitor for nausea, vomiting, hypotension, tachycardia, cardiac arrhythmias.	Provides information on hydration status. These are signs and symptoms of water intoxication; they must be differentiated from other problems.
	Monitor FHR by continuous electronic fetal monitoring. Obtain 15-minute tracing prior to beginning induction to evaluate fetal status; *do not* start infusion or advance rate (if induction has already begun) if FHR is not in range of 120–160 beats/min, if decelerations are present, or if variability decreases.	Will provide continuous data regarding fetal response to induction.

Induction of Labor (*continued*)

Nursing Diagnosis	Nursing Interventions	Rationale	Evaluation
	Evaluate maternal BP and pulse before beginning induction and then before each increase in infusion rate; do not advance infusion rate in presence of maternal hypertension or hypotension or radical changes in pulse rate.	To establish baseline data and to assess client response in induction; client status may change rapidly.	
	Evaluate contraction frequency, duration, and intensity prior to each increase in infusion rate.	Evaluates uterine response to induction.	
	Do not increase rate of infusion if contractions are every two to three minutes, lasting 40–60 seconds, with moderate intensity.	Desired effect has been obtained. Further increase in rate may produce hypertonic labor pattern (contractions with frequency of less than two minutes, for example more than five contractions in ten min-	

utes or a duration of longer
than 75–90 seconds).

Discontinue oxytocin infusion if:

1. Contractions are more
   frequent than every two
   minutes.
2. Contraction duration
   exceeds 75–90
   seconds.
3. Uterus does not relax
   between contractions.

Uterus is being overstimulated
and serious complications may
develop for woman and fetus.
Ruptured uterus or abruptio
placentae can result from drug-
induced tumultuous labor.
(Note: Terms hyperstimulation, hypertonic labor pattern,
and tumultuous labor are used
interchangeably.)
Contractions lasting over 90
seconds with decreased resting tone may result in fetal
hypoxia.

Increase oxytocin IV infusion rate every 20 minutes
until adequate contractions
are achieved; do *not* exceed an infusion rate of
20–40 mU/min.
(Note: protocols directing
how often oxytocin is in-
creased may vary from

Uterine response to oxytocin
may be individualized.

(*continued*)

Induction of Labor (*continued*)

Nursing Diagnosis	Nursing Interventions	Rationale	Evaluation
	30–60 minutes. See American College of Obstetrics and Gynecology [ACOG 1988] guidelines and agency protocol.)		
	Check infusion pump to assure oxytocin is infusing; check whether pump is on, chamber refills and empties, level of fluid in IV bottle becomes lower; if problem is found, correct it, and restart infusion at beginning dose. Check main IV site frequently. Check piggy-back connection to primary tubing to assure solution is not leaking.	Oxytocin may not be infusing due to pump, mechanical, or human error.	
	Evaluate cervical dilatation by vaginal examination	When cervix responds by stretching or pulling, *do not*	

(*continued*)

with each oxytocin dosage increase after labor is established.

increase oxytocin dosage; overdosage may occur, causing rapid labor with possible cervical lacerations and fetal damage; when there is no change in the cervix, additional oxytocin is needed.

Monitor FHR continuously (normal range is 120–160/min).

O_2 deficiency may occur over a long period of time; in cases of placental insufficiency or cord compression, compensated tachycardia may be evoked.

In episodes of bradycardia (<120 beats/min) lasting for more than 30 seconds, administer O_2 by face mask at 6–10 L/min.

Stop oxytocin infusion. Position woman on left side if quick recovery of FHR does not occur.

Carefully evaluate fetal tachycardia (>160 beats/min).

Persistent fetal tachycardia causes more prominent O_2 deficiency (hypoxia) and CO_2 increase in fetal blood. Vasoconstriction occurs, with increased fetal blood flow

Sustained tachycardia may necessitate discontinuation of oxytocin infusion.

Induction of Labor (continued)

Nursing Diagnosis	Nursing Interventions	Rationale	Evaluation
	Assess for presence of meconium staining. Notify physician/CNM.	through coronary arteries, brain, and placenta; this increased demand on myocardial performance leads to cardiac decompensation if oxygen exchange is impaired and hypoxia continues. Fetal hypoxia may also cause central vasomotor center to release adrenal catecholamines; at term, this enhances depolarization of cardiac pacemaker cells, which will result in direct bradycardia. Bradycardia or subsequent reflex tachycardia temporarily remedies the O_2 deficiency.	
Nursing Diagnosis: Pain related to uterine contractions	Provide support to woman as she uses breathing techniques.	Contractions may build up more quickly with oxytocin induction and may be more painful.	The woman maintains breathing pattern and a sense of control during labor.

Client Goal: The woman will maintain her breathing pattern and a relaxed state during contractions.	Encourage use of effleurage, back rub, and other supportive measures. Assess need for analgesia or anesthesia.	Techniques help maintain relaxation and thereby decrease pain sensation. After labor is well established, analgesia or epidural anesthesia may be given without delaying progress.

Nursing Care Plan
Infant with Acquired
Immunodeficiency Syndrome (AIDS)

Client Assessment

Nursing History

Maternal

History of drug abuse or needle sharing

Sexual partner or partners with a positive HIV antibody test or ELISA test

Physical Examination

Complete physical examination—Variable findings and symptoms depending on the type of infection

Diagnostic Studies

ELISA—Detects HIV antibody. May take six months to convert to seropositive.

Newborns may have HIV antibodies from maternal infection

Western Blot test—To confirm ELISA test

Immunoglobin studies—to detect increased levels of IgG and IgM, depressed levels of T4 and T4:T8 ratio

Hemoglobin and hematocrit—Detect anemia

Nursing Diagnosis	Nursing Interventions	Rationale	Evaluation
Infections: High risk related to perinatal exposure and immunoregulation suppression *Client Goal:* Infant will not develop infection while in birthing area	Assess infant for signs of ongoing infection such as: • Failure to thrive • Weight loss over 10% at time of diagnosis • Temperature instability • More than three diarrheal episodes a day • Hepatosplenomegaly-palpate once a day for continued enlargement • Lethargy	Signs and symptoms of infection and inflammation may persist prior to definitive AIDS diagnosis. Decreased activity and lethargy can indicate sepsis.	At-risk infant is identified and remains free of opportunistic infections.
	Assess for opportunistic diseases such as: Herpes simplex lasting more than one month Cytomegalovirus disease Lymphoid interstitial pneumonia Viral, fungal, or protozoal infections	Opportunistic infections occur because of immune system suppression.	

(continued)

Infant with Acquired Immunodeficiency Syndrome (AIDS), (*continued*)

Nursing Diagnosis	Nursing Interventions	Rationale	Evaluation
	Maintain universal precautions—especially until baby has had first bath—when changing diapers, drawing blood or doing heel sticks, and suctioning newborn.	Universal precautions protect care givers from infant's body secretions. Also newborn is protected from other infectious agents.	
Altered nutrition: less than body requirements related to formula intolerance and inadequate intake.	Assess for residuals, abdominal distention (abdominal girth measurements) prior to each feeding. Obtain accurate intake and output (weigh diapers).	Feeding intolerance causes gastric residuals, increasing abdominal girth and dehydration.	Baby has steady weight gain and follows normal growth curve.
Client Goal: Baby will gain weight and progress on normal growth curve.	Monitor stools for amount, type, consistency, and any change in pattern. Check stools for occult blood and reducing substances. Provide small frequent feedings.	Loose stools and presence of reducing substances may indicate feeding intolerance. Occult blood indicates irritation or ulceration of bowel mucosa.	

Altered parenting related to diagnosis of AIDS and fear of future outcome *Client Goal:* Parents will express fears and begin to bond with their infant.	Assess cause of parents' fear by • Providing time for expression of concerns • Determine parents' understanding about AIDS Provide information about AIDS as to cause, signs of HIV in infants, current and experimental treatment modalities, support groups, and community resources.	Lack of information and distorted perception about AIDS may increase parents' fears. Accurate information about AIDS reduces fear. Access to community services and participation in support groups provides assistance with coping with a potentially critically ill child.	Parents verbalize their fears, hold and talk with newborn, and carry out infant caretaking activities.

Nursing Care Plan
Newborn of a
Substance–Abusing Mother

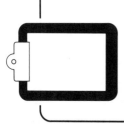

Client Assessment

Nursing History

Type and amount of drug(s) consumed by mother during each month of pregnancy

Type and amount of prenatal care

Prior history of addiction and treatment

Maternal disease/infection such as placenta previa, hypertension, bacterial and TORCH infections, HIV

Physical Examination

Withdrawal symptoms: hyperactivity, jitteriness, irritability, shrill high-pitched cry, vomiting, diarrhea, weak suck, stuffy nose, frequent sneezing, yawning, tachycardia, hypertension, apnea. With cocaine, withdrawal pattern may be unpredictable or may be asymptomatic with only subtle behavioral state organization problems. Disturbed sleep-wake cycle and rhythm at 24 to 28 hr.

Diagnostic Studies

Toxicology screen—Identify drug(s) and drug levels in mother and infant blood and urine

Serum electrolyte (Na, K, Ca)—Detect losses from vomiting, diarrhea, detect causes of neurologic symptoms or seizures

Glucose

Serial capillary gases

seropositive and sexually transmitted diseases

Preterm labor and birth

CBC and blood culture—Detect sepsis

Urine specific gravity—high due to dehydration.

Nursing Diagnosis	Nursing Interventions	Rationale	Evaluation
Altered sleep pattern disturbance related central nervous system excitation secondary to drug withdrawal *Client Goal:* Babies at risk for withdrawal will be identified early and normal rest/sleep patterns will be established throughout withdrawal period.	Assess for withdrawal symptoms including: frequent sneezing and yawning, restlessness, high-pitched shrill cry, hypertonicity, vomiting or diarrhea, wakefulness Provide calming techniques including: Swaddle infant tightly in side-lying or prone position with small pillow supporting back. Provide quiet, dim environment for rest	Most addicted newborns will show symptoms of withdrawal as early as 12 hr after birth. Begins with jitteriness, hyperactivity and wakefulness; progressing to GI symptoms and seizures. Early identification allows for early intervention and prevention of complications. Positioning provides for rest and discourages hyperactivity and increases comfort while reducing stimuli. Quiet environment decreases external stimuli and therefore infant's irritability.	Baby is free from jitteriness and has normal sleep-wake behaviors.

(*continued*)

Newborn of a Substance-Abusing Mother (*continued*)

Nursing Diagnosis	Nursing Interventions	Rationale	Evaluation
	Schedule tests or treatments to avoid stress.	Planned care allows for maximum rest and reduce external stimuli.	
	Hold, rock, and cuddle infant. Use touching, patting, smiling, and talking to infant. Use infant snugglies for closeness.	Holding infant as often as possible promotes comfort and cuddling quiets and comforts infant. These activities promote close contact.	
	Provide pacifier or position baby so that baby can get hand to mouth.	Hand to mouth activity or pacifier satisfies increased need to suck during withdrawal.	
	Administer medications for withdrawal as ordered such as paregoric, chlorpromazine, valium, phenobarbital; observe for effectiveness and side effects.	Pharmacologic agents alleviate withdrawal symptoms.	

Altered nutrition: less than body requirements related to withdrawal symptoms *Client Goal:* Baby will not lose more than 2% weight, will take feeding without vomiting, aspiration or fatigue, and will gain weight.	Assess for increased nutritional needs because of gestational age, weight, uncoordinated suck and swallow, vomiting, diarrhea, and regurgitation. Provide appropriate nutrition: Initiate IV feedings until stable.	Infants of drug-addicted mothers tend to be SGA and premature. CNS stimulation causes hyperactivity leading to poor feeding, GI hypermotility and irritation leading to inability to retain or absorb nutrients. Oral feeding an irritable infant with possible seizures may foster aspiration.	Infant gains approximately 1 oz per day and has vigorous suck reflex.
	Supplement oral or gavage feedings with intravenous intake per orders. Give small, frequent feedings of high caloric formula; may start feedings at one-half strength every 3 hours.	SGA infants need 110–120 cal/kg/day for optimal nutrition. Smaller feedings facilitate nutritional intake.	
	Check for residuals after oral or gavage feedings; reduce feeding volume if residuals are high. As hy-	Prevents vomiting from overfeeding while still providing IV fluids according to infant's tolerance.	

(*continued*)

Newborn of a Sustance-Abusing Mother (*continued*)

Nursing Diagnosis	Nursing Interventions	Rationale	Evaluation
	peractivity decreases, increase feedings as tolerated. Place on right side with back support or on abdomen after feedings.	Position decreases vomiting, regurgitation and distention.	
Knowledge deficit related to feelings of inadequacy or inability to care for infant. *Client Goal:* Mother will touch, hold infant and develop confidence in her ability to provide safe newborn care.	Identify mother's knowledge needs and readiness for learning. Provide information including: 1. Signs and symptoms of baby's withdrawal, current condition, and rationale for treatment 2. Newborn capabilities and developmental behaviors	Assessment provides information regarding mother's ability to care for infant. Provides information about parent's understanding of baby's behavior and how to care for the baby with symptoms. Assists parents to be realistic about infant's progress.	Mother has bonded with infant; parents are involved in care and have realistic expectations for their baby.

3. Newborn's need for appropriate stimulation as well as rest depending on infant's cues

Mother needs to adjust infant interaction based on infant's cues to foster development.

4. Physical care needs such as feeding, bathing, clothing, and holding

This information helps mother provide for safe infant care.

Encourage and support positive mothering behaviors with infant.

Increases mother's feelings of competence in her parenting abilities.

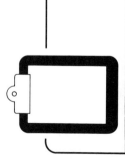

Nursing Care Plan
Newborn with Jaundice

Client Assessment

Nursing History

Maternal

ABO incompatibility

Rh negative

Diabetes

Presence of infection, such as syphilis, cytomegalovirus, rubella, toxoplasmosis

Presence of familiar blood dyscrasias such as sphero-cytosis, G-6-PD deficiency

Medications: Novobiocin, sulfonamides, and salicylates interfere with conjugation or compete for serum albumin-binding sites

Physical Examination

Generalized edema with pleural and pericardial effusion

Pallor or jaundice noted in first 24–36 hours

May have enlargement of spleen or liver

Changes in behavior (lethargy, irritability), tremors

Dark, concentrated urine

Hypoactive bowel sounds

Hypotonia

Presence of hematomas or large bruises (assess for other signs of enclosed bleeding)

Excessive ecchymosis or petechiae

Meconium passage may be delayed

Number and outcome of previous pregnancies

Condition at birth and current health status of other children

Paternal

Rh factor—negative or positive

Birth

Enlarged placenta (larger than one-seventh of neonate's weight)

Delayed clamping of umbilical cord

Traumatic birth

Neonate

Enclosed hemorrhage, hematoma, large bruises, intra-cranial bleeding

Bacterial and/or viral infections can affect liver and thus decrease glucuronyl transferase activity

Polycythemia (central hematocrit of 65% or more)

Biliary atresia, cystic fibrosis (inspissated bile)

Congenital hypothyroidism

Conditions that decrease available albumin-binding sites:

1. Fetal or neonatal asphyxia decreases binding affinity of bilirubin to albumin.

Diagnostic Studies

Coombs' test—direct on baby, indirect on mother's blood

Total bilirubin level

Indications for exchange transfusion:

In ABO incompatibility, serum bilirubin levels greater than 20 mg/dL (full-term) and 15 mg/dL (preterm)

In Rh incompatibility, serum bilirubin greater than 20 mg/dL (term) greater than 15 mg/dL (large preterms), and greater than 13 mg/dL (less than 1250 g preterms)

Total serum protein (provides measure of binding capacity)

Complete blood cell count (CBC)—assess anemia and polycythemia

Peripheral smear—evaluate red blood cells for immaturity or abnormality

Blood glucose

CO_2 combining power

Reticulocyte count

Kleihauer-Betke test

Transcutaneous jaundice meter

(continued)

Newborn with Jaundice (*continued*)

Client Assessment

2. Chilling and hypoglycemia create fatty acids to compete for binding sites.

3. Preterm neonates tend to have lower serum albumin levels and therefore less albumin to bind to.

Nursing Diagnosis	Nursing Interventions	Rationale	Evaluation
Impaired tissue integrity related to predisposing factors associated with hyperbilirubinemia	Evaluate baby's history for predisposing factors for hyperbilirubinemia.	Early identification of risk factors enables the nurse to monitor babies for early signs of hyperbilirubinemia. Acidosis, hypoxia, hypothermia, etc increase the risk of hyperbilirubinemia at lower bilirubin levels.	Baby's jaundice is identified early.
Client Goal: Babies at risk for jaundice and early signs of jaundice will be identified.	Observe color of amniotic fluid at time of rupture of membranes.	Amber-colored amniotic fluid is indicative of hyperbilirubinemia.	

Nursing Diagnosis	Intervention	Rationale	Expected Outcome
	Assess baby for developing jaundice in daylight if possible.	Early detection is affected by nursery environment. Artificial lights (with pink tint) may mask beginning of jaundice.	
	1. Observe sclera.	Most visible sign of hyperbilirubinemia is jaundice noted in skin, sclera, or oral mucosa. Onset is first seen on face.	
	2. Observe skin color and assess by blanching.	Blanching the skin leaves a yellow color to the skin immediately after pressure is released.	
	3. Check oral mucosa, posterior portion of hard palate, and conjunctival sacs for yellow pigmentation in dark-skinned newborns.	Underlying pigment of dark-skinned people may normally appear yellow.	
	Report jaundice occurring within 24 hours of birth.		
Injury: High risk related to reabsorption of bilirubin	Initiate feedings as soon as possible, at least within	Early feeding stimulates digestive enzymes involved in	Baby tolerates feedings with minimal regurgitation; (continued)

Newborn with Jaundice (*continued*)

Nursing Diagnosis	Nursing Interventions	Rationale	Evaluation
secondary to decreased stooling	four to six hr after birth or per protocol.	establishing gut bacterial flora and decreased enterohepatic circulation.	active bowel sounds are present in all four quadrants; meconium stool is passed within 24 hours.
Client Goal: Baby will start feedings within four to six hr after birth, have active bowel sounds, and begin to pass meconium stools.			
Fluid volume deficit secondary to phototherapy	Offer feedings every two to four hr. Do not skip feedings	Adequate hydration increases peristalsis and excretion of bilirubin.	Baby tolerates oral feedings and is adequately hydrated as indicated by good skin turgor, six to eight wet diapers per day, and maintenance of weight.
Client Goal: Baby will have good skin turgor, clear amber urine output of 1–3 mL/kg/hr, six to eight wet diapers/day, and will maintain weight.	Provide 25% extra fluid intake. Offer water between breast- or bottle-feedings.	Replace fluid losses due to watery stools, if under phototherapy.	
	Assess for dehydration:	Phototherapy treatment may cause liquid stools and in-	
	1. Poor skin turgor		

(continued)

Intervention	Rationale
2. Depressed fontanelles 3. Sunken eyes 4. Decreased urine output 5. Weight loss 6. Changes in electrolytes	creased insensible water loss, which increases risk of dehydration.
Monitor intake and output. Weigh diapers before discarding. Check specific gravity every eight hr. Record urine color and frequency. Record number and characteristics of stools.	
Weigh daily. Report signs of dehydration.	Prevents fluid overload.
Administer IV fluids 1. Monitor flow rates. 2. Assess insertion site for signs of infection.	IV fluids may be used if baby is dehydrated or in presence of other complications. IV may be started if exchange transfusion is to be done.

Newborn with Jaundice (*continued*)

Nursing Diagnosis	Nursing Interventions	Rationale	Evaluation
Injury: High risk related to use of phototherapy *Client Goal:* Baby will not have any corneal irritation/drainage, skin breakdown, or major fluctuations in temperature.	Cover baby's eyes with eye patches while under phototherapy lights. Cover testes/penis in male infants.	Protects retina from damage due to high intensity light and testes from damage from heat.	Baby's eyes are protected at all times while under the phototherapy lights, no corneal irritation occurs; baby maintains a stable temperature.
	Make certain that eyelids are closed prior to applying eyepatches. Ensure patches do not slip down over nose.	Prevents corneal abrasions. Blocked nose causes upper airway obstruction and apnea.	
	Remove baby from under phototherapy and remove eye patches during feedings.	Provides visual stimulation and facilitates attachment behaviors.	
	Inspect eyes every eight hours for conjunctivitis, drainage, and corneal abrasions due to irritation from eye patches.	Prevents or facilitates prompt treatment of purulent conjunctivitis.	

Administer thorough perianal cleansing with each stool or change of perianal protective covering.	Frequent stooling increases risk of skin breakdown. Prevents infection.
Provide minimal coverage—only of diaper area.	Provides maximal exposure. Shielded areas become more jaundiced, so maximum exposure is essential.
Use paper face mask after removing nose strip.	Metal strip can burn baby's skin when heated by the lights.
Avoid the use of oily applications on the skin.	
Reposition baby every two hours.	Provides equal exposure of all skin areas and prevents pressure areas.
Observe for bronzing of skin.	Bronzing is related to use of phototherapy with increased direct bilirubin levels or liver damage; may last for two to four months.
Place baby approximately 18 inches from light source.	Ensures correct exposure to the phototherapy lights.

(continued)

Newborn with Jaundice (*continued*)

Nursing Diagnosis	Nursing Interventions	Rationale	Evaluation
	Place Plexiglas™ shield between baby and light.	Hypothermia and hyperthermia are common complications of phototherapy. Hypothermia results from exposure to lights, subsequent radiation, and convection losses.	
	Monitor baby's skin and core temperature frequently until temperature is stable.	Hyperthermia may result from the increased environmental heat.	
	Check axillary temperature with readings on servo-controlled unit on Isolette.	Additional heat from phototherapy lights frequently causes a rise in the baby's and the Isolette's temperatures. Fluctuations in temperature may occur in response to radiation and convection.	
	Regulate Isolette temperature as needed.		

			Baby's neurologic status is within normal limits.

Sensory/perceptual alterations related to neurologic damage secondary to kernicterus	Monitor any neurologic/behavioral changes in baby by taking vital signs every two hr. Report any changes promptly.	Baby may develop green, watery stools and green urine due to excretion of bilirubin byproducts.	
Client Goal: Baby will not show signs of altered biorhythms, hypotonia, temperature instability, spasticity, lethargy, poor sucking reflex.	Closely assess infant's daily patterns to detect notable changes in food ingestion, bowel and urine and sleeping and waking rhythms, irritability.	Changes in biologic rhythms caused by phototherapy are unclear and may indicate signs of worsening condition.	
	Report signs of worsening condition (kernicterus): 1. Hypotonia, lethargy, poor sucking reflex, hypertonicity 2. Spasticity and opisthotonus 3. Temperature instability 4. Gradual appearance of extrapyramidal signs 5. Impaired or absent hearing	Deposition of bilirubin in brain leads to development of symptoms of kernicterus. Note: Treatment may be more aggressive in presence of neonatal complications such as asphyxia, respiratory distress, metabolic acidosis, hypothermia, low serum protein, sepsis, signs of CNS deterioration (Avery 1987).	

(continued)

Newborn with Jaundice (*continued*)

Nursing Diagnosis	Nursing Interventions	Rationale	Evaluation
	Monitor laboratory studies as indicated:		
	1. Direct and indirect bilirubin		
	2. CO_2		
	3. Reticulocyte count		
	4. Hematocrit and hemoglobin (H&H), total serum protein		
Knowledge deficit related to causes of and care of baby with hyperbilirubinemia	Provide explanation of:	Parents may not understand what is happening or why.	Parents understand the process and treatment of jaundice and reasons for interruption of breast-feeding.
	1. Infant's condition		
Client Goals: Parents will be informed of baby's disease process, rationale for treatments, and expected outcome.	2. Treatment modalities, causative and contributing factors of jaundice and hyperbilirubinemia	Physician preference of treatment modalities may vary. Parents may not understand why their newborn is not receiving a treatment that another with the same condition is receiving.	

(*continued*)

Mother will understand the reason for temporary discontinuation of breast-feeding, how to pump her breasts, and how to reinstate breast-feeding.	3. Reasons that mother may be asked to cease breast-feeding temporarily	The etiology of breast milk jaundice remains uncertain. The serum bilirubin levels begin to fall within 48 hr after discontinuation of breast-feeding.
		Opinion of physicians varies regarding the need for discontinuing breast-feeding.
	Assist mother to pump her breasts to maintain her milk supply.	Mother may need support and information to restart breast-feeding.
	Give explanation of equipment being used and changes in bilirubin levels. Allow parents an opportunity to ask questions; reinforce or clarify information as needed.	If breast-feeding is temporarily discontinued, assess mother's knowledge of pumping her breasts and provide information and support as needed.
	Teach parents signs of jaundice (example: yellow tinge to skin or sclera) and to report them to the health care team.	Parents know when to report recurrence of jaundice and importance of follow-up.

Newborn with Jaundice (*continued*)

Nursing Diagnosis	Nursing Interventions	Rationale	Evaluation
Altered parenting: High risk related to parenting a baby with jaundice	Encourage parents to provide tactile stimulation during feeding and diaper changes.	Neonate has normal needs for tactile stimulation.	Parents are involved in the care of their baby and the bonding process occurs.
Client Goals: Parents will provide care and stimulation for their baby.	Provide cuddling and eye contact during feedings and talk to baby frequently.	Provides comforting and decreases sensory deprivation.	
	Encourage parents to come into nursery or bring baby to mother's room for feedings and to touch their baby. Provide opportunities for parents to express feelings.	Presence of equipment may discourage parents from interacting with neonate.	

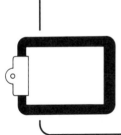

Nursing Care Plan
Newborn with
Respiratory Distress Syndrome

Client Assessment

Nursing History

Preterm delivery

Gestational history: Recent episodes of fetal or intrapartal stress (maternal hypotension, bleeding, maternal and resultant fetal oversedation), severe fetal lung circulation compromise

Neonatal history: Birth asphyxia resulting in acute hypoxia, exposure to hypothermia

Familial tendency

Low Apgar score, requiring bag and mask resuscitation in birthing area

Diagnostic Studies

Lung profile to determine lung maturity is done on amniotic fluid (for fetuses predisposed to RDS) as follows:

- Lecithin/Sphingomyelin: Ratio of 2:1 or more indicates pulmonary maturity.
- Phosphatidylglycerol (PG): Elevated at 35 weeks' gestation

Arterial blood gases (indicating respiratory failure): PaO_2 less than 50 mm Hg while breathing 100% O_2, and PCO_2 above 60 mm Hg

(continued)

Newborn with Respiratory Distress Syndrome (*continued*)

Nursing Diagnosis	Nursing Interventions	Rationale	Evaluation
Physical Examination At birth or within two hours, rapid development initially of tachypnea (over 60 respirations/min), expiratory grunting (audible), or subcostal/intercostal retractions Followed by flaring of nares on inspiration, cyanosis and pallor, signs of increased air hunger (apneic spells, hypotonus), rhythmic movement of body and labored respirations, chin tug Auscultation: Initially breath sounds may be normal; then decreased air exchange with harsh breath sounds and, upon deep inspiration, rales; later a low-pitched systolic murmur indicates patent ductus Increasing oxygen concentration requirements to maintain adequate PO₂ levels		Potassium levels increase as potassium is released from injured alveolar cells. X-ray: Diffuse reticulogranular density bilaterally, with air-filled tracheobronchial tube outlined by opaque lungs (air bronchogram); atelectasis/hypoexpansion in severe cases. Clinical course worsens first 24–48 hours after birth and persists for more than 24 hours Dextrostix	

Nursing Diagnosis	Nursing Interventions	Rationale	Evaluation
Nursing Diagnosis: Impaired gas exchange related to inadequate lung surfactant	Determine baseline of respiratory effort, ventilatory adequacy—observation of chest wall movement, skin,	Alveoli of normal infant remain stable during expiration due to presence of surfactant. Alveoli of infant with RDS lack	Baby's respirations are 30–50 per minute without apnea, PaO₂ is between 50–70 mm Hg.

(*continued*)

Client Goals: Baby's respirations will be 30–50/min, regular, and without apneic periods. Baby's oxygen requirement and work of breathing will diminish.	mucous membranes, color; estimation of degree and equality of air entry by auscultation, arterial blood gases, and pH determination.	surfactant and collapse with expiration. Values used to determine adequate oxygenation—normal PaO_2 50–70 mm Hg. Adequate ventilation—normal $PaCO_2$ 35–45 mm Hg. Acid-base balance—normal pH 7.35–7.45.
Baby's need for assisted ventilation will be noted early.	Maintain on respiratory and cardiac monitors—note rates every 30–60 min or more often as indicated by the severity of infant's distress. Check and calibrate all monitoring and measuring devices every eight hr. Calibrate oxygen devices to 21% and 100% O_2 concentrations.	Alveolar atelectasis and intrapulmonary shunting results in poor gas exchange, hypoxemia, hypercarbia, and acid-base derangements. Grunting, a compensatory mechanism, increases transpulmonary pressure, overcomes high surface tension, forces and prevents atelectasis, and thus enables improved oxygenation and a rise in PaO_2. It is the sound of the glottis closing to stop exhalation of air by forcing it against the vocal cords.

Newborn with Respiratory Distress Syndrome (*continued*)

Nursing Diagnosis	Nursing Interventions	Rationale	Evaluation
	Provide warmed air (89°F to 93°F) 31.7°C to 33.9°C and humidified (40% to 60%) oxygen.	Humidified oxygen prevents mucosal dryness.	
	Monitor oxygen concentrations at least every hour.	Maintains constant level.	
	Administer oxygen by oxygen hood (a small transparent head hood that contains an inlet and carbon dioxide outlet) (NCP12).	Provides a constant oxygen environment. Incubators are not recommended for long-term oxygen delivery since the concentration is difficult to regulate and fluctuates when portholes are opened for care giving.	

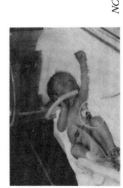

NCP12-1 Infant in oxygen hood

Avoid hood touching infant's face.	Contact with infant's face may cause apnea by stimulating facial nerve.
Maintain stable oxygen concentration by increasing or decreasing oxygen by 5%–10% increments and then obtain arterial blood gases.	Stable concentration of oxygen is necessary to maintain PaO_2 within normal limits (50–70 mm Hg). Sudden increase or decrease in O_2 concentration may result in disproportionate increase or decrease in PaO_2 due to vasoconstriction in response to hypoxemia.
Monitor:	Observations of clinical condition are taken serially for comparison and changes.
1. Color (pink), cyanosis (central or acrocyanosis), duskiness, pallor	Observations should be taken while infant is receiving oxygen and with any oxygen adjustment.
2. Respiratory effort (evaluation at rest), rate of respirations, patterns (apnea, periodic breathing), quality (easy, unlabored; abdominal, labored), auscultation (site of breath sounds—	

(continued)

Newborn with Respiratory Distress Syndrome (continued)

Nursing Diagnosis	Nursing Interventions	Rationale	Evaluation
	overall or part of lung fields—describe quality of breath sounds every one to two hr), accompanying sounds with respiratory effort (change from previous observations)		
	3. Activity—less active, flaccid, lethargic, unresponsive, increased activity, restless, irritable; inability to tolerate exertion, crying, sucking, or nursing care activity		
	4. Circulatory response (evaluate at rest); rate, regularity, and rhythm		

(*continued*)

of heart rate; periods of bradycardia; alterations of blood pressure

Return O_2 concentration to previous levels if there is deterioration in neonate's condition or drop below desired transcutaneous oxygen monitor (TCM) levels.

Repeat arterial blood gases (keep PaO_2 50–70 mm Hg). Gases should be done within 15–20 min after any change in ambient O_2 concentration or after inspiratory or expiratory pressure changes.

Record and report clinical observations and action taken.

Any deterioration of clinical condition with oxygen adjustments (usually a decrease in ambient oxygen concentration) indicates inability of neonate to compensate for hypoxia.

Newborn with Respiratory Distress Syndrome (*continued*)

Nursing Diagnosis	Nursing Interventions	Rationale	Evaluation
	Maintain stable environment prior to collection of arterial blood gas sample:		
	1. Maintain constant O_2 concentration at least 15–20 min before sample.	Accurate arterial blood determinations are essential in management of any infant receiving oxygen, because presence or absence of cyanosis is unreliable.	
	2. Avoid any disturbances of infant 15 min before gases are drawn.	Crying or struggling may cause hyperventilation or breath holding and may increase shunting of blood.	
	Do not suction; if suction is absolutely necessary, delay blood sample.		
	Maintain temperature of sample (pH should be measured at body temperature).	Use of temporal, radial, or brachial arteries takes skill, is time-consuming, and may have serious consequences;	

(*continued*)

Provide arterial blood gas setup (a 3-mL syringe with heparinized solution and a heparinized tuberculin syringe) to obtain blood sample.

After blood sample is taken, recheck flow through line to assure patency and prevent establishment of clot.

Replace blood used to clear line.

Use heparinized flush solution before restarting IV solution to prevent clots in the line.

With transcutaneous PO_2 or pulse oximeter, monitor continuously or every hour and record. Calibrate sen-

therefore, most common technique for sampling is through umbilical artery catheter.

Total blood volume of infant is small; blood removed to clear catheter must be returned to prevent hypovolemia, anemia.

Transcutaneous monitors and pulse oximeter measure percentage of oxygen in inspired air, ensures FIO_2 concentra-

Newborn with Respiratory Distress Syndrome (*continued*)

Nursing Diagnosis	Nursing Interventions	Rationale	Evaluation
	sor each shift and rotate sensor position every 3–4 hr.	tions and accuracy of readings. Rotating sensor prevents skin burns. Electrode sites include chest, abdomen, and inner thigh. Oxygen diffuses through the skin from capillaries directly beneath the skin and can then be measured. Oximeter is preferred because it doesn't produce heat.	
	Assess need for assisted ventilatory measures. Criteria for assisted ventilation: 1. Apnea 2. Hypoxia (PaO_2 <50 mm Hg) 3. Hypercarbia ($PaCO_2$ >60 mm Hg)	Application of CPAP or PEEP produces same stabilization force on alveoli as grunting does and produces same effect—improved oxygenation and rise in PaO_2.	

4. Respiratory acidosis (pH <7.20)

Altered nutrition: less than body requirements related to increased metabolic needs of stressed infant	Have ventilatory support equipment available. Administer ventilator care per agency protocol.	Delivery of CPAP or PEEP can only be done by use of nasal prongs, nasopharyngeal tube, or oral intubation.	Baby maintains normal glucose levels, follows normal weight curves, and is tolerating oral feedings.
Client Goals: Baby will not have greater than 2% weight loss, will have greater than 40 mg % glucose, and will progress to oral feedings.	Maintain IV rate at prescribed levels, usually 65 to 80 mL/kg/day	This is the needed rate for initial caloric intake.	
	Maintain IV rate at prescribed level; record type and amount of fluid infused hourly. Use infusion pump. Observe vital signs for signs of too-rapid infusion. Maintain normal urine output (1–3 mL/kg/hr). Maintain specific gravity of urine between 1.006 and 1.012. Take daily weights.	Fluids are provided to sick neonate by intravenous route and are calculated to replace sensible and insensible water losses as well as evaporative losses due to tachypnea. Overload of circulatory system by too much or too rapid administration of fluid causes pulmonary edema and cardiac embarrassment that may be fatal.	

(continued)

Newborn with Respiratory Distress Syndrome (*continued*)

Nursing Diagnosis	Nursing Interventions	Rationale	Evaluation
	Manage route of IV administration. With umbilical catheter: Protect catheter from strain or tension. Restrain as necessary. Prevent dislodgement of catheter. Always keep catheter and stopcock on top of bed linens so they are easily visible.	Greater nutritional fluid is required because of energy needed to cope with stress. Stressed infants are predisposed to hypoglycemia because of increased metabolic demands as well as reduced glycogen stores and decreased ability to convert fat and protein to glucose.	
	Observe for occlusion of vessels by clot and for vasospasm—discoloration of skin, discoloration of toes or feet (blanching or cyanosis). If discoloration occurs, contralateral foot may be wrapped with	Vasospasm in unwrapped foot will be relieved by treatment, and the discoloration will disappear and toes will be pink. If discoloration persists, clot may be occluding vessel—catheter must be removed, or loss of extremity is possible.	

(continued)

warm cloth, but this is controversial. Removal of catheter is preferred.

Observe for signs of infection or sepsis: temperature instability, drainage, redness or foul odor from cord, lethargy, irritability, vomiting, poor feeding, hypotonia.

Peripheral IV in scalp or extremity vein: Prepare equipment, insert IV in vein, and restrain infant.

If vessel chosen is an artery, it pulsates. Place peripheral IV in vein (which doesn't pulsate).

Very small arteries may not pulsate and arterial area will blanch if saline is infused.

Maintain proper placement of IV.

Ability to aspirate blood and/or easily inject small amount of saline indicates patent IV. Infiltration is evaluated by area of edema and redness about

Newborn with Respiratory Distress Syndrome (*continued*)

Nursing Diagnosis	Nursing Interventions	Rationale	Evaluation
		site, inability to obtain blood on aspiration, or difficulty in injecting solution.	
	Provide total parenteral nutrition (TPN) when indicated.	TPN is used as nutritional alternative if bowel sounds are not present and infant remains in acute distress.	
	Advance as soon as possible from intravenous to oral feedings. Gavage or nipple feedings are used, and IV is used as supplement (discontinued when oral intake is sufficient) (see Procedure 31–1).		
	Provide adequate caloric intake: amount of intake, type of formula, route of administration, and need for supplementation of intake by other routes.	Calories are essential to prevent catabolism of body proteins, and metabolic acidosis due to starvation or inadequate caloric intake.	

Infection: High risk related to invasive procedures. *Client Goals:* Baby will maintain a stable temperature and blood pressure and will be free from infection.	Monitor for hypocalcemia. Monitor for hypoglycemia: Dextrostix below 45 mg/dL, urine screening for glucose. See section on sepsis nursing care. Pay careful attention to infection control by cleaning and replacing nebulizers/humidifiers at least every 24 hr; use sterile tubing and replace ever 24 hr; use sterile distilled water.	Hypocalcemia and hypoglycemia result from delayed or inadequate caloric intake and stress. Decreased lung expansion predisposes to atelectasis and secondary superimposed infections. The warm, moist environment found in Isolettes and with O_2 equipment promotes growth of microorganisms.	Baby's temperature and blood pressure are within normal limits and are stable; no signs of infection are present.
Ineffective thermoregulation related to increased respiratory effort secondary to RDS	Observe infant for temperature instability and signs of increased oxygen consumption (need for increased O_2 concentration) and metabolic acidosis.	Cold stress increases oxygen consumption and promotes pulmonary vasoconstriction. This leads to hypoxia and acidosis, which further depress surfactant production.	Baby's temperature was within normal limits. Signs of cold stress are absent or minimized.

(continued)

Newborn with Respiratory Distress Syndrome (*continued*)

Nursing Diagnosis	Nursing Interventions	Rationale	Evaluation
Client Goals: Baby will maintain a stable temperature. Baby will not become hypoglycemic, cyanotic, or have periods of bradycardia or apnea.	Maintain neutral thermal environment.	Cold stress leads to chemical thermogenesis (burning brown fat to maintain body temperature), which increases O_2 needs in an already compromised infant.	
	Use servocontrol to maintain constant temperature regulation.		
	Warm all inspired gases. Place a thermometer in the oxygen hood and document the temperature of the delivered gas with vital signs. Oxyhood and Isolette temperature should be maintained in the infant's neutral thermal range.	Cold air/oxygenation blown in face of newborn is source of cold stress and is stimulus for increased consumption of oxygen and increased metabolic rate.	

Place thermometer in line of ventilatory circuit and maintain inspired gas at 34°C to 35°C.

Use heat shields for small infants.

Heat shields will prevent heat loss by convection and reduce insensible water losses.

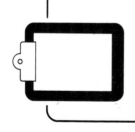

Nursing Care Plan
Non-English-Speaking Woman
at First Prenatal Visit

Nursing History:

1. Assess degree of communication possible. Determine if the woman understands some English, even if her verbal skills are limited.

2. Gather basic information as possible about course of pregnancy, estimated gestational age, sensitivity to medications, existing problems or concerns.

Physical Examination:

1. Vital signs, height and weight, general appearance.

2. Observe for signs of confusion, fear, anxiety.

Diagnostic Studies:

1. Urinalysis

2. CBC

3. Rubella titer, hepatitis screen if indicated.

4. Other lab work as appropriate.

Nursing Diagnosis Goals	Nursing Interventions	Rationale	Evaluation
Nursing Diagnosis: Impaired verbal communication related to lack of understanding of care giver's language. *Client Goal:* The woman will have an opportunity to share information	Arrange for an interpreter—family member, friend, or staff person—to be present at this visit and subsequent visits as needed.	For effective ongoing communication, a shared language is essential.	The woman is comfortable communicating through the interpreter as evidenced by her willingness to answer questions and provide information and by her expressions of acceptance of the process.
Nursing Diagnosis: Impaired social interaction related to differing cultural practices and expectations between client and nurse. *Client Goal:* The woman will discuss her expectations.	Ask the woman to describe her expectations of the health care system. Ask her about customs and culturally specific practices that are important to her. Ask her to describe any practices that are specifically forbidden in her culture.	To provide effective, culturally sensitive care the nurse must gather information about acceptable and proscribed activities for the woman and her family.	The woman is able to discuss her expectations of the health care system and identify cultural practices that are important to her. She shows no evidence of fear or emotional distress about prenatal practices common to this country. *(continued)*

Non-English-Speaking Woman at First Prenatal Visit (*continued*)

Nursing Diagnosis	Nursing Interventions	Rationale	Evaluation
	Describe procedures usually performed during a prenatal visit and discuss her feelings about them. Postpone any nonessential procedures to a subsequent visit if she appears overloaded.		
Nursing Diagnosis: Impaired social interaction related to culturally specific expectations of the role of the partner in the pregnancy and birth. *Client Goal:* The woman will have an opportunity to discuss her wishes regarding her partner's involvement.	Ask the woman about her partner's and her expectations of his degree of involvement. Is it preferable to them for him to be the primary support person, or do they prefer that a family member or close friend fill that role?	The role of the partner is often culturally specific and may vary greatly. The nurse should recognize this and respect the couple's wishes.	The woman is able to express her preferences about the partner's degree of involvement clearly and specifically.

| Nursing Diagnosis: Knowledge deficit related to a lack of information about the changes associated with pregnancy and about prenatal care practices in this country. | Provide basic information about pregnancy and prenatal care. Plan additional sessions as needed so that the woman is not overwhelmed with information. Provide opportunities for questions and clarification. If possible provide printed information in the woman's language. | All pregnant women have the right to clear, accurate information in order to be active participants in their health care. | The woman is able to ask questions and discuss areas of interest. She is willing to return for regular prenatal care. |
| *Client Goal:* The woman will gain information regarding pregnancy changes and prenatal care. | Establish a mutually acceptable method for her to contact a care giver if she has questions or problems, or in an emergency. | | |

Nursing Care Plan
Pregnancy-Induced Hypertension (PIH) (Preeclampsia-Eclampsia)

Client Assessment

Nursing History

1. Identification of predisposing factors in client history:
   a. Primigravida
   b. Presence of diabetes mellitus
   c. Multiple pregnancy
   d. Hydramnios
   e. Gestational trophoblastic disease
   f. Preexisting vascular or renal disease

Physical Examination

1. Blood pressure elevated (compared with baseline if possible)
2. Presence of edema as indicated by weight gain, puffy hands and feet; requires ongoing assessment for development of periorbital or facial edema
3. Presence of hyperreflexia and clonus

Diagnostic Studies

1. Evaluate urinary output for quantity and specific gravity.
2. Urine for urinary protein:
   1 g protein/24 hr = 1–2+;
   5 g protein/24 hr = 3–4+.
3. Hematocrit: Elevation of hematocrit implies hemoconcentration, which occurs as fluid leaves the

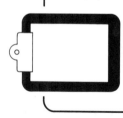

g. Adolescent or older maternal age

4. Presence of headache, visual disturbances, drowsiness, epigastric pain

5. Observe any vaginal bleeding, abdominal tenderness, or signs of labor

intravascular space and enters the extravascular space.

4. BUN: Not usually elevated except in women with cardiovascular or renal disease.

5. Blood uric acid appears to correlate well with the severity of the preeclampsia-eclampsia (Note: Thiazide diuretics can cause significant increases in uric acid levels).

Nursing Diagnosis	Nursing Interventions	Rationale	Evaluation
Nursing Diagnosis: Fluid volume deficit related to fluid shift from intravascular to extravascular space secondary to vasospasm	Assess BP every 1–4 hr, using same arm, with woman in same position.	Blood pressure can fluctuate hourly; BP increases as a result of increased peripheral resistance due to peripheral vasoconstriction and arteriolar spasm.	Woman's edema decreases, urine output remains normal, proteinuria decreases, and hematocrit is within normal limits.
	Weigh daily; gain of 1 kg/wk or more in second trimester or ½ kg/wk or more in third trimester is suggestive of PIH.	Weight gain and edema are due to sodium and water retention.	

(continued)

Pregnancy-Induced Hypertension (PIH) (Preeclampsia-Eclampsia) (continued)

Nursing Diagnosis	Nursing Interventions	Rationale	Evaluation
Client Goal: Fluid volume deficit will be controlled and intravascular volume will be maintained as evidenced by decreased edema, adequate urine output, normal specific gravity, decreased proteinuria, and improved hematocrit.	Assess edema: +(1+) Minimal; slight edema of pedal and pretibial areas ++(2+) Marked edema of lower extremities +++(3+) Edema of hands, face, lower abdominal wall, and sacrum ++++(4+) Anasarca with ascites	Decreased plasma colloid osmotic pressure causes movement of fluid from the intravascular to extravascular space.	
	Maintain on bed rest. Encourage left lateral recumbent position.	Bed rest produces an increase in GFR.	

Maintain normal salt intake (4–6 g/24 hr)	Normal salt intake is now advised, but excessive salt intake may make the condition worse.
Report urine output < 30 mL/hr or urine specific gravity > 1.040.	Renal plasma flow and glomerular filtration are decreased in PIH. Increasing oliguria indicates a worsening condition.
Test urine for protein hourly or as ordered. Maintain in-dwelling catheter.	Proteinuria results from swelling of the endothelium of the glomerular capillaries.
Evaluate hematocrit levels regularly.	Decreased intravascular fluid volume leads to increased hematocrit level because of change in proportion of RBCs to volume of fluid.
Provide adequate protein: 1.5 g/kg/24 hr for incipient and mild preeclampsia.	Plasma proteins affect movement of intravascular and extravascular fluids.

(continued)

Pregnancy-Induced Hypertension (PIH) (Preeclampsia-Eclampsia) (*continued*)

Nursing Diagnosis	Nursing Interventions	Rationale	Evaluation
Nursing Diagnosis: Knowledge deficit related to PIH, its treatment, and the implications for her and her unborn child	Discuss PIH, its implications for client and fetus/neonate.	Illness and hospitalization during pregnancy is usually unanticipated and may cause a major disruption in a couple's life. With thorough information they are better able to understand the condition and its implications.	Woman is able to discuss PIH, its therapy and implications, and she cooperates with the care regimen.
	Explain purpose and importance of treatment measures.		
Client Goal: Woman will clearly understand her condition and its implications as evidenced by her ability to discuss PIH and its therapy and her cooperation with the treatment regimen.	Work with woman and support person to plan ways for the family to deal with the woman's hospitalization.		
Nursing Diagnosis: Injury: High risk related to possibility of convulsion secondary to cerebral vasospasm or edema.	Monitor knee, ankle, and biceps reflexes and clonus.	Hyperreflexia indicates central nervous system (CNS) irritability.	No seizures develop; client's condition improves.
	Promote bed rest. Encourage woman to rest quietly in a darkened, quiet room.	Rest reduces external stimuli.	
	Limit visitors.		

Client Goal: Woman will not develop seizures, and signs that her condition is worsening will not develop.

Administer magnesium sulfate per physician order:

1. IV dose: 4 g loading dose $MgSO_4$ followed by continuous infusion at a rate of 2 g/hr.

2. IM dose: 10 g of 50% $MgSO_4$ injected deep IM (½ in the upper outer quadrants of each buttock) using a 20-gauge, 3-inch needle. (1.0 mL of 2% lidocaine may be added to the syringe to decrease the discomfort.)

Monitor magnesium levels frequently to prevent overdose (either 2 hours after beginning infusion or prior to next IM dose).

Before administering subsequent doses of magnesium sulfate, check reflexes

Magnesium sulfate is a cerebral depressant; it also reduces neuromuscular irritability and causes vasodilation and drop in BP.

Therapeutic blood level is 4–7 mEq/L.

Knee jerk disappears when magnesium sulfate blood levels are 7 to 10 mEq/L.

(continued)

Pregnancy-Induced Hypertension (PIH) (Preeclampsia-Eclampsia) (*continued*)

Nursing Diagnosis	Nursing Interventions	Rationale	Evaluation
	(knee, ankle, biceps), respirations and urine output.	Toxic signs and symptoms develop with increased blood levels; respiratory arrest can be associated with blood levels of 10 to 15 mEq/L.	
	Do not give magnesium sulfate if:		
	1. Reflexes are absent.	Cardiac arrest can occur if blood levels are 30 mEq/L.	
	2. Respirations are < 12/min	Kidneys are only route for excretion of magnesium sulfate.	
	3. < 100 mL urine output in past four hours		
	Have calcium gluconate available.	Calcium gluconate is antidote for magnesium sulfate.	
	Maintain seizure precautions:		
	1. Keep room quiet, darkened.	Quiet reduces stimuli.	
	2. Have emergency equipment available—O$_2$, suction, padded tongue blade.		

(continued)

3. Pad side rails.

Padding protects client.

4. Educate other care givers regarding the possibility of convulsions and appropriate actions.

Provide supportive care during convulsion:

1. Place tongue blade or airway in patient's mouth, if can be done without force.

Acts to maintain airway and to prevent patient from biting tongue

2. Suction nasopharynx as necessary.

Removes mucus and secretions

3. Administer oxygen.

Promotes oxygenation

4. Note type of seizure and length of time it lasts.

Precipitous labor may start during seizures.

After seizure, assess for uterine contractions.

Assess fetal status.

Continuous fetal monitoring is necessary to identify fetal stress.

Pregnancy-Induced Hypertension (PIH) (Preeclampsia-Eclampsia) (*continued*)

Nursing Diagnosis	Nursing Interventions	Rationale	Evaluation
Nursing Diagnosis: Injury: High risk to fetus related to inadequate placental perfusion secondary to vasospasm or possible abruptio placentae.	Encourage mother to assume a side-lying position.	Side-lying position avoids pressure on vena cava and promotes optimum placental perfusion.	Fetus develops normally and IUGR is avoided. Fetus tolerates stress of labor well.
Client Goal: Fetus will tolerate the stress of maternal condition without injury as evidenced by normal intrauterine growth, reactive NST, and/or negative CST.	Evaluate results of serial fetal assessments such as NST, CST, ultrasound, biophysical profile.	Fetal assessment determines fetal status and ability to withstand stress of labor, as well as fetal maturity.	
	Report any signs of abruptio placentae such as uterine tenderness, vaginal bleeding, change in fetal activity, change in fetal heart rate, sustained abdominal pain.	Vasospasm and high blood pressure of PIH increase the risk of abruptio placentae.	
	If labor begins, monitor fetus closely with electronic fetal monitor. Report evidence of late decelerations.	Because of decreased placental perfusion due to vasospasm, fetus may have difficulty tolerating the stress of labor and cesarean birth may be necessary.	

Nursing Diagnosis:
Injury: High risk related to development of hematologic and hepatic abnormalities secondary to the HELLP syndrome

Client Goal: Woman will not develop injury from the development of complications, as evidenced by normal hemoglobin levels, absence of signs of anemia, normal liver function tests, and adequate platelet count.

1. Obtain blood samples as ordered to evaluate hemoglobin and hematocrit, SGOT, SGPT, and platelet count.

2. Monitor test results and report abnormal findings.

3. Report signs of hemolytic anemia including pallor, fatigue, anorexia, and dyspnea.

4. Report signs of liver dysfunction including nausea and vomiting, right upper quadrant pain, jaundice, and malaise.

5. Report signs of developing DIC immediately. Signs include epistaxis, petechiae, hematuria, bleeding gums, GI tract bleeding, and retinal or conjunctival hemorrhages.

HELLP syndrome refers to hemolysis of RBCs (causing signs of anemia), elevated liver enzymes because of liver damage (causing jaundice, etc) and low platelet count related to severe vasospasm and developing DIC.

Woman does not develop signs of hematologic and hepatic complications.

Nursing Care Plan
Puerperal Infection

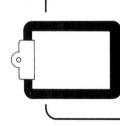

Nursing History

1. Predisposing health factors include the following:
   a. Malnutrition
   b. Anemia
   c. Debilitated condition
2. Predisposing factors associated with labor and birth including the following:
   a. Prolonged labor
   b. Hemorrhage
   c. Premature and/or prolonged rupture of membranes
   d. Soft tissue trauma
   e. Invasive techniques (eg, internal monitoring, frequent vaginal exams)

    (4) Rapid pulse (tachycardia)
    (5) Lower abdominal pain or uterine tenderness
    (6) Lochia—appearance varies depending on causative organism: may appear normal, be profuse, bloody, and foul smelling, may be scant and serosanguineous to brownish and foul smelling
    (7) Severe afterpains
    (8) Vomiting, diarrhea
    (9) Uterine subinvolution

3. Pelvic cellulitis (parametritis)
   a. Signs and symptoms of severe infection (see previous discussion of endometritis)

f. Operative procedures

g. Maternal exhaustion

Physical Examination

1. Localized episiotomy infections may present with the following signs and symptoms:

   a. Complaints of unusual degree of discomfort, localized pain

   b. Reddened edematous lesion

   c. Purulent drainage, sanguineous drainage

   d. Failure of skin edges to approximate

   e. Fever (generally below 38.3C or 101F)

   f. Dysuria with or without dysuria

2. Endometritis

   a. Mild case may be asymptomatic or characterized only by low-grade fever, anorexia, and malaise

   b. More severe cases may demonstrate:

      (1) Fever of 101°F–103°F+ (38.3°C to 39.4°C)

      (2) Anorexia, extreme lethargy

      (3) Chills

   b. Severe abdominal pain, usually lateral to the uterus on one or both sides and apparent with both abdominal palpation and pelvic examination

   c. Possible abscess formation; dependent on location; may be palpated vaginally, rectally, or abdominally

4. Puerperal peritonitis

   a. Symptoms just described plus severe abdominal pain

   b. Abdominal rigidity, guarding, rebound tenderness

   c. Possible vomiting and diarrhea

   d. Tachycardia, shallow respirations, anxiety, restlessness

   e. Marked bowel distention if paralytic ileus develops, absent bowel sounds

Diagnostic Studies

1. Elevated white blood count (WBC), although it may be within normal puerperal limits (15,000–30,000/mm^3) initially

2. Culture of intrauterine material to reveal causative organism

3. Urine culture to rule out an asymptomatic urinary tract infection (should be normal)

4. Elevated sedimentation rate

5. Bimanual examination

6. Ultrasonography

(continued)

Puerperal Infection (*continued*)

Nursing Diagnosis	Nursing Interventions	Rationale	Evaluation
Injury: High risk related to the spread of infection	Evaluate history for factors that would retard wound healing.	Careful evaluation of client history enables the nurse to identify those women who are at risk for infection and for delayed wound healing.	Therapy and supportive measures are effective and woman does not suffer injury from infection.
Client Goal: Woman will not suffer injury from infection as evidenced by: return of temperature to normal range, WBC count in normal range for postpartum client. If localized infection—decreased redness, edema, ecchymosis, drainage; wound edges approximated. If systemic infection—absence of malaise, uterine	Employ principles of medical asepsis in hand washing and disposal of contaminated material by client and care giver. Promote normal wound healing by using: 1. Sitz baths two to four times daily for 10–15 min or surgigator 2. Peri-care following elimination 3. Frequent changing of peri-pads 4. Early ambulation	Infection may be spread through direct contact with bacteria on hands, contaminated material, etc. Warm water is cleansing, promotes healing through increased vascular flow to affected area, and is soothing to woman. Peri-care promotes removal of urine and fecal contaminants from perineum. Changing pads frequently decreases the media for bacterial growth. Ambulation promotes drainage of lochia. These nu-	

tenderness, foul-smelling lochia, fever, elevated WBC, abdominal pain, chills, lethargy, tachycardia, abdominal rigidity.

5. Diet high in protein and vitamin C, iron
6. Fluid intake to 2000 mL/day

...trients are essential for satisfactory wound healing.

Evaluate degree of healing using the REEDA scale. Report signs and symptoms of wound infection, including:

1. Redness
2. Edema
3. Excessive pain
4. Inadequate approximation of wound edges
5. Purulent drainage
6. Fever, anorexia, malaise

REEDA scale provides consistent, objective tool for evaluation of wound healing. Wound infection produces characteristic signs and symptoms that reflect the body's response to the invading organism.

Obtain culture from wound site and administer antibiotics, per physician order.

Increase wound drainage by:

1. Assisting physician in opening wound for drainage, when indicated

Antibiotic therapy based on knowledge of causative organism is treatment of choice for localized infection.

(continued)

Puerperal Infection (*continued*)

Nursing Diagnosis	Nursing Interventions	Rationale	Evaluation
	2. Anticipating packing of a cavity greater than 2–3 cm with iodoform gauze	Abscesses may develop when infected material accumulates in closed body cavity. Iodoform packing maintains patency of opening so drainage can continue.	
	Report signs of progressive infection such as uterine subinvolution, foul-smelling lochia, uterine tenderness, severe lower abdominal pain, fever, elevated WBC, malaise, chills, lethargy, tachycardia, nausea and vomiting, abdominal rigidity.	More severe infections such as endometritis, pelvic cellulitis, or peritonitis can develop and produce characteristic signs as the body responds systematically to the invading pathogens.	
	Administer IV fluids and antibiotics as ordered	IV fluids maintain adequate hydration; antibiotics are the treatment of choice to combat the infection.	

(*continued*)

Maintain semi-Fowler's position.	Promotes comfort and helps prevent spread of infection.
Monitor vital signs, especially temperature, every four hr and more frequently if they are significantly abnormal. Note temperature trends.	Tachycardia and fever occur because the body's metabolic rate increases in response to its efforts to combat infection. A profound systemic infection can produce septic shock with ↓ blood pressure (BP) and ↑ respirations.
Monitor intake and output, urine specific gravity, and level of hydration as ordered.	Vigorous fluid and electrolyte therapy is necessary not only because of vomiting and diarrhea, but also because both fluid and electrolytes become sequestered in lumen and wall of bowel.
Maintain continuous nasogastric suction per physician order and assess bowel sounds.	Continuous nasogastric suction is used to decompress the bowel when paralytic ileus complicates the course and results in cessation of gastrointestinal (GI) motility.

Puerperal Infection (*continued*)

Nursing Diagnosis	Nursing Interventions	Rationale	Evaluation
	Transfer woman to intensive care if indicated by her condition.	Woman with peritonitis is in critical condition, and quality of nursing care this patient receives will weigh the balance between recovery and demise.	
Pain related to the presence of infection	Promote comfort by:	Comfort is essential to enable the woman to rest and recover.	Woman states she is free of pain. She is able to rest well and is coping emotionally with her infection.
Client Goal: Woman will obtain relief of pain as evidenced by her verbal expressions of comfort, ability to sleep, reduction in tachycardia.	1. Ensuring adequate periods of rest 2. Minimizing disturbing environmental stimuli 3. Judicious use of analgesics and antipyretics 4. Providing emotional support 5. Using supportive nursing measures such as back rubs, instruction in relaxation techniques,	External environmental stimuli may increase pain perceptions. Plan rest periods to increase client's emotional reserve.	

Altered parenting: High risk related to delayed parent-infant attachment secondary to woman's malaise and other symptoms of infection

Client Goal: Woman will bond with her infant as evidenced by her ability to feed her infant successfully, her involvement in her infant's care, her demonstration of affectionate behaviors, and her expressions of positive thoughts about her baby.

maintenance of cleanliness, provision of diversional activities

Promote and maintain mother-infant interaction:

1. Provide opportunities for the mother to see and hold her infant.

2. Encourage the mother to feed the infant if she feels able. Assist mother with feeding when IV is in place.

3. If breast-feeding mother is unable to nurse, assist her in pumping her breasts to maintain milk production.

Critically ill woman may become very depressed not only from disease process but also because her anticipated postpartal course is now denied to her, and she may interpret this as a failure of her ability to mother her infant.

Success at infant feeding generally enhances the woman's outlook and encourages mother-infant interaction.

The woman bonds well with her newborn and altered parenting is avoided.

(continued)

Puerperal Infection (*continued*)

Nursing Diagnosis	Nursing Interventions	Rationale	Evaluation
	4. Encourage partner/support person to discuss infant with woman and to become involved in infant's care if the woman is not able to do so.	Assists woman to feel involved with her infant and reassures her that her baby is receiving care and love.	
	5. Provide pictures of the infant for the mother's bedside.		
	6. Encourage verbalization of anxieties, fears, and concerns.		
	Assess breast-feeding infant's mouth for signs of thrush, a common side effect of antibiotics taken by the mother. Treatment should be initiated, but breast-feeding need not be stopped.	Thrush, a monilial infection caused by *Candida albicans*, often occurs when normal oral flora are destroyed by antibiotic therapy.	

Knowledge deficit related to a lack of understanding of condition and its treatment *Client Goal:* Woman will be able to discuss her condition, its treatment, and her care needs following discharge.	Provide information regarding predisposing factors, signs and symptoms, and treatment. Discuss the value of a nutritious diet in promoting healing. Review hygiene practices such as correct wiping after voiding, hand washing, etc, to prevent the spread of infection. Discuss home care routines following postpartal infection.	Women have the right and responsibility to be actively involved in their own health care to the extent that they are able. To be an active participant the woman needs appropriate information.	Woman is able to describe her condition and its implications. She cooperates with therapy and asks appropriate questions.

Nursing Care Plan
Regional Anesthesia—Lumbar Epidural

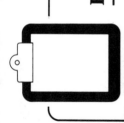

Client Assessment

Nursing History

Maternal information

1. Allergies to drugs (especially anesthetic agents)
2. Psychologic status
   a. What kind of anesthesia does woman want and what kind will she accept?
   b. Does she understand the procedure?
   c. What does she expect it to accomplish?
   d. Is she able to cope with the labor process, and can she follow directions?
3. Prenatal preparation and education
   a. Type of childbirth classes
   b. Degree of involvement in preparation classes
4.
3. Quality of contractions
   a. Frequency
   b. Duration
   c. Intensity
4. Vaginal examination to determine
   a. Status of cervix
      (1) Dilatation
      (2) Effacement
   b. Maternal-fetal pelvic relationship
      (1) Presentation and position
      (2) Station of presenting part
   c. Rate of progress in labor
5. Determination whether site to be used for injection is free from infection

4. Presence of disease states
   a. Cardiovascular disorders
   b. Pulmonary disorders
   c. CNS disorders
   d. Metabolic problems
5. Course of current pregnancy
6. Support person available
7. When did she last eat or take fluids
8. What other drugs has she taken recently

Fetal information

1. Gestational age
   a. Calendar dates
   b. Ultrasound
2. Status of fetus
   a. Stability of FHR
   b. Result of assessments of fetal well-being

Physical Examination

1. Maternal vital signs and FHR to establish baselines
2. Estimation of pregnant uterus (Leopold's maneuver to determine fetal size, presentation, and position)

Diagnostic Studies

1. Screening lab tests for coagulation disorders (Nicholson et al 1990)

TEST	NORMAL VALUE
Bleeding time	1 to 5 minutes
Platelet count	150,000 to 400,000 μL
Thrombin time	16 to 20 seconds
Partial thromboplastin time	24 to 36 seconds
Prothrombin time	11 to 12 seconds

2. Fetal scalp blood samples if fetal distress occurs

Analysis of Nursing Priorities

1. Maintaining a safe environment for the mother and fetus
2. Continuous monitoring of maternal status to detect and treat potential problems
3. Continuous monitoring of fetal status for same reason
4. Promoting thorough understanding of procedure through education of both parents

(continued)

Regional Anesthesia—Lumbar Epidural (*continued*)

Nursing Diagnosis	Nursing Interventions	Rationale	Evaluation
Nursing Diagnosis: Knowledge deficit related to regional anesthetic and analgesia	Determine current knowledge level.	Determination of woman's current knowledge level and factors that affect learning allows nurse to provide individualized teaching.	Woman is able to discuss the regional block and has no further questions.
Client Goal: Woman will be able to discuss the regional block, as measured by ability to verbalize: • Type of regional block • Expected effect • Possible adverse effects • Alternatives to regional block • Expected nursing care	Evaluate factors related to learning such as primary language spoken, ability to hear and interpret information, and/or presence of anxiety, which may affect ability to process information. Provide information regarding: • Reason for the block • Effect of the block • Possible side effects	Understanding of the anticipated effects, side effects, and nursing care will help woman be informed and participate in decision making.	

- Possible alternative pain relief measures
- Associated nursing care that may be expected

Nursing Diagnosis: Injury: High risk related to hypotension secondary to vasodilation and pooling of blood in the extremities

Client Goal: Woman will not experience hypotension as measured by: Blood pressure (BP) remains above 90/60. Pulse remains in 60–80 range.

Have legal consents signed. Have woman empty bladder.
Begin intravenous fluids. Initiate intravenous infusion.

Hydrate the woman receiving an epidural block with 500–1000 mL fluid prior to procedure.
Dextrose-free solution is recommended.

Position woman correctly for procedure (see text for proper positioning for individual procedures).

Regional anesthesia interferes with woman's urge to void. Intravenous fluids maintain adequate hydration and provide systemic access in the event of maternal hypotension or other untoward events.

Increased intravenous fluid intake increases blood volume and increases cardiac output to help minimize hypotension. Rapid infusion of fluids containing dextrose causes fetal hyperglycemia with rebound hypoglycemia in the first two hours after birth.

Woman remains normotensive. FHR is between 120 and 160; accelerations are present with fetal movement; no variable or late deceleration.

(continued)

Regional Anesthesia—Lumbar Epidural (*continued*)

Nursing Diagnosis	Nursing Interventions	Rationale	Evaluation
	Assess maternal status:		
	1. Obtain baseline vital signs before any anesthetic agent is given.	Baseline reading allows more complete evaluation of maternal status.	
	2. Monitor blood pressure every five min for 30 min following administration of anesthetic agent.	Hypotension is a frequent complication of regional anesthesia.	
	3. Monitor pulse and respiration.	Pulse may slow following spinal anesthesia due to decreased venous return, decreased venous pressure, and decreased right heart pressure. Respiratory paralysis is a potential complication of regional anesthesia.	

Monitor fetal status:

1. Use fetal monitoring to establish a baseline reading of FHR.
2. Monitor FHR continuously.

Observe, record, and report complications of anesthesia, including hypotension, fetal distress, respiratory paralysis, changes in uterine contractility, decrease in voluntary muscle effort, trauma to extremities, nausea and vomiting, loss of bladder tone, and spinal headache.

Observe, record, and report symptoms of hypotension, including systolic pressure <100 mm Hg or a 25% fall in systolic pressure, apprehension, restlessness, dizziness, tinnitus, headache.

Maternal hypotension may interfere with fetal oxygenation and is evidenced by fetal bradycardia.

(*continued*)

Regional Anesthesia—Lumbar Epidural (*continued*)

Nursing Diagnosis	Nursing Interventions	Rationale	Evaluation
	Institute treatment measures:		
	1. Place woman with head flat and foot of bed elevated.	Gravity increases venous filling of the heart and the pulmonary blood volume; the result is an increase in stroke volume and cardiac output with a rise in blood pressure.	
	2. Increase IV fluid rate.	Blood volume increases and circulation improves.	
	3. Administer O_2 by face mask.	Oxygen content of circulating blood increases.	
	4. Administer vasopressors as ordered.	Vasoconstriction occurs; vasopressors are not used in pregnant women unless absolutely necessary because they may further compromise the fetus.	

Specific interventions for treatment of hypotension following peridural anesthesia:

1. Raise knee gatch on bed.

2. Manually displace uterus laterally to left. — Increases venous return (vena cava is usually to the right).

3. Administer O_2 by face mask at 6–10 L/min. — Face mask is preferred because woman in labor breathes through her mouth.

4. Increase rate of IV fluids.

5. Keep woman supine for 5–10 min following administration of block to allow drug to diffuse bilaterally; after 5–10 min position woman on side.

(continued)

Regional Anesthesia—Lumbar Epidural (*continued*)

Nursing Diagnosis	Nursing Interventions	Rationale	Evaluation
	Specific interventions for hypotension following spinal anesthesia:	BP drops following spinal anesthesia, probably because of paralysis of the sympathetic vasoconstrictor fibers to blood vessels.	Maternal hypotension causes decreased blood circulation to fetus and results in fetal hypoxia.
	1. Administer O$_2$ by face mask at 6–10 L/min.		Amide group of anesthetic agents (bupivacaine, mepivacaine, and lidocaine) have potential to produce direct fetal myo-
	2. Manually displace uterus to left.	Increases venous return.	
	3. Increase rate of IV fluids.		
	4. Place legs in stirrups.		
		Observe, record, and report fetal bradycardia (FHR <120/min) and loss of beat-to-beat variability.	
		Institute treatment measures for maternal hypotension. (Note: Paracervical blocks commonly cause a drop in FHR for a short period.)	

Nursing Diagnosis: Decreased cardiac output related to sympathetic blockade	Monitor uterus for onset of a contraction	Uterine contraction during injection of anesthetic agent may increase upward spread to a higher level than desired.
Client Goal: Woman remains normotensive as measured by BP in 110/80 to 138/88 range.	Converse with woman during test dose.	Altered sensorium may indicate a complication.
	Assist with injection and taping of catheter.	Catheter must be securely taped to prevent displacement.
	Monitor maternal BP, pulse, and respiration every five minutes for 20–30 minutes.	Local anesthetic agent causes sympathetic blockade, may cause other complications. Regimen must also be followed after every reinjection.
Nursing Diagnosis: Impaired gas exchange in fetus due to anesthetic agent	Observe, record, and report symptoms of hypotension: BP <100 mm Hg or 25% fall in systolic pressure, nausea, and apprehension.	Maternal hypotension will decrease oxygenation of fetus. Early detection and immediate treatment decrease hypoxia in fetus.
		FHR remains 120–160, with average variability, and no late or variable decelerations.

cardial depression; bradycardia may be caused by reduced placental blood flow. Woman is normotensive.

(*continued*)

Regional Anesthesia—Lumbar Epidural (*continued*)

Nursing Diagnosis	Nursing Interventions	Rationale	Evaluation
Client Goal: FHR is 120–160, with average variability, no late or variable decelerations or accelerations with fetal movement or scalp stimulation.	If hypotension occurs institute treatment measures:		
	1. Place woman with head flat and foot of bed elevated, left lateral position.	Gravity increases venous return to heart, increasing pulmonary blood volume; result is an increase in stroke volume and cardiac output with a rise in BP.	
	2. Increase IV fluid rate.	Blood volume increases and circulation improves.	
	3. Administer O$_2$ by face mask at 6–10 L/min.	Increases oxygen content of circulating blood.	
	4. Administer vasopressor as ordered.	Vasoconstriction occurs; used only when BP cannot be maintained by other means.	
	Monitor BP and pulse following birth.	Hypotension due to anesthetic agent may be delayed in onset.	

	Explain possible delayed effects of anesthetic agents on fetus.	Anesthetic agents may produce neonatal neurobehavioral effects that could interfere with bonding.
	Assist woman to assume left lateral position.	Left lateral position prevents compression of vena cava, assisting venous return from extremities.
	Monitor and record BP and pulse every 5 minutes initially and then every 15 minutes.	Early detection and treatment of hypotension can minimize effect on the fetus.
	Monitor FHR continuously.	Local anesthetic agents may cause loss of variability and late decelerations.
Nursing Diagnosis: Altered patterns of urinary elimination related to effects of epidural	Assess bladder and encourage woman to void at frequent intervals.	Urinary retention frequently accompanies epidural block; client may be unaware of need to void. Woman's bladder remains empty, no bladder distention is present.

(*continued*)

Regional Anesthesia—Lumbar Epidural (continued)

Nursing Diagnosis	Nursing Interventions	Rationale	Evaluation
Client Goal: Woman will have normal urinary elimination as measured by: • Bladder is not distended. • Urination occurs without difficulty. • No urinary retention is present.	Catheterize if necessary.	Client has been overhydrated and distention may (1) impede progress of labor, (2) increase chance of bladder trauma, and (3) cause lack of postpartum bladder tone. Anesthetic agents may decrease frequency of contractions. Return of uncomfortable contractions is an indication of need for reinjection of epidural catheter. Optimal time is prior to the return of painful contractions.	
Nursing Diagnosis: Injury: High risk related to decreased motor control	Assess progress of labor: increase in frequency and duration of contractions, observe for increase in show, perform vaginal examinations.	Woman who chooses epidural wants to experience and participate in labor and birth.	

(continued)

Client Goal: The woman's extremities will be supported during movement. The woman will verbalize need for assistance as measured by her using the call light to request assistance when ambulating.	Inform woman of progress in labor. Provide reassurance throughout labor. During second stage of labor coordinate woman's pushing effort with increased uterine pressure of contractions.	Loss of sensation may decrease awareness of the urge to push and the ability to push. Pushing without contraction will be ineffective and cause maternal exhaustion.	The woman's extremities are supported during movement. Woman asks for assistance during ambulation in early postpartum period.
	Assist with "sitting dose" reinjection for birth.	Additional anesthesia is necessary for perineal relaxation, birth, and episiotomy repair.	
	Support extremities during movement. Position legs securely in stirrups (or on table for cesarean delivery).	Epidural block should not produce motor paralysis but the client may not have full control of extremities.	
	Ensure woman understands need for assistance with ambulation.	Motor control of the legs may be weak following epidural. Ambulation is delayed until complete sensation and ability to control legs has returned.	

Regional Anesthesia—Lumbar Epidural (continued)

Nursing Diagnosis	Nursing Interventions	Rationale	Evaluation
Nursing Diagnosis: Injury: High risk related to toxic systemic reaction	Observe for and report symptoms of toxic reaction: excitement, disorientation, incoherent speech, muscle twitching, nausea and vomiting, and convulsions or severe reactions of sudden loss of consciousness, severe hypotension, bradycardia, respiratory depression, and cardiac arrest.	Larger volume of anesthetic agent used with epidural increases likelihood of toxic reaction.	
Client Goal: Woman will remain free of signs and symptoms of toxic systemic reaction as measured by no evidence of:			Woman remains free of signs and symptoms.
● Excitement			
● Disorientation			
● Incoherent speech	Small, more frequent doses of analgesic agent are recommended to avoid severe reactions.		
● Nausea			
● Vomiting			
● Loss of consciousness			
● Severe hypotension	Institute treatment immediately:	Immediate treatment will lessen the effects of toxic systemic reactions on fetus.	
● Bradycardia	1. Support ventilation.		
● Respiratory or cardiac arrest	2. Increase IV fluids.		

3. Administer muscle relaxant for convulsions as ordered.

4. Be prepared for respiratory and cardiac resuscitation.

Nursing Care Plan
Small-for-Gestational-Age Newborn

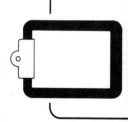

Client Assessment

Nursing History

Maternal factors:

Vascular—PIH, chronic hypertension, advanced diabetes

Preexisting diseases—heart disease, alcoholism, narcotic addiction, sickle cell anemia, PKU

Primiparity, smoking, lack of prenatal care, low socioeconomic level, very young or old

Environmental factors—high altitude, x-rays, maternal drug use (antimetabolics, anticonvulsants)

Physical Examination

Large-appearing head in proportion to chest and abdomen

Loose dry skin

Scarcity of subcutaneous fat, with emaciated appearance

Long, thin appearance

Sunken abdomen

Sparse scalp hair

Anterior fontanelle may be depressed

May have vigorous cry and appears alert

Birth weight below tenth percentile

Diagnostic Studies

Blood glucose and Dextrostix/Chemstrip

Hematocrit

Total bilirubin level

Calcium levels

Chest x-rays

Placental factors—infarcts, placenta previa

Fetal factors:
Congenital infections
Multiple pregnancy
Inborn errors of metabolism
Chromosomal syndrome

Nursing Diagnosis	Nursing Interventions	Rationale	Evaluation
Impaired gas exchange related to aspiration of meconium. *Client Goal:* Baby's respirations will be 30–50/min with no periods of apnea, intermittent cyanosis, sternal retractions, grunting, or nasal flaring.	Auscultate breath sounds every four hr. Suction endotracheal tube every three to four hr. Give oxygen prior to suction as needed. Ensure chest physiotherapy is done as indicated. Observe for worsening signs of respiratory distress such as generalized cyanosis; worsening retractions, grunting, and nasal flaring, as evidenced by	In utero, hypoxia causes relaxation of anal sphincter and reflex gasping of meconium. Maintain airway patency.	Baby's respirations are 30 to 50 per minute without apnea, retractions, grunting or nasal flaring.

(continued)

Small-for-Gestational-Age Newborn (*continued*)

Nursing Diagnosis	Nursing Interventions	Rationale	Evaluation
	Silverman respiratory index; sustained tachypnea; apnea episodes; inequality of breath sounds; presence of rales and rhonchi.		
	Administer oxygen per order for relief of respiratory distress signs and treatment of meconium aspiration, infant resuscitation.		
	Implement treatment plan by respiratory distress.		
	Monitor blood glucose levels every eight hours until stable or by Dextrostix/Chemstrip within one to two hr after birth and frequently for two to three days.	Respiratory distress increases consumption of glucose.	

Hypothermia related to decreased subcutaneous fat *Client Goal:* Baby will maintain skin temperature between 36.1°C and 36.7°C (97–98°F).	Provide neutral thermal zone (NTZ) range for infant based on postnatal weight.	Neutral thermal environment charts used for preterm baby must be altered for SGA newborns.	Baby's temperature is maintained between 36.1°C and 36.7°C.
	Use skin probe to maintain skin temperature at 36.1°–36.7°C.	Diminished subcutaneous fat and a large body surface compared to body weight predispose SGA baby to thermoregulation problems.	
	Obtain axillary temps and compare to registered skin probe temp every two to three hrs. and PRN. If discrepancy exists, evaluate potential cause.	Discrepancies between axillary and skin probe monitor temp may be due to mechanical causes or the burning of brown fat.	
	Adjust and monitor incubator or radiant warmer to maintain skin temperature.		
	Minimize heat losses and prevent cold stress by:	SGA infant has increased heat loss due to decreased available brown fat stores for heat production and less fat insulation.	

(continued)

Small-for-Gestational-Age Newborn (*continued*)

Nursing Diagnosis	Nursing Interventions	Rationale	Evaluation
	1. Warming and humidifying oxygen without blowing over face in order to avoid increasing oxygen consumption		
	2. Keeping skin dry		
	3. Keeping Isolettes, radiant warmers, and cribs away from windows and cold external walls and out of drafts		
	4. Avoiding placing infant on cold surfaces such as metal treatment tables, cold x-ray plates		
	5. Padding cold surfaces with diapers and using radiant warmers during procedures		

Nursing Diagnosis / Client Goal	Nursing Interventions	Rationale	Evaluation
	6. Warming blood for exchange transfusions.		
Injury: High risk to tissues related to decreased glycogen stores and impaired gluconeogenesis	Monitor for signs and symptoms of cold stress: decreased temperature, lethargy, pallor.	Cold stress increases oxygen requirements.	
Client Goal: Baby will have blood glucose of greater than 40 mg/dL, no signs of respiratory distress, and will be alert and active.	Monitor blood glucose per SGA protocol and report values < 40 mg/dL.	Combined with depletion of glycogen stores, impaired gluconeogenesis predisposes SGA infants to profound hypoglycemia within first two days of life.	Baby's blood glucose is greater than 40 mg/dL, baby is alert and active.
	Observe, record, and report signs of hypoglycemia: cyanosis, lethargy, jitteriness, seizure activity, and apnea.	Hypoglycemia causes CNS irritability.	
	Notify physician if values are low. Monitor vital signs every two hr PRN.		
	Initiate feeding schedule for SGA newborns per agency protocol. Monitor blood glucose.	Frequent monitoring of blood glucose assists in identifying decreasing glucose levels.	

(continued)

Small-for-Gestational-Age Newborn (*continued*)

Nursing Diagnosis	Nursing Interventions	Rationale	Evaluation
	Provide glucose intake either through early enteral feeding (before four hr) or by IV per physician's order. See further discussion of hypoglycemia on p 1035.	Provision of glucose through early feedings (begin before four hr of age), or IV, maintains needed glucose levels.	
	Record input and output, monitor IV rate and site hourly.	Decreasing glucose is reflected in lethargy, decreased appetite.	
Altered nutrition: less than body requirements related to SGA's increased metabolic rate	Initiate test water feeding at one hr of age, then proceed to 5% glucose/water. Move early to formula feeding every two to three hr.	Sterile water is desirable for first feedings because it causes fewer pulmonary complications in the presence of aspiration of feeding.	Baby receives 120–150 cal/kg/day, maintains weight with expected gain pattern, takes formula without tiring.
Client Goal: Baby will not lose more than 2% weight, will take formula without tiring, and will gain weight.	Supplement oral feedings with intravenous intake per orders. Monitor intake and output every four hours or more frequently.	SGA newborns require more calories/kg for growth because of increased metabolic activity and oxygen consumption secondary to increased percentage of body weight made up by visceral organs.	

(*continued*)

Use concentrated formulas that supply more calories in less volume, such as Similac 24.	Small, frequent feedings of high caloric formula are used because of limited gastric capacity and decreased gastric emptying.
Promote growth by providing caloric intake of 120–150 cal/kg/day in small amounts. Monitor and record signs of respiratory distress or fatigue occurring during feedings.	Small, frequent feedings decrease fatigue associated with feeding.
Supplement gavage, bottle or breast feedings with intravenous therapy per physician order until oral intake is sufficient to support growth.	Adequate nutritional intake promotes growth and prevents such complications as metabolic catabolism and hypoglycemia.
Begin bottle- or breast–feeding slowly, such as bottle- or breast–feed once per day, bottle- or breast–feed once per shift, and then bottle- or breast–feed every other feeding.	Gavage feedings require less energy expenditure on the part of the newborn.

Small-for-Gestational-Age Newborn (*continued*)

Nursing Diagnosis	Nursing Interventions	Rationale	Evaluation
	Monitor daily weight with anticipation of small amount of weight loss when bottle- or breast-feedings start.	Bottle- or breast–feeding, an active rather than passive intake of nutrition, requires energy expenditure, burning of calories, and potential weight loss.	
Altered tissue perfusion related to increased blood viscosity	Obtain central hematocrit on admission	Exact etiology of polycythemia in SGA is not known but is thought to be a physiologic response to chronic hypoxia with increased erythropoietin production.	Baby's hemoglobin is less than 22 g/dL, hematocrit is less than 65%, and there are no signs of respiratory distress.
Client Goals: Baby's hemoglobin will be less than 22 g/dL, hematocrit less than 65%; baby will show no signs of respiratory distress, cyanosis, or tachycardia.	Monitor, record, and report symptoms, including: 1. Decrease in peripheral pulses, discoloration of extremity, alteration in activity or neurologic depression, renal vein	Polycythemia is defined as a central venous hematocrit above 65% – 70% in the first week of life. Hyperviscosity is resultant "thickness" of red-cell rich blood so that its ability to perfuse the tissues is dis-	

thrombosis with decreased urine output, hematuria, or proteinuria in thromboembolic conditions	turbed due to thickness and decrease in deformability of cells. Symptoms are caused by poor perfusion of tissues.
2. Tachycardia or congestive heart failure	
3. Respiratory distress syndrome, cyanosis, tachypnea, increased oxygen need, labored respirations, or hemorrhage in respiratory system	
Watch for other signs of increased hematocrit such as hyperbilirubinemia Monitor bilirubin levels every eight hr.	As the increased red blood cells begin to break down, hyperbilirubinemia may present.
Assist with partial plasma exchange.	Partial plasma exchange decreases blood volume and blood viscosity to less than 60%.

(continued)

Small-for-Gestational-Age Newborn (*continued*)

Nursing Diagnosis	Nursing Interventions	Rationale	Evaluation
Altered parenting: High risk related to prolonged separation of baby and parents secondary to illness.	Include parents in determining infant's plan of care and encourage their participation. Encourage parents to visit frequently. Provide opportunities for parents to touch, hold, talk to, and care for infant. Determine the type and amount of appropriate sensory stimulation and implement sensory stimulation program.	Parent-infant bonding begins in first few hours or days following birth of an infant. SGA infants experience prolonged periods of separation from their parents, which necessitates intervention to ensure parent-infant bonding. Emotional support of the psychologic well-being of family, including positive parent-infant bonding and sensory stimulation of infant, is important.	Baby's parents have bonded with their infant, are involved in their infant's care, and have realistic expectations about their baby.
Client Goals: Baby's parents will touch, hold, and participate in the baby's care and talk about the future of their baby.			
Knowledge deficit (parental) concerning care of newborn at home	Prepare for discharge by instructing parents in such areas as feeding techniques, formula preparation (including bottle sterilization), and breast-feeding;	Parents should receive the same postpartum teaching as any parent taking a new infant home. Parents need to understand the changes to expect in color	Baby's parents verbalize how to take care of their baby at home and know when to return for follow-up and when to call their health care provider.
Client Goals: Baby's parents will ask about taking			

her or him home and will participate in discharge planning, attend necessary classes on infant care, and ask about when to call the doctor and follow-up needs.

bathing, diapering, and hygiene; rectal temperature monitoring; administration of vitamins; sibling rivalry; care of complications and preventing exposure to infections; normal elimination patterns, expected weight gain patterns, normal reflexes and activity, and how to promote normal growth and development without being overprotective; returning for continued medical care; and availability of community resources if indicated.

of the infant's stool and number of bowel movements plus odor from bottle- or breast-feeding in order to avoid unnecessary concern. Preterm infants usually do not require referral to community agencies such as visiting nurse associations unless there is a specific problem requiring assistance. Infants with congenital abnormalities, feeding problems, or resolving complications with infections, or mothers unable to cope with defective infants are examples of conditions requiring referral to community resources.

Nursing Care Plan
Thromboembolic Disease

Client Assessment

Nursing History

1. Predisposing factors include the following:
   a. Increased maternal age
   b. Obesity
   c. Increased parity
   d. Prolonged labor with associated pressure of the fetal head on the pelvic veins
   e. PIH
   f. Heart disease
   g. Hypercoagulability of the early puerperium
   h. Anemia
   i. Immobility
   j. Hemorrhage
   k. Previous history of venous thrombosis

Physical Examination

1. Superficial thrombophlebitis
   a. Tenderness along the involved vein
   b. Areas of palpable thrombosis
   c. Warmth and redness in the involved area
2. Deep venous thrombosis (DVT)
   a. Positive Homan's sign (pain occurs when foot is dorsiflexed while leg is extended)
   b. Tenderness and pain in affected area
   c. Fever (initially low, followed by high fever and chills)
   d. Edema in affected extremity
   e. Pallor and coolness in affected limb
   f. Diminished peripheral pulses
   g. Increased potential for pulmonary embolus

2. Initiating factors may include the following:
   a. Trauma to deep leg veins due to faulty positioning for delivery
   b. Operative delivery, including cesarean birth
   c. Abortion
   d. Postpartal pelvic cellulitis

Diagnostic Studies

Thrombophlebitis

a. Doppler ultrasonography demonstrates increased circumference of affected extremity
b. Occlusive cuff IPG
c. Venography confirms diagnosis

Nursing Diagnosis	Nursing Interventions	Rationale	Evaluation
Injury: High risk related to obstructed venous return *Client Goal:* Client will not experience any injury, as evidenced by absence of pain, edema, and pallor; pulses will be palpable; ambulation will be possible; and anticoagulant overdose will be avoided.	Report signs and symptoms of developing thrombo-phlebitis (see client assessment section of nursing care plan). Maintain bed rest and warm, moist soaks as ordered, with legs elevated. For DVT, administer intra-venous heparin as ordered, by continuous intravenous drip, heparin lock, or sub-cutaneously including the following:	Early detection of developing thrombophlebitis permits prompt treatment. As the thrombus increases in size, signs of obstruction also increase. Bed rest is ordered to de-crease possibility that portion of clot will dislodge and cause pulmonary embolism. Warmth promotes blood flow to affected area. Elevation of legs decreases edema and prevents venous stasis.	The woman recovers fully and injury is avoided.

(continued)

Thromboembolic Disease (*continued*)

Nursing Diagnosis	Nursing Interventions	Rationale	Evaluation
	1. Monitor IV or heparin lock site for signs of infiltration.	Heparin does not dissolve clot but is administered to prevent further clotting. It is safe for breast-feeding mothers because heparin is not secreted in mother's milk.	
	2. Obtain Lee-White clotting times or partial thromboplastin time (PTT) per physician order and review prior to administering heparin.		
	3. Observe for signs of anticoagulant overdose with resultant bleeding, including the following: a. Hematuria b. Epistaxis c. Ecchymosis d. Bleeding gums		
	4. Provide protamine sulfate, per physician	Protamine sulfate is heparin antagonist, given intravenously,	

(*continued*)

order, to combat bleeding problems related to heparin overdosage.

which is almost immediately effective in counteracting bleeding complications caused by heparin overdose.

Immediately report the development of any signs of pulmonary embolism, including the following:

1. Sudden onset of severe chest pain, often located substernally
2. Apprehension and sense of impending catastrophe
3. Cough (may be accompanied by hemoptysis)
4. Tachycardia
5. Fever
6. Hypotension
7. Diaphoresis, pallor, weakness
8. Shortness of breath
9. Neck vein engorgement

Pulmonary embolism is major complication of deep venous thrombosis / thrombophlebitis. Signs and symptoms may occur suddenly and require immediate emergency treatment; prognosis is related to size and location of embolism.

Thromboembolic Disease (*continued*)

Nursing Diagnosis	Nursing Interventions	Rationale	Evaluation
	10. Friction rub and evidence of atelectasis upon auscultation		
	Initiate or support any emergency treatment.		
	Initiate progressive ambulation following the acute phase; provide properly fitting elastic stockings prior to ambulation for management of superficial thrombophlebitis and DVT.	Elastic stockings or "TEDs" help prevent pooling of venous blood in lower extremities.	
	For DVT, obtain prothrombin time (PT) and review prior to beginning warfarin. Repeat periodically per physician order.	PT is the test most commonly used to monitor the blood of clients receiving warfarin. Warfarin sodium (Coumadin) inhibits Vitamin K-dependent activation of clotting factors II, VII, IX, and X. Goal of treatment is to maintain prothrombin time (PT) at 1.5 to 2 times normal.	

Pain related to tissue hypoxia and edema secondary to vascular obstruction	Administer analgesics as ordered for relief of pain. Provide supportive nursing comfort measures such as back rubs, provision of quiet time for sleep, diversional activities.	Analgesics act to relieve pain and enable the woman to rest. Aspirin or ibuprofen products are contraindicated, as they inhibit platelet adhesiveness. Acetaminophen may be ordered by the physician.	Woman states that pain is relieved and that she is able to rest comfortably.
Client Goal: Woman will obtain relief of pain as evidenced by verbal expressions of comfort and ability to rest and sleep.	Maintain limb in elevated position.	Elevation of affected limb promotes venous return and helps decrease edema.	
Potential altered parenting related to decreased maternal-infant interaction secondary to bed rest and IVs	Maintain mother-infant attachment when mother is on bed rest:	Maternal-infant attachment is enhanced by frequent contact and opportunities to interact.	Woman successfully develops bonds of attachment with her infant.
Client Goal: Woman will develop bonds of attachment with her infant as evidenced by her ability to feed her infant successfully, her involvement in her infant's care, her demonstra-	1. Provide frequent contacts for mother and infant; modified rooming-in is possible if the crib is placed close to the mother's bed and nurse checks often to help mother lift or move infant.		

(continued)

Thromboembolic Disease (*continued*)

Nursing Diagnosis	Nursing Interventions	Rationale	Evaluation
tion of affectionate behaviors, and verbal expressions of positive thoughts about her baby.	2. Encourage mother to feed baby. Breast–feeding mothers may nurse; for acutely ill mothers it may be necessary to pump the breasts. 3. Provide photos of infant if contact is limited.		
Altered family processes related to illness of family member *Client Goal:* Woman and her family will cope effectively with her illness as evidenced by frequent visits from partner (and other family members, including siblings), verbalized plans for handling family	1. Encourage woman to express her concerns to her partner. Assist couple in planning ways to manage while woman is hospitalized and after her discharge. 2. Encourage partner or support person to bring other children to hospital to visit mother and meet new sibling.	Illness of any family member impacts the entire family. This is especially true when the family situation is such that the mother is the primary nurturer and she is absent. Family members attempt to continue their own roles while also assuming the tasks of the missing member. This can result in crisis.	Woman expresses assurance that family misses her but is coping effectively. Family is able to discuss plans for coping following the woman's discharge.

tasks and for coping when woman is discharged, and expressions of assurance by woman that the family will deal effectively with her illness.

Knowledge deficit related to the DVT/thrombophlebitis, its treatment, preventive measures, and the medication, warfarin

Client Goal: Woman will understand her condition, its treatment, and long-term implications as evidenced by her ability to discuss the condition and answer questions about her care and responsibilities.

3. Encourage partner or support person to bring in family pictures. Encourage phone calls.
4. Contact social services if indicated to obtain additional assistance for family if needed.

1. Discuss ways of avoiding circulatory stasis such as avoiding prolonged standing or sitting; avoiding crossing legs.
2. Review need to wear support stockings and to plan for rest periods with legs elevated.

In the presence of DVT, discuss the following:

1. The use of warfarin, its side effects, possible interactions with other

Such discussion is essential to help the woman understand the condition, her medication, and its implications. She must have a clear understanding to be able to provide effective self-care.

Woman is able to discuss her condition, its treatment, preventive measures, and long-term implications.

(continued)

Thromboembolic Disease (*continued*)

Nursing Diagnosis	Nursing Interventions	Rationale	Evaluation
	medications, and need to have dosage assessed through periodic checks of the prothrombin time.		
	2. Discuss signs of bleeding, which may be associated with warfarin sodium and which need to be reported immediately, including the following: a. Hematuria b. Epistaxis c. Ecchymosis d. Bleeding gums e. Rectal bleeding		
	3. Monitor menstrual flow—bleeding may be heavier.		

4. Review need for woman to eat a consistent amount of leafy green vegetables (lettuce, cabbage, brussels sprouts, broccoli) every day.

Foods are high in vitamin K and will affect balance between dose of warfarin and PT.

5. Instruct woman to report *any* bleeding that continues more than 10 minutes.

6. Instruct woman to do the following:
   a. Routinely inspect body for bruising
   b. Carry Medic Alert card indicating she is on anticoagulant therapy
   c. Use electric razor to avoid scratching skin, use *soft* bristle tooth brush
   d. Avoid alcohol intake or keep intake at minimum

(*continued*)

Thromboembolic Disease (*continued*)

Nursing Diagnosis	Nursing Interventions	Rationale	Evaluation
	e. Not to take any other drugs without checking with physician f. Note that stools may change color to pink, red, or black as a result of anticoagulant use		

Nursing Care Plan
Unplanned Adolescent Pregnancy

Nursing History:
Note age and subjective symptoms of pregnancy, LMP, gravida, parity, menstrual history. Note client's perception of pregnancy and anxiety level. Identify family structure.

Physical Examination:
Pelvic examination to assess for uterine changes associated with pregnancy.

Diagnostic Studies:
Urine hCG

Nursing Diagnosis Goals	Nursing Interventions	Rationale	Evaluation
Nursing Diagnosis: Anxiety related to fear of parental reaction secondary to unplanned adolescent pregnancy.	Encourage the adolescent to express her own feelings and concerns, including her perception regarding parental response to the pregnancy.	Helps to identify specific areas of concerns where guidance in problem solving is needed. Health care providers must listen carefully, which means previous clarification of own	The adolescent will begin to realistically identify the potential reactions of her parents to her pregnancy.

(continued)

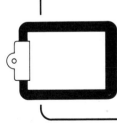

Unplanned Adolescent Pregnancy (*continued*)

Nursing Diagnosis	Nursing Interventions	Rationale	Evaluation
Client Goal: The adolescent will reduce her anxiety by identifying a support system to help her in her decision-making process. She will understand, however, that the final decision about maintenance of the pregnancy or pregnancy termination should be hers.		values and beliefs regarding pregnancy termination, and not impose values on client. If unable not to superimpose own values in client, need to refer to more objective counseling source.	
	In those states where appropriate, reassure client that decision to share news of pregnancy with parents is hers. Confidentiality of health care providers is required.	Most states do not require parental notification if abortion is chosen. In addition, it is important to investigate the possibility of incest with the young adolescent, especially when adolescent is evasive and uncomfortable about discussing sexual partner.	
	Encourage her to identify a support system in helping her make a decision about	Important for adolescent to have support from significant individuals in her life in mak-	

	Interventions	Rationale
	how to deal with her unplanned pregnancy.	ing decision and for follow-up support. This is essential if she plans to maintain the pregnancy.
Nursing Diagnosis: Anxiety related to decisional conflict secondary to handling unplanned pregnancy.	Assess relationship with sexual partner and explore possible consequences in contacting him.	The adolescent may want her sexual partner involved in the decision but may be concerned about parental reaction to his involvement.
Client Goal: The adolescent will understand the alternatives in dealing with her unplanned pregnancy as she begins to cope effectively with her conflict.	If adolescent accompanied by a parent, important to visit with adolescent initially by herself to assess her concerns without the presence of parents.	May be only way to find out how adolescent feels and any special concerns she has. If under 14, important to explore family relationships since incest is a concern in the early adolescent.
	Present the alternatives: terminating pregnancy, maintaining the pregnancy and keeping the baby, maintaining the pregnancy and placing the baby for adoption.	Most adolescents have probably not thought through all the alternatives available in dealing with an unplanned pregnancy.
		The client will begin to effectively evaluate the consequences in her life of each alternative response to her pregnancy.

(*continued*)

Unplanned Adolescent Pregnancy (*continued*)

Nursing Diagnosis	Nursing Interventions	Rationale	Evaluation
	With each alternative, explore with the client her perception of projected consequences as it relates to her situation in life.	It is important to assess the client's perception of projected consequences in her own life in order to help her do more effective problem solving in arriving at a decision most comfortable for her.	
	Identify agency resources for help for each of the alternatives.	Most adolescents are unaware of resources available to support them in the choices they may make, especially if they decide to maintain their pregnancy and give the baby up for adoption.	
Nursing Diagnosis: Knowledge deficit related to induced abortion. *Client Goal:* The adolescent will be able to describe the procedure	Assess client's perceptions and knowledge about induced abortion.	Clients frequently have many misconceptions about induced abortions. Important to clarify misconceptions before explaining procedure involved.	The adolescent can describe the abortion process and its consequences. In addition, she understands the importance of an early decision if this option is chosen.

involved with an induced abortion, and the importance of an early decision if this alternative is chosen.

Explain what to expect with an abortion done in first trimester including procedure, where it is done, what most women experience, etc.	The adolescent is usually unaware of what is actually involved with an abortion, physical consequences, and what to expect regarding the products of conception in first trimester.
Discuss how second trimester abortions differ.	Adolescent may not realize that all factors related to induced abortion change as pregnancy progresses.
Discuss cost considerations related to an abortion.	Adolescents often have unrealistic ideas about health costs. Cost considerations may be an important factor in the adolescent's decision to share news of pregnancy with parents if parental notification not required by state law.
Explain state law requirements related to parental notification with induced abortion.	Most states do not require parental notification, but this may change in the future.

(continued)

Unplanned Adolescent Pregnancy (*continued*)

Nursing Diagnosis	Nursing Interventions	Rationale	Evaluation
	Discuss with adolescent the importance of her feeling comfortable with her final decision regarding her pregnancy, recognizing that some ambivalence would be experienced with any of the decisions. In addition, if leaning toward termination of pregnancy, safest when done as early in the pregnancy as possible.	Most adolescents are unaware of the limited timeframe in which a first trimester abortion can be done, especially if they have delayed confirmation of their pregnancy. If delayed too long, procedure for a first-trimester abortion may not be a choice.	
	Encourage her to examine closely her own values and beliefs about abortion.	Important for her to understand examination of her beliefs is important in her comfort with her decision, not the beliefs and values of her parents or peers, which may be in conflict with hers.	

Common Abbreviations in Maternal-Newborn Nursing

ABC	Alternative birthing center *or* airway, breathing, circulation
Accel	Acceleration of fetal heart rate
AC	Abdominal circumference
ACD	Acetate citrate dextrose
AFAFP	Amniotic fluid alpha fetoprotein
AFP	α-fetoprotein
AFV	Amniotic fluid volume
AGA	Average for gestational age
AID or AIH	Artificial insemination donor (H designates mate is donor)
AIDS	Acquired Immune Deficiency Syndrome
AP	Anterior posterior
ARBOW	Artificial rupture of bag of waters
AROM	Artificial rupture of membranes
BAT	Brown adipose tissue (brown fat)
BBT	Basal body temperature
BL	Baseline (fetal heart rate baseline)
BMR	Basal metabolic rate
BOW	Bag of waters
BP	Blood pressure
BPD	Biparietal diameter *or* Bronchopulmonary dysplasia
BPM	Beats per minute
BSE	Breast self examination
BSST	Breast self-stimulation test
CC	Chest circumference *or* Cord compression
cc	cubic centimeter
CDC	Centers for Disease Control
C–H	Crown-to-heel length
CHF	Congestive heart failure
CID	Cytomegalic inclusion disease
CMV	Cytomegalovirus
cm	centimeter
CNM	Certified nurse-midwife
CNS	Central nervous system
CPAP	Continuous positive airway pressure
CPD	Cephalopelvic disproportion *or* Citrate-phosphate-dextrose

CPR	Cardiopulmonary resuscitation
CRL	Crown-rump length
C/S	Cesarean section or (C-section)
CST	Contraction stress test
CT	Computerized tomography
CVA	Costovertebral angle
CVP	Central venous pressure
CVS	Chorionic villus sampling
D&C	Dilatation and curettage
decels	deceleration of fetal heart rate
DFMR	Daily fetal movement response
DIC	Disseminated intravascular coagulation
dil	dilatation
DM	Diabetes mellitus
DRG	Diagnostic related groups
DTR	Deep tendon reflexes
ECHMO	Extracorporal membrane oxygenator
EDB	Estimated date of birth
EDC	Estimated date of confinement
EDD	Estimated date of delivery
EFM	Electronic fetal monitoring
EFW	Estimated fetal weight
ELF	Elective low forceps
epis	Episiotomy
FAD	Fetal activity diary
FAS	Fetal alcohol syndrome
FB	Finger breadth
FBD	Fibrocystic breast disease
FBM	Fetal breathing movements
FBPP	Fetal biophysical profile
FBS	Fetal blood sample *or* fasting blood sugar test
FECG	Fetal electrocardiogram
FFP	Fresh frozen plasma
FHR	Fetal heart rate
FHT	Fetal heart tones
FL	Femur length
FM	Fetal movement
FMAC	Fetal movement acceleration test
FMD	Fetal movement diary
FMR	Fetal movement record
FPG	Fasting plasma glucose test
FRC	Female reproductive cycle
FSH	Follicle-stimulating hormone
FSI	Foam stability index
G or grav	Gravida

GDM	Gestational diabetes mellitus
GFR	Glomerular filtration rate
GI	Gastrointestinal
GTPAL	Gravida, term, preterm, abortion, living children; a system of recording maternity history
GYN	Gynecology
HA	Head-abdominal rates
HAI	Hemagglutination-inhibition test
HC	Head compression
hCG	Human chorionic gonadotrophin
hCS	Human chorionic somatomammotrophin (same as hPL)
HMD	Hyaline membrane disease
hMG	Human menopausal gonadotrophin
hPL	Human placental lactogen
HVH	Herpes virus hominis
ICS	Intercostal space
IDDM	Insulin-dependent diabetes mellitus (Type I)
IDM	Infant of a diabetic mother
IGT	Impaired glucose tolerance
IGTT	Intravenous glucose tolerance test
IPG	Impedance phlebography
IUD	Intrauterine device
IUFD	Intrauterine fetal death
IUGR	Intrauterine growth retardation
LADA	Left-acromion-dorsal-anterior
LADP	Left-acromion-dorsal-posterior
LBW	Low birth weight
LDR	Labor, delivery and recovery room
LGA	Large for gestational age
LH	Luteinizing hormone
LMA	Left-mentum-anterior
LML	Left mediolateral (episiotomy)
LMP	Last menstrual period *or* Left-mentum-posterior
LMT	Left-mentum-transverse
LOA	Left-occiput-anterior
LOF	Low outlet forceps
LOP	Left-occiput-posterior
LOT	Left-occiput-transverse
L/S	Lecithin/sphingomyelin ratio
LSA	Left-sacrum-anterior
LSP	Left-sacrum-posterior
LST	Left-sacrum-transverse
LTV	Long-term variability

MAS	Meconium aspiration syndrome *or* Movement alarm signal
mec	Meconium
mec st	Meconium stain
M & I	Maternity and Infant Care Projects
mL	milliliter
ML	Midline (episiotomy)
MLE	Midline echo
MRI	Magnetic resonance imaging
MSAFP	Maternal serum alpha fetoprotein
multip	Multipara
NANDA	North American Nursing Diagnosis Association
NEC	Necrotizing enterocolitis
NGU	Nongonococcal urethritis
NIDDM	Noninsulin-dependent diabetes mellitus (Type II)
NIH	National Institutes of Health
NP	Nurse practitioner
NPO	Nothing by mouth
NSCST	Nipple stimulation contraction stress test
NST	Nonstress test *or* nonshivering thermogenesis
NSVD	Normal sterile vaginal delivery
NTD	Neural tube defects
NTZ	Neutral thermal zone
OA	Occiput anterior
OB	Obstetrics
OCT	Oxytocin challenge test
OF	Occipitofrontal diameter of fetal head
OFC	Occipitofrontal circumference
OGTT	Oral glucose tolerance test
OM	Occipitomental (diameter)
OP	Occiput posterior
OTC	Over-the-counter drugs
p	Para
Pap smear	Papanicolaou smear
PBI	Protein-bound iodine
PDA	Patent ductus arteriosus
PEEP	Positive end-expiratory pressure
PG	Phosphatidyglycerol *or* Prostaglandin
PI	Phosphatidylinositol
PID	Pelvic inflammatory disease
PIH	Pregnancy-induced hypertension
Pit	Pitocin
PKU	Phenylketonuria
PMI	Point of maximal impulse

PPHN	Persistent pulmonary hypertension
Preemie	Premature infant
Primip	Primapara
PROM	Premature rupture of membranes
PTT	Partial thromboplastin test
PUBS	Percutaneous umbilical blood sampling
RADA	Right-acromion-dorsal-anterior
RADP	Right-acromion-dorsal-posterior
RDA	Recommended dietary allowance
RDS	Respiratory distress syndrome
REEDA	Redness, edema, ecchymosis, discharge (or drainage), approximation (a system for recording wound healing)
REM	Rapid eye movements
RIA	Radioimmune assay
RLF	Retrolental fibroplasia
RMA	Right-mentum-anterior
RMP	Right-mentum-posterior
RMT	Right-mentum-transverse
ROA	Right-occiput-anterior
ROM	Rupture of membranes
ROP	Right-occiput-posterior, or retinopathy of prematurity
ROT	Right-occiput-transverse
RRA	Radioreceptor assay
RSA	Right-sacrum-anterior
RSP	Right-sacrum-posterior
RST	Right-sacrum-transverse
SFD	Small for dates
SGA	Small for gestational age
SIDS	Sudden infant death syndrome
SMB	Submentobregmatic diameter
SOAP	Subjective data, objective data, analysis, plan
SOB	Suboccipitobregmatic diameter
SRBOW	Spontaneous rupture of the bag of waters
SROM	Spontaneous rupture of the membranes
STD	Sexually transmitted disease
STS	Serologic test for syphilis, Sexually transmitted serology
STV	Short-term variability
SVE	Sterile vaginal exam
TC	Thoracic circumference
TCM	Transcutaneous monitoring
TORCH	Toxoplasmosis, rubella, cytomegalovirus, herpesvirus hominis type 2

TSS	Toxic shock syndrome
ū	umbilicus
u/a	urinalysis
UA	Uterine activity
UAC	Umbilical artery catheter
UAU	Uterine activity units
UC	Uterine contraction
UPI	Uteroplacental insufficiency
U/S	Ultrasound
UTI	Urinary tract infection
VBAC	Vaginal birth after cesarean
VDRL	Venereal Disease Research Laboratories
WBC	White blood cell
WIC	Supplemental food program for Women, Infants, and Children

Conversion of Pounds and Ounces to Grams

Conversion of Pounds and Ounces to Grams

POUNDS	0	1	2	3	4	5	6	7	8	9	10	11	12	13	14	15
0	—	28	57	85	113	142	170	198	227	255	283	312	340	369	397	425
1	454	482	510	539	567	595	624	652	680	709	737	765	794	822	850	879
2	907	936	964	992	1021	1049	1077	1106	1134	1162	1191	1219	1247	1276	1304	1332
3	1361	1389	1417	1446	1474	1503	1531	1559	1588	1616	1644	1673	1701	1729	1758	1786
4	1814	1843	1871	1899	1928	1956	1984	2013	2041	2070	2098	2126	2155	2183	2211	2240
5	2268	2296	2325	2353	2381	2410	2438	2466	2495	2523	2551	2580	2608	2637	2665	2693
6	2722	2750	2778	2807	2835	2863	2892	2920	2948	2977	3005	3033	3062	3090	3118	3147
7	3175	3203	3232	3260	3289	3317	3345	3374	3402	3430	3459	3487	3515	3544	3572	3600
8	3629	3657	3685	3714	3742	3770	3799	3827	3856	3884	3912	3941	3969	3997	4026	4054
9	4082	4111	4139	4167	4196	4224	4252	4281	4309	4337	4366	4394	4423	4451	4479	4508
10	4536	4564	4593	4621	4649	4678	4706	4734	4763	4791	4819	4848	4876	4904	4933	4961
11	4990	5018	5046	5075	5103	5131	5160	5188	5216	5245	5273	5301	5330	5358	5386	5415
12	5443	5471	5500	5528	5557	5585	5613	5642	5670	5698	5727	5755	5783	5812	5840	5868
13	5897	5925	5953	5982	6010	6038	6067	6095	6123	6152	6180	6209	6237	6265	6294	6322
14	6350	6379	6407	6435	6464	6492	6520	6549	6577	6605	6634	6662	6690	6719	6747	6776
15	6804	6832	6860	6889	6917	6945	6973	7002	7030	7059	7087	7115	7144	7172	7201	7228
16	7257	7286	7313	7342	7371	7399	7427	7456	7484	7512	7541	7569	7597	7626	7654	7682
17	7711	7739	7768	7796	7824	7853	7881	7909	7938	7966	7994	8023	8051	8079	8108	8136
18	8165	8192	8221	8249	8278	8306	8335	8363	8391	8420	8448	8476	8504	8533	8561	8590
19	8618	8646	8675	8703	8731	8760	8788	8816	8845	8873	8902	8930	8958	8987	9015	9043
20	9072	9100	9128	9157	9185	9213	9242	9270	9298	9327	9355	9383	9412	9440	9469	9497
21	9525	9554	9582	9610	9639	9667	9695	9724	9752	9780	9809	9837	9865	9894	9922	9950
22	9979	10007	10036	10064	10092	10120	10149	10177	10206	10234	10262	10291	10319	10347	10376	10404

OUNCES (column headers, 0–15)

Cervical Dilatation Assessment Aid

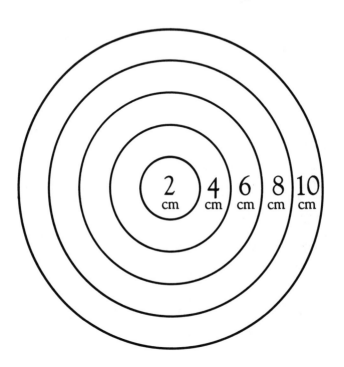

*Actions and Effects of Selected Drugs During Breast–Feeding**

Anticholinergics

Atropine: May cause hyperthermia in the newborn; may decrease maternal milk supply

Anticoagulants

Coumarin derivatives (Warfarin): May cause bleeding problems; should be discontinued in mother or breast–feeding temporarily halted if infant to have surgery

Heparin: Relatively safe to use; check PTT

Phenindione (Hedulin): Passes easily into breast milk; neonate may have increased pro time and PTT

Antihistamines
May cause decreased milk supply; infant may become drowsy, irritable, or have tachycardia

Antimetabolites
Unknown, probably long-term anti-DNA effect on the infant; potentially very toxic

Antimicrobials

Ampicillin: Skin rash, candidiasis, diarrhea

Chloramphenicol: Possible bone marrow suppression; Gray syndrome; refusal of breast

Methacycline: Possible inhibition of bone growth; may cause discoloration of the teeth; use should be avoided

Sulfonamides: May cause hyperbilirubinemia; use contraindicated until infant over 1 month old

Penicillin: Possible allergic response; candidiasis

Metronidazole (Flagyl): Posssible neurologic disorders or blood dyscrasias; delay breast–feeding for 12 to 24 hours after last dose

Aminoglycosides: May cause ototoxicity or nephrotoxicity if given for more than two weeks

*Based on data from Hill WC: Drugs contraindicated during pregnancy and lactation. *Medical Times* 1987; 115 (June):132. Riordan J: *A Practical Guide to Breastfeeding.* St. Louis: Mosby, 1983, pp 140–145. Spencer RT, et al: *Clinical Pharmacology and Nursing Management,* 2nd ed. Philadelphia: Lippincott, 1986, p 1016.

Tetracycline: Long-term use and large doses should be avoided; may cause tooth staining or inhibition of bone growth

Antithyroids

Thiouracil: Contraindicated during lactation; may cause goiter or agranulocytosis

Barbiturates
May produce sedation

Phenothiazines: May produce sedation

Bronchodilators

Aminophylline: May cause insomnia or irritability in the infant

Caffeine
Excessive consumption may cause jitteriness

Cardiovascular

Propranolol (Inderal): May cause hypoglycemia; possibility of other blocking effects

Quinidine: May cause arrhythmias in infant

Reserpine (Serpasil): Nasal stuffiness, lethargy, or diarrhea in infant

Corticosteroids
Adrenal suppression may occur with long-term administration of doses greater than 10 mg/day.

Heavy metals

Gold: Potentially toxic

Mercury: Excreted in the milk and hazardous to infant

Hormones

Androgens: Suppress lactation

Oral contraceptives: Decrease milk supply; may alter milk composition; may cause gynecomastia in male infants

Thyroid hormones: May mask hypothyroidism

Laxatives

Cascara: May cause diarrhea in infant

Milk of magnesia: Relatively safe

Phenolphthalein: May cause diarrhea in infant

Narcotic analgesics

Codeine: Accumulation may lead to neonatal depression

Meperidine: May lead to neonatal depression

Morphine: Long-term use may cause newborn addiction

Nonnarcotic analgesics

Salicylates: Safe after first week of life

Acetaminophen: Relatively safe for short-term analgesia

Propoxyphene (Darvon): May cause sleepiness and poor nursing in infant

Radioactive materials for testing

Gallium citrate (^{67}G): Insignificant amount excreted in breast milk; no nursing for 2 weeks

Iodine: Contraindicated; may affect infant's thyroid gland

^{125}I: Discontinue nursing for 48 hours

^{131}I: Nursing should be discontinued until excretion is no longer significant; after a test dose, nursing may be resumed after 24 to 36 hours; after a treatment dose, nursing may be resumed after 2 to 3 weeks

$^{99}Technetium$: Discontinue nursing for 48 hours (half-life = 6 hours)

Sedatives/Tranquilizers

Diazepam (Valium): May accumulate to high levels; may increase neonatal jaundice; may cause sedation

Lithium carbonate: Contraindicated; may cause neonatal flaccidity and hypotonia

Chlordiazepoxide (Librium): Use with caution after infant one week old

Selected Maternal-Newborn Laboratory Values

Normal Maternal Laboratory Values

Test	Non-pregnant Values	Pregnant Values
Hematocrit	37%–47%	32%–42%
Hemoglobin	12–16 gm/dL*	10–14 gm/dL*
Platelets	150,000–350,000/mm³	Significant increase three to five days after birth (predisposes to thrombosis)
Partial thromboplastin time (PTT)	12–14 seconds	Slight decrease in pregnancy and again in labor (placental site clotting)
Fibrinogen	250 mg/dL	400 mg/dL
Serum Glucose:		
Fasting	70–80 mg/dL	65 mg/dL
2-hour postprandial	60–110 mg/dL	Less than 140 mg/dL
Total protein	6.7–8.3 gm/dL	5.5–7.5 gm/dL
White blood cell total	4500–10,000/mm³	5000–15,000/mm³
Polymorphonuclear cells	54%–62%	60%–85%
Lymphocytes	38%–46%	15%–40%

*at sea level

Normal Neonatal Laboratory Values

Test	Normal Values
Hematocrit	51% to 56%
Hemoglobin	16.5 gm/dL (cord blood)
Platelets	150,000–400,000/mm^3
White blood cell total	18,000/mm^3
White blood cell differential:	
Bands	1600/mm^3 (9%)
Polymorphonuclear (segs)	9400/mm^3 (52%)
Eosinophils	400/mm^3 (2.2%)
Basophils	100/mm^3 (0.6%)
Lymphocytes	5500/mm^3 (31%)
Monocytes	1050/mm^3 (5.8%)
Serum glucose	40–80 mg/dL
Serum electrolytes:	
Sodium	135–147 mEq/L
Potassium	4–6 mEq/L
Chloride	90–114 mEq/L
Carbon dioxide	15–25 mEq/L
Bicarbonate	18–23 mEq/L
Calcium	7–10 mg/dL

APPENDIX F

Universal Precautions

The Centers for Disease Control recommend "*universal blood and body fluid precautions,*" now referred to simply as "*universal precautions,*" in the care of *all* clients, especially those in emergency care settings, in which the risk of blood exposure is increased and the infection status of the client is unknown. Under universal precautions, blood and certain body fluids of *all* clients are considered potentially infectious for human immunodeficiency virus (HIV), hepatitis B virus (HBV), and other blood-borne pathogens.

The CDC (1989, p. 9) recommends that these precautions apply to blood and to body fluids containing visible blood, as well as semen and vaginal secretions; to tissues, and to the following fluids: cerebrospinal fluid, synovial fluid, pleural fluid, peritoneal fluid, pericardial fluid, and amniotic fluids. **Blood is the single most important source of HIV, HBV, and other blood-borne pathogens in the health care setting**. Universal precautions do not apply to nasal secretions, sputum, saliva (except in the dental setting, where saliva is likely to be contaminated with blood), sweat, tears, urine, feces, and vomitus unless they contain visible blood. However, current infection control practices, already in existence, include the use of gloves for digital examination of mucous membranes and endotracheal suctioning, and hand washing after exposure to saliva. These practices should minimize the risk, if any, for salivary transmission of HIV and HBV (*MMWR*, 1988, p. 379).

The following specific precautions are recommended to reduce the risk of exposure to potentially infective materials:

- Refrain from all direct client care and from handling client-care equipment if you have exudative lesions or weeping dermatitis. Resume care when the condition is resolved.

Hand Washing Wash your hands thoroughly with warm water and soap (a) immediately, if contaminated with blood or other body fluids to which universal precautions apply, or potentially contaminated articles; (b) between clients; and (c) immediately after gloves are removed, even if the gloves appear to be intact. When hand washing facilities are not available, use a waterless antiseptic hand cleaner in accordance with the manufacturer's directions.

Gloves

- Wear gloves when touching blood and body fluids containing blood, as well as when handling items or surfaces soiled with blood or body fluids as mentioned above.

- Change gloves between client contacts.

- Use sterile gloves for procedures involving contact with normally sterile areas of the body.

- Use examination gloves for procedures involving contact with mucous membranes, unless otherwise indicated, and for other client care of diagnostic procedures that do not require the use of sterile gloves.

- When performing phlebotomy (venipuncture) wear gloves (a) if you have cuts, scratches, or other breaks in the skin; (b) in situations where hand contamination with blood may occur, e.g., with an uncooperative client; and (c) when you are learning phlebotomy techniques.

- Wear gloves when performing finger and/or heel sticks on infants and children.

- Do not wash or disinfect surgical or examination gloves for reuse. Washing with surfactants may cause *wicking*, i.e., the enhanced penetration of liquids through undetected holes in the glove. Disinfecting agents may cause deterioration.

- Use general-purpose gloves (e.g., rubber household gloves) for housekeeping chores involving potential blood contact and for instrument cleaning and decontamination procedures. Utility gloves may be decontaminated and re-used, but should be discarded if they are peeling, cracked, or discolored, or if they have punctures, tears, or other evidence of deterioration.

Other Protective Barriers

- Wear masks and protective eyewear (glasses, goggles) or face shields to protect the mucous membranes of your mouth, nose, and eyes during procedures that are likely to generate droplets of blood or other body fluids to which universal precautions apply.

- Wear a disposable plastic apron or gown during procedures that are likely to generate splatters of blood or other body fluid (e.g., peritoneal fluid) and soil your clothing.

- Place mouthpieces, resuscitation bags, or other ventilation devices, in areas where the need for emergency mouth-to-mouth resuscitation is predictable—even though saliva has not been implicated in HIV transmission.

- Wear disposable impervious shoe covering where there is massive blood contamination on floors and wear gloves to remove them.

Needles and Sharps Disposal   To prevent injuries, place used disposable needle-syringe units, scalpel blades, and other sharp items in puncture-resistant containers for disposal. Discard used needle-syringe units **uncapped** and **unbroken**. Place puncture-resistant containers as close as practicable to use areas.

Laundry   Handle soiled linen as little as possible and with minimum agitation to prevent gross microbial contamination of the air and of persons handling the linen. Place linen soiled with blood or body fluids in leakage-resistant bags at the location where it is used.

Specimens   Put all specimens of blood and listed body fluids in well-constructed containers with secure lids to prevent leakage during transport. When collecting specimens, take care to avoid contaminating the outside of the container.

Blood Spills

- Use a chemical germicide that is approved for use as a hospital disinfectant to decontaminate work surfaces after there is a spill of blood or other applicable body fluids. In the absence of a commercial germicide, a solution of sodium hypochlorite (household bleach) in a 1:100 dilution is effective.
- Wear gloves during cleaning and decontaminating procedures. Before decontaminating areas, first remove visible material with disposable towels or other appropriate means that prevent direct contact with the body fluid. Make sure plastic bags are available to remove contaminated items from spill sites.
- Brush-scrub contaminated boots and leather goods with soap and hot water.

Infective Wastes

- Follow agency policies for disposal of infective waste, both when disposing of, and when decontaminating, contaminated materials.

- Carefully pour bulk blood, suctioned fluids, and excretions containing blood and secretions, down drains that are connected to a sanitary sewer.

Sources   U.S. Department of Health and Human Services, Public Health Service, Update: Universal precautions for prevention of transmission of human immunodeficiency virus, hepatitis B virus, and other blood-borne pathogens in health care settings, *Morbidity and Mortality Weekly Report*, June 24, 1988; 37: 377–382, 387–388; *Morbidity and Mortality Weekly Report*, June 23, 1989, 38/No. S-6: 9–18.

RESOURCE DIRECTORY

This Resource Directory lists associations, support groups, and other organizations that can provide information or other assistance to maternal-newborn nurses and their clients. The resources are organized by topic, usually with brief descriptions of their services. Since many of these organizations have branches or chapters throughout North America, we recommend that you refer to your telephone directory for the location of the local branch.

GENERAL INFORMATION RESOURCES

National Center for Health Statistics (NCHS)
(*produces vital and health statistics for the United States*)
Scientific and Technical
Information Branch
Department of Health
and Human Services
6525 Belcrest Rd.
Hyattsville, MD 20782
(301) 436-8500

National Health Information Center
working through The Office of Disease Prevention and Health Promotion
(*provides information on health organizations and publications; selected diseases; Medicare, Medicaid and other insurances*)
P.O. Box 1133
Washington, DC 20013-1133
(301) 565-4167; (800) 336-4797

National Institute of Child Health and Human Development (NICHD)
National Institutes of Health
9000 Rockville Pike
Bldg. 31A, Room 2A32
Bethesda, MD 20892
(301) 496-5133

National Library of Medicine (NLM)
(*collects and disseminates biomedical information; publishes indexes of journal and research literature related to biomedical fields*)
Public Information Office
8600 Rockville Pike
Bethesda, MD 20894
(301) 496-6308
(800) 272-4787

National Maternal and Child Health Clearinghouse
(*provides information and publications regarding maternal/child health, nutrition, pregnancy, etc.*)
38th & R. St., NW
Washington, DC 20057
(202) 625-8410

National Technical Information Service (NTIS)
(*source of specialized social, scientific, business, and economic information, mostly originated or sponsored by federal agencies*)
Department of Commerce
5285 Port Royal Road
Springfield, VA 22161
(703) 487-4600

Office of Research for Women's Health
National Institute of Health
9000 Rockville Pike
Bldg. 1, Room 201
Bethesda, MD 20892
(301) 402-1770

Public Health Service
200 Independence Avenue, SW,
Rm. 719H
Washington, DC 20201
(202) 245-6867

ONLINE COMPUTER SERVICES

BRS Information Technologies
1200 Route 7
Latham, NY 12110
(800) 289-4277; (518) 783-1161

DIALOG Information Services, Inc.
3460 Hillview Avenue
Palo Alto, CA 94304
(800) 334-2564
(415) 858-2700

National Library of Medicine
MEDLARS Management Section
Bldg. 38A, Room 4N-421
8600 Rockville Pike
Bethesda, MD 20894
(800) 638-8480

RESOURCES BY TOPIC

ABORTION

National Abortion Federation
(*provides information and referrals for abortion services*)
1436 U Street, NW
Suite 103
Washington, DC 20009
(202) 667-5881; (800) 772-9100

National Abortion Rights Action League
(*pro-choice political action group*)
1101 14th Street, NW, 5th floor
Washington, DC 20005
(202) 408-4600

National Right to Life Committee
(*pro-life political action group*)
419 7th Street, NW
Suite 500
Washington, DC 20004
(202) 626-8800

Planned Parenthood Federation of America
810 Seventh Avenue
New York, NY 10019
(212) 541-7800; (800) 829-7732
See also Family Planning

ADOPTION

AASK (Aid to the Adoption of Special Kids)
(*provides assistance to families who adopt older and handicapped children*)
3530 Grand Avenue
Oakland, CA 94610
(415) 451-1748; (800) 232-2751

Adoptees' Liberty Movement Association (ALMA) Society
(*provides assistance for adopted children to locate natural parents and for natural parents to locate relinquished children*)
P.O. Box 154
Washington Bridge Station
New York, NY 10033
(212) 581-1568

Child Welfare Administration
(*provides information on adoption, foster care, and child abuse*)
80 Lafayette
New York, NY 10013
(212) 266-2000

Child Welfare League of America

(*provides information about adoption, especially of children with special needs*)
4 41st, NW, Suite 310
Washington, DC 20001-2085
(202) 638-2952

AIDS (ACQUIRED IMMUNE DEFICIENCY SYNDROME)

American Foundation for AIDS Research (AmFar)

(*provides funding for scientific research, education, and clinical trials. Does not provide general information*)
1515 Broadway St., Suite 3601
New York, NY 10036-8901
(212) 719-0033

American Social Health Association

Home Office
P.O. Box 13827
RTP, NC 27709

AIDS INFORMATION HOTLINE

(800) 342-AIDS

SIDA Hotline

(*provides AIDS information in Spanish*)
(800) 344-7432

TTY/TTD Hotline

(*provides AIDS information for the deaf*)
(800) 243-7889

Community Health Education Core

(*conducts research and maintains an extensive research library on women's health and HIV prevention*)
Columbia University School of Public Health
722 W. 168th Street
Box 29
New York, NY 10032
(212) 740-7292

National AIDS Clearinghouse

(*provides treatment directory*)
P.O. Box 6003
Rockville, MD 20849-6003
(800) 458-5231
for information regarding clinical trials:
(800) TRIALS-A

Shanti Project

(*provides counseling and assistance to individuals with AIDS*)
525 Howard St.
San Francisco, CA 94105
(415) 777-2273
See also Sexually Transmitted Infections

ALCOHOL ABUSE

Al-Anon/Alateen

P.O. Box 862
Midtown Station
New York, NY 10018
(212) 302-7240; (800) 344-2666

Alcoholics Anonymous

P.O. Box 459
Grand Central Station
New York, NY 10017
(212) 686-1100

National Clearinghouse for Alcohol and Drug Information

P.O. Box 2345
Rockville, MD 20852
(301) 468-2600; (800) 729-6686

Victim Outreach Program Mothers Against Drunk Drivers (MADD)

(*operates Victim Outreach Program to aid victims through the court process. Conducts research*)
P.O. Box 541688
Dallas, TX 75354-1688
(214) 744-6233

Women for Sobriety, Inc.
(*support group for women with drinking problem*)
P.O. Box 618
Quakertown, PA 18951
(215) 536-8026; (800) 333-1606

BIRTH CONTROL

See Family Planning

BIRTH DEFECTS

American Cleft Palate Association
(*provides information about cleft palates and cleft palate centers and parent support groups*)
1218 Grandview Ave.
Pittsburgh, PA 15211
(412) 481-1376

Cystic Fibrosis Foundation
2250 N. Druid Hills Rd.
Suite 275
Atlanta, GA 30329
(404) 325-6973; (800) 476-4483

Institutes for the Achievement of Human Potential
(*resource for parents with brain-injured children*)
8801 Stenton Avenue
Philadelphia, PA 19118
(215) 233-2050

March of Dimes Birth Defects Foundation
Public Health Education Foundation
1275 Mamaroneck Avenue
White Plains, NY 10605
(914) 428-7100

Spina Bifida Association of America
(*provides information and support to parents of infants with neural tube defects*)
1700 Rockville Pike
Suite 250
Rockville, MD 20852
(800) 621-3141
See also Down Syndrome; Genetic Disorders; Sickle Cell Anemia

BREAST CANCER

Reach to Recovery
(*support program for women who have undergone mastectomies as a result of breast cancer*)
American Cancer Society
19 W. 56th St.
New York, NY 10019
(212) 586-8700
See also Cancer

BREAST–FEEDING

Health Education Associates
(*provides continuing education programs for health professionals on breast-feeding management*)
211 South Easton Road
Glenside, PA 19038
(215) 876-2220

Human Lactation Center
(*limited to research on international infant/maternal feeding practices. No information provided*)
666 Sturges Highway
Westport, CT 06880
(203) 259-5995

La Leche League International

(*provides information about breast–feeding and support for breast–feeding mothers*)
9616 Minneapolis Avenue,
P.O. Box 1209
Franklin, IL 60131-8209
(708) 455-7730; (800) 525-3243
                                    LaLeche

Lact-Aid

(*provides services, literature, and supplies to promote breast–feeding*)
P.O. Box 1066
Athens, TN 37371-1066
(615) 744-9090
See also Childbirth; Infant Health, Maternal Health

Lactation Consultants Association, Ltd. (ILCA)

P.O. Box 4031
University of Virginia Station
Charlottesville, VA 22903

CANCER

American Cancer Society National Office

1599 Clifton Rd., NE
Atlanta, GA 30329
(404) 320-3333; (800) 227-2345

Cancer Information Service, Cancer Inquiries

(*provides cancer information for the general public*)
National Cancer Institute
900 Wisconsin Ave.
Bethesda, MD 20814
(301) 496-5583
(*to access regional offices for cancer information in English or Spanish:*)
(800) 4-CANCER
See also Breast Cancer; DES Exposure; Smoking

CESAREAN BIRTH

C/SEC, Inc. (Cesarean/Support Education and Concern)

(*provides information about cesarean birth*)
22 Forest Road
Framingham, MA 01701
(508) 877-8266

VBAC (Vaginal Birth After Cesarean)

10 Great Plain Terrace
Needham, MA 01292

CHILD ABUSE

C. Henry Kempe National Center for Prevention and Treatment of Child Abuse and Neglect

(*publishes a newsletter with information on prevention and treatment of child abuse*)
University of Colorado Medical Center
Department of Pediatrics
1205 Oneida Street
Denver, CO 80220
(303) 321-3963

Clearinghouse on Child Abuse and Neglect Information

Office of Child Development
P.O. Box 1182
Washington, DC 20013
(703) 821-2086

National Committee for Prevention of Child Abuse (NCPCA)

(*provides literature on child abuse prevention programs*)
332 South Michigan Avenue
Suite 1600
Chicago, IL 60604
(312) 663-3520

CHILD HEALTH AND DEVELOPMENT

Canadian Institute of Child Health
410 Laurier Avenue
Suite 803
West Ottawa, Ont. K1R 7T6

National Center for Education in Maternal and Child Health
38th and R Streets, NW
Washington, DC 20057
(202) 625-8400

National Institute of Child Health and Human Development (NICHD)
9000 Rockville Pike
Bldg. 31, Room 2A32
Bethesda, MD 20892
(301) 496-4000

Family Resource Clearinghouse
Child Development Center
Box 85
Metropolitan State College
P.O. Box 173362
Denver, CO 80217
(303) 556-8362
See also Infant Health

CHILDBIRTH

American Foundation for Maternal and Child Health, Inc.
(*clearinghouse for scientific information on obstetrical care*)
439 E. 51st Street
New York, NY 10002
(212) 759-5510

Birth: Issues in Prenatal Care and Education
(quarterly journal)
(*publisher also provides directory of instructional materials for childbirth educators*)
Blackwell Scientific Publications, Inc.
3 Cambridge Center, Suite 208
Cambridge, MA 02142

International Childbirth Education Association
(*provides information to educators and consumers on childbirth education*)
P.O. Box 20048
Minneapolis, MN 55420
(612) 854-8660

Maternity Center Association
(*freestanding birth center that provides information and advocacy functions*)
48 East 92nd Street
New York, NY 10028
(212) 369-7300

National Association of Parents and Professionals for Safe Alternatives in Childbirth
(*provides information and support for alternatives in birth experiences*)
Rt. 1, Box 646
Marble Hill, MO 63764
(314) 238-2010

National Association of Childbearing Centers
(*organization that provides information and suggests guidelines for birth centers*)
3123 Gottschall Road
Perkiomenville, PA 18074
(215) 234-8068

Family Resource Clearinghouse
Box 85
Metropolitan State College
P.O. Box 173362
Denver, CO 80217
(303) 556-8362
See also Cesarean Birth;
Childbirth Education/
Preparation; Home Birth

CHILDBIRTH EDUCATION/ PREPARATION

American Academy of Husband-Coached Childbirth
(*provides information on the Bradley method of childbirth*)
P.O. Box 5224
Sherman Oaks, CA 91413
(818) 788-6662;
(800) 42-BIRTH within CA
(800) 423-2397 outside CA

American Society for Psychoprophylaxis in Obstetrics
(*provides information about the Lamaze method of childbirth*)
1101 Connecticut Ave., NW
Suite 700
Washington, DC 20036
(202) 857-1128; (800) 368-4404

Association for Childbirth at Home (ACHI)
(*provides information to parents, educators, midwives, and physicians on safe home birth*)
P.O. Box 430
Glendale, CA 91209
(213) 667-0839

Childbirth Graphics, Ltd.
(*provides audiovisual and other types of teaching aids for childbirth education*)
P.O. Box 20540
Rochester, NY 14602-0540
(716) 272-0300; FAX (716) 272-0716

Read Natural Childbirth Foundation, Inc.
(*provides information about the Dick-Read method of childbirth*)
P.O. Box 956
San Rafael, CA 94915
(415) 456-8462
See also Cesarean Birth;
Childbirth; Home Birth

CIRCUMCISION

American Academy of Pediatrics
(*report on circumcision available for a minimal fee*)
P.O. Box 927 141 Northwest
Point Blvd.
Elk Grove, IL 60009-0927
(708) 228-5005

Childbirth Education Foundation
(*Eastern area contact for No—CIRC promotes reform in childbirth practices, especially in the treatment of the newborn*)
P.O. Box 5
Richboro, PA 18954
(212) 357-2792

National Organization of Circumcision Information Resource Center (No-CIRC)
(*western area contact*)
P.O. Box 2512
San Anselmo, CA 94960
(415) 488-9883

CONGENITAL DISORDERS/ DEFECTS

See Birth Defects; Genetic Disorders

CONTRACEPTION

See Family Planning

COUNSELING SERVICES

Family Service America
(*organization of local family
counseling agencies throughout
North America*)
11700 Westlake Park Drive
Milwaukee, WI 53224
(414) 359-1040

Women in Transition (WIT)
(*provides counseling
information and referrals for
women in distress and transition
because of divorce, widowhood,
and separation*)
125 S. 9th St., Suite 502
Philadelphia, PA 19107
(215) 922-7500; (215) 922-7177

DES (DIETHYLSTILBESTROL) EXPOSURE

**Cancer Information Service,
Cancer Inquiries**
(*provides information to DES
mothers and daughters*)
National Cancer Institute
900 Wisconsin Ave.
Bethesda, MD 20814
(301) 496-5583
(*to access regional offices for
cancer information in English
or Spanish*:)
(800) 4-CANCER

DES Action
(*provides information on DES
and the DES cancer network*)
1615 Broadway, Suite 510
Oakland, CA 94612
(415) 465-4011

DOWN SYNDROME

**National Association for
Down's Syndrome (NADS)**
(*provides information about
Down syndrome*)
1800 Dempster
Park Ridge, IL 60068-1146
(708) 823-7550; (800) 232-6372

**National Down's Syndrome
Society Hotline**
666 Broadway
New York, NY 10012
(800) 221-4602; in New York
(212) 460-9330
See also Birth Defects; Genetic
Disorders

FAMILY

**Displaced Homemakers
Network**
(*national advocacy group for
women over 35 who have lost
their primary means of support
through death, divorce, or
disabling of spouse*)
1411 K Street, NW
Suite 930
Washington, DC 20005
(202) 628-6767

Fathers for Equal Rights
P.O. Box 010847
Flagler Station
Miami, FL 33101
(305) 895-6351

Family Service America
(*provides counseling and
assistance to families*)
11700 Westlake Park Drive
Milwaukee, WI 53223
(414) 359-1040

Parenthood After Thirty
(*provides information and
programs for professionals and
individuals who have delayed
childbearing*)
451 Vermont
Berkeley, CA 94707
(415) 524-6635

Parents Without Partners
(*support group for single
parents*)
8807 Colesville Road
Silver Spring, MD 20910
(301) 588-9354; (800) 637-7974

Step Family Foundation
333 West End Ave.
New York, NY 10023
(212) 877-3244

FAMILY PLANNING

Association of Voluntary Sterilization, Inc. (AVS)
(provides information on sterilization and referral service)
79 Madison Ave.
New York, NY 10168
(212) 351-2500

Couple to Couple League International, Inc. (CCL)
(teaches natural family planning techniques; publishes manual on the symptothermal method, The Art of Natural Family Planning)
P.O. Box 111184
Cincinnati, OH 45211
(513) 661-7612

Planned Parenthood Federation of America
810 Seventh Avenue
New York, NY 10019
(212) 541-7800; (800) 829-7732

Family Life Information Exchange
P.O. Box 37299
Washington, DC 20013-7299
(301) 585-6636

FOOD AND NUTRITION

See Nutrition

GENETIC DISORDERS

National Center for Education in Maternal and Child Health
(provides educational services and technical assistance to organizations, agencies, and individuals with interests in maternal and child health issues)
38th & R Streets, NW
Washington, DC 20057
(202) 625-8400

HAZARDOUS WASTES

See Environmental Hazards

HEARING-IMPAIRED CHILDREN

American Society for Deaf Children
(provides education and support to parents of hearing-impaired children)
814 Thayer Avenue
Silver Springs, MD 20910
(301) 585-5400; (800) 942-ASDC

International Organization for the Education of the Hearing Impaired
(provides information on speech and oralism in newborns and information regarding "at risk" infants. Grants financial assistance for the funding of hearing aids, speech therapy, etc. for parents of hearing-impaired children under 5 years)
% Alexander Graham Bell Association for the Deaf
3417 Volta Pl., NW
Washington, DC 20007
(202) 337-5220

HOME BIRTH

Association for Childbirth at Home, International
P.O. Box 430
Glendale, CA 91209
(213) 667-0839
See also Childbirth

INFANT DEATH

Compassionate Friends
(self-help organization offering friendship and understanding to bereaved parents and siblings due to the death of a child of any age for any reason)
P.O. Box 3696
Oak Brooks, IL 60522-3696
(708) 990-0010

SHARE (Source of Help in Airing and Resolving Experiences)
(*support group for parents who have suffered loss of newborn baby*)
% St. John's Hospital
800 E. Carpenter Street
Springfield, IL 62769
(217) 525-5675
See also Sudden Infant Death Syndrome

INFANT HEALTH

American Foundation for Maternal and Child Health
(*clearinghouse for research on the perinatal period*)
439 E. 51st St.
New York, NY 10022
(212) 759-5510

American Red Cross
(*offers classes to prepare expectant parents for care and nurturing of infant*)
431 18th St., NW
Washington, DC 20006
(202) 737-8300

National Center for Clinical Infant Programs
(*promotes optimum development and mental health for infants and their families*)
2000 14th St., N.
Suite 380
Arlington, VA 22201
(703) 528-4300
See also Child Health

INFERTILITY

American Fertility Foundation
2140 11th Ave., S.
Suite 200
Birmingham, AL 35205-2800
(205) 933-8494

Fertility Research Foundation (FRF)
(*provides medical and consultation services for infertile couples; publishes journals,* Fertility Review *and* Infertility)
1430 Second Avenue
Suite 103
New York, NY 10021
(212) 744-5500

Resolve, Inc.
5 Water Street
Arlington, MA 02174
(617) 643-2424

Test-tube Fertilization
Eastern Virginia Medical School
Norfolk General Hospital
The Howard and Georgeanna Jones Institute for Reproductive Medicine
825 Fairfax Avenue
Norfolk, VA 23507
(804) 446-8948

INTRAUTERINE PROCEDURES

National Institute for Child Health and Human Development (NICHD)
9000 Rockville Pike
Bldg. 31, Room 2A32
Bethesda, MD 20892
(301) 496-4000

LEGAL CONCERNS

National Center on Women and Family Law
(*collects information on battered women, child support, and custody*)
799 Broadway
Room 402
New York, NY 10003
(212) 674-8200

Reproductive Freedom Project
American Civil Liberties Union
132 West 43rd Street
New York, NY 10036

MATERNAL HEALTH

Maternal Health Society
Box 46563, Station G
Vancouver, B.C. V6R 4G8

National Center for Education in Maternal and Child Health
38th and R Streets, NW
Washington, DC 20057
(202) 625-8400
See also Childbirth; Pregnancy; Women's Health

MEDICAL ORGANIZATIONS

American Academy of Family Physicians
8880 Ward Parkway
Kansas City, MO 64114
(816) 333-9700

American Academy of Pediatrics
141 Northwest Point Blvd.
Elk Grove Village, IL 60007
(312) 569-2025; (800) 433-9016

American College of Obstetricians and Gynecologists
409 12th St., SW
Washington, DC 20024
(202) 638-5577

American Medical Association
515 N. State St.
Chicago, IL 60610
(312) 464-5000

Society of Obstetricians and Gynaecologists of Canada
1785 Alta Vista Dr.
Suite 102
Ottawa, Ont. K1G 3Y6
(613) 521-4192

MEDICATIONS (PRESCRIPTION AND OVER-THE-COUNTER)

Food and Drug Administration (FDA)
Office of Consumer Affairs
Public Inquiries
5600 Fishers Lane (HFE-20)
Rockville, MD 20857
(301) 443-5006
See also Consumer Information

MIDWIFERY

The Farm
(*offers lay midwifery program; published midwifery handbook,* Spiritual Midwifery; *publishes periodical* The Birth Gazette)
P.O. Box 35, The Farm
Summertown, TN 38483
(615) 964-3574
See also Nurse-Midwifery

MULTIPLE BIRTH

Center for the Study of Multiple Birth
333 East Superior Street
Suite 464
Chicago, IL 60611
(312) 266-9093

National Organization of Mothers of Twins Clubs, Inc.
P.O. Box 23188
Albuquerque, NM 87198-1188
(505) 275-0955

NURSE-MIDWIFERY

American College of Nurse Midwives
1522 K Street, NW
Suite 1000
Washington, DC 20005
(202) 289-0171

Journal of Nurse-Midwifery
(periodical)
Elsevier Science Publishing Co.,
Inc.
655 Ave. of the Americas
New York, NY 10010
(212) 989-5800

**Midwives Alliance of North
America**
(*organization of nurse and lay
midwives in the United States
and Canada*)
P.O. Box 1121
Bristol, VA 24203-1121
(615) 764-5561

NURSING ORGANIZATIONS

**American Association of
Nurse Anesthetists (AANA)**
216 W. Higgins Rd.
Park Ridge, IL 60068
(708) 692-7050

**American Nurses Association
and Foundation**
1101 14th Street, NW
Suite 200
Washington, DC 20005
(202) 789-1800

Canadian Nurses Association
50 The Driveway
Ottawa, Ont. 4 Canada

**Nurses Association of the
American College of
Obstetricians and
Gynecologists (NAACOG)**
409 12th St., SW
Washington, DC 20024-2191
(202) 638-0026

**National League for Nursing
(NLN)**
350 Hudson St.
New York, NY 10014
(212) 989-9393
See also Nurse-Midwifery

NUTRITION

**American Institute
of Nutrition**
9650 Rockville Pike
Bethesda, MD 20814
(301) 530-7050

**Food and Drug
Administration (FDA)**
Office of Consumer Affairs
Public Inquiries
5600 Fishers Lane (HFE 20)
Rockville, MD 20857
(301) 443-5006

OBESITY

See Nutrition; Weight Control

OCCUPATIONAL HEALTH

**Clearinghouse for
Occupational Safety and
Health Information**
National Institute for
Occupational Safety and Health
4676 Columbia Parkway
Cincinnati, OH 45226
(513) 533-8236

PREGNANCY

**COPE (Coping with the
Overall Pregnancy/Parenting
Experience)**
530 Tremont Street
Boston, MA 02116
(617) 357-5588
See also Childbirth; Family
Planning; Maternal Health;
Women's Health

PREMENSTRUAL SYNDROME

See also Women's Health

RAPE

See telephone directory for local Rape Centers

Women Against Rape
P.O. Box 02084
Columbus, OH 43202
(614) 291-9751
See also Sexual Abuse
and Assault

SELF-CARE

Medical Self-Care Magazine
(periodical)
P.O. Box 1000
Point Reyes, CA 94956
(415) 663-8462

SEX EDUCATION

Center for Population Options
(*develops programs and material to educate teenagers on sex and sexual responsibility*)
1025 Vermont Ave., NW
Suite 210
Washington, DC 20005
(202) 347-5700; FAX (202) 347-2263

Planned Parenthood Federation of America
810 Seventh Avenue
New York, NY 10019
(212) 541-7800; (800) 829-7732
See also Family Planning

SEXUAL ABUSE AND ASSAULT

Child Assault Prevention (CAP) Project
Women Against Rape
P.O. Box 02084
Columbus OH 43202
(614) 291-9751

National Committee for Prevention of Child Abuse
332 S. Michigan Avenue
Suite 1600
Chicago, IL 60604
(312) 663-3520

Voices in Action, Inc.
(*provides a communication and peer support network for victims of incest and those affected by it*)
P.O. Box 148309
Chicago, IL 60614
(312) 327-1500

SEXUALLY TRANSMITTED INFECTIONS

Center for Prevention Services
(*Conducts research. Provides information to physicians.*)
Centers for Disease Control
1600 Clifton Road, NE
Atlanta, GA 30333
Physicians ONLY call: (404) 639-3311
STD Hotline: (800) 227-8922

V.D. National Hotline
(800) 227-8922
See also AIDS; Sex Education

SICKLE CELL ANEMIA

Center for Sickle Cell Disease
2121 Georgia Avenue, NW
Washington, DC 20059
(202) 806-7930

SMOKING

The following organizations provide information about the effects of smoking as well as how to quit smoking. See the white pages of telephone directory for local chapters.

American Cancer Society
19 W. 56th St.
New York, NY 10019
(212) 586-8700

American Heart Association
7320 Greenville Avenue
Dallas, TX 75231
(214) 373-6300

American Lung Association
1740 Broadway
New York, NY 10019
(212) 315-8700

SUDDEN INFANT DEATH SYNDROME (SIDS)

Loyola University
(*maintains scientific research center for the investigation of SIDS*)
2160 S. 1st Ave.
Maywood, IL 60153
(708) 531-3000

National Sudden Infant Death Syndrome Clearinghouse (NSIDSC)
8201 Greensboro Dr.
Suite 600
McLean, VA 22102
(703) 821-8955, ext. 361
See also Infant Death

TOXIC SUBSTANCES

See Environmental Hazards

WEIGHT CONTROL

The following groups provide information about weight control and support for their members. See the white pages of telephone directory for local chapters.

Overeaters Anonymous
383 Van Ness Ave.
Suite 1601
Torrance, CA 90501
(213) 618-8835

TOPS (Take Off Pounds Sensibly)
P.O. Box 07360
4575 S. Fifth Street
Milwaukee, WI 53207-0360
(414) 482-4620

Weight Watchers International, Inc.
Jericho Atrium
500 North Broadway
Jericho, NY 11753-2196
(516) 939-0400
See also Nutrition

WOMEN'S HEALTH

Boston Women's Health Book Collective
(*publishes* Our Bodies, Ourselves, *a well-known book on women's health*)
240 Elm St.
Summerville, MA 02144-2935
(617) 625-0271

Coalition for Homelessness
(*Advocates for the rights of the homeless. Provides education regarding homelessness*)
126 Hyde
San Francisco, CA 94102
(415) 346-3740

Community Health Education Core
(*conducts research and maintains an extensive research library on women's health, as well as HIV prevention*)
Columbia University School of Public Health
722 W. 168th Street
Box 29
New York, NY 10032
(212) 740-7292

Office of Research for Women's Health
National Institute of Health
9000 Rockville Pike
Bldg. 1, Room 201
Bethesda, MD 20892
(301) 402-1770

National Action Forum for Older Women at Stony Brook: A Center for the Health and Housing Concerns of Women Over 40
(*promotes an improved quality of life for women in midlife and older; publishes a newsletter,* Forum)

National Women's Health Network
(*provides information about and is involved in legislative action for women's health issues*)
1325 G St., NW
Washington, DC 20005
(202) 347-1140

Women's Sports Foundation
(*provides information about women's sports, physical fitness, and related topics*)
(800) 227-3988
See also Childbirth; Family Planning; Maternal Health; Occupational Health

INDEX